Frontal Seizures and Epilepsies in Children

Fondazione Pierfranco e Luisa Mariani ONLUS
viale Bianca Maria 28
20129 Milan, Italy

Telephone: +39 02 795458
Fax: +39 02 76009582
e-mail: publications@fondazione-mariani.org
www.fondazione-mariani.org

Frontal Seizures and Epilepsies in Children

Edited by
Anne Beaumanoir, Frederick Andermann,
Patrick Chauvel, Laura Mira and Benjamin Zifkin

Mariani Foundation Paediatric Neurology Series: 11
Series Editor: Maria Majno

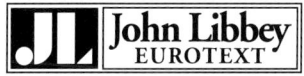

ISSN 0969-0301
ISBN 2-7420-0483-1

Cover illustration: William Turner, A Colour Wash Underpainting (1819)
from *Como and Venice Sketchbook*.
© *Tate, London 2003*.

Published by

Éditions John Libbey Eurotext
127, avenue de la République, 92120 Montrouge, France.
Tél.: 33 (0)1 46 73 06 60; Fax: 33 (0)1 40 84 09 99
e-mail: contact@john-libbey-eurotext.fr
http//www.john-libbey-eurotext.fr

© 2003 John Libbey Eurotext. All rights reserved.

Unauthorized duplication contravenes applicable laws.

Il est interdit de reproduire intégralement ou partiellement le présent ouvrage sans autorisation de l'éditeur ou du Centre Français d'Exploitation du Droit de Copie, 20, rue des Grands-Augustins, 75006 Paris.

Contents

Chapter 1	Functional anatomy of the prefrontal cortex *Joaquín M. Fuster*	1
Chapter 2	Cognitive development and the frontal lobe *Federica Lucchelli*	11
Chapter 3	Epileptogenesis in the frontal lobe *Giuliano Avanzini*	19
Chapter 4	Cognitive evoked potentials in the study of frontal lobe executive functions and their maturation *Luis García-Larrea*	33
Chapter 5	The neuroethological interpretation of motor behaviours in 'nocturnal-hyperkynetic-frontal seizures': emergence of 'innate' motor behaviours and role of central pattern generators *Carlo Alberto Tassinari, Elena Gardella, Stefano Meletti and Guido Rubboli*	43
Chapter 6	Natural history of frontal lobe epilepsies *Fabienne Picard and Anne de Saint Martin*	49
Chapter 7	Can we classify frontal lobe seizures? *Patrick Chauvel*	59
Chapter 8	Dorsolateral frontal lobe seizures: validity and usefulness of compartmentalization *François Dubeau*	65
Chapter 9	Cingulate and mesial frontal seizures *Adriana Magaudda and Carol di Perri*	83
Chapter 10	Reflex frontal lobe epilepsies *Jean-Pierre Vignal and Louis Maillard*	93
Chapter 11	Frontal lobe epilepsy in infancy *Olivier Dulac, Jean-Paul Rathgeb and Perrine Plouin*	107

Chapter 12	Ictal video-EEG features in children with nocturnal frontal lobe seizures *Paolo Tinuper*	113
Chapter 13	Generalized epilepsies and frontal lobe epilepsies in children *Charlotte Dravet*	121
Chapter 14	Acquired epileptic frontal syndrome in children *Thierry Deonna, Anne-Lise Ziegler and Eliane Roulet-Perez*	133
Chapter 15	Neuropsychology of frontal lobe epilepsy in children *Maryse Lassonde, Hannelore C. Sauerwein and Maria-Teresa Hernandez*	147
Chapter 16	Functional imaging of frontal lobe epilepsies *John S. Duncan*	159
Chapter 17	Magnetic resonance imaging in the diagnosis of frontal lobe epilepsy in children *Nadia Colombo, Alberto Citterio, Laura Tassi, Stefano Francione, Giorgio Lo Russo and Giuseppe Scialfa*	177
Chapter 18	Electroclinical semeiology of frontal lobe seizures in infants and children: contribution of intracranial video EEG recording *Martine Fohlen, Claude Jalin and Olivier Delalande*	187
Chapter 19	Secondary bilateral synchrony: significant EEG pattern in frontal lobe seizures *Anne Beaumanoir and Laura Mira*	195
Chapter 20	Medical treatment of frontal lobe seizures in children *Paola Costa, Daniela Valseriati, Andréa Van Lierde, Pierangelo Veggiotti and Piernanda Vigliano*	207
Poster 1	Neuropsychological aspects of frontal lobe epilepsy *Francesca Maria Battaglia, Maria Giuseppina Baglietto, Roberto Gaggero, Maria Cirrincione, Eleonora Garbarino and Edvige Veneselli*	215
Poster 2	Genetics of autosomal dominant nocturnal frontal lobe epilepsy *Maria Teresa Bonati, Rosanna Asselta, Stefano Duga, Romina Combi, Massimo Malcovati, Luigi Ferini-Strambi, Marco Zucconi, Alessandro Oldani, Maria Luisa Tenchini and Leda Dalprà*	219
Poster 3	Continuous spike and wave activity during slow sleep and acquired epileptic frontal syndrome: long-term follow-up in two patients *Stefania Maria Bova, Elisa Granocchio, Cristiano Termine, Cristina Tebaldi, Pierangelo Veggiotti and Giovanni Lanzi*	223
Poster 4	Neuropsychological profile in children with frontal lobe epilepsy *Michele Roccella and Marco Bonanno*	227

Chapter 1

Functional anatomy of the prefrontal cortex

Joaquín M. Fuster

*Neuropsychiatric Institute and Brain Research Institute, University of California,
760 Westwood Plaza, Los Angeles, CA 90024, USA*
joaquinf@ucla.edu

Summary

The prefrontal cortex is the association cortex of the frontal lobe. It develops late, phylogenetically as well as ontogenetically. Its lateral and medial regions play important roles in emotional and social behaviour. The lateral prefrontal areas constitute the highest stage in the cortical hierarchy of executive memory. Their networks of neuron assemblies represent schemas of sequential action, past and planned. The performance of a sequence of actions is a continuous process of temporal integration. Temporal integration is a major function of the lateral prefrontal cortex. It is based on the mediation of cross-temporal contingencies between the action plan, the goal and the individual acts of the sequence. The prefrontal cortex controls four cognitive operations that mediate those contingencies: selective attention, working memory, preparatory set and monitoring. The results of microelectrode studies indicate that: (i) temporal integration involves transactions in prefrontal cortex between neurons that engage in working memory and neurons that engage in preparatory set; (ii) working memory consists of the temporary activation, for prospective action, of a cortical network of long-term memory; and (iii) this temporary activation is sustained by reverberation of neuronal activity within that network.

To understand the functional anatomy of the prefrontal cortex, it is indispensable to distinguish its role as a store of long-term executive memory from its role in cognitive operations. The first, representational, role consists of a vast array of overlapping and intersecting networks widely distributed in all prefrontal regions (Fig. 1). These networks represent the long-term memory of actions of the organism upon its internal and external environments. The networks have been formed in the course of repeated interactions of the organism with those environments. That process of memory network formation is based on changes in synaptic strength between prefrontal cell assemblies, probably in accord with Hebbian principles. Medial and orbital prefrontal regions contain networks that represent patterns of emotional, social and visceral action. The lateral prefrontal region, on the other hand, contains networks that represent structured actions in the behavioural, linguistic and cognitive domains. Networks of all three prefrontal regions – medial, orbital and lateral – are interconnected so that, in the aggregate, they represent complex patterns of action with several aspects (e.g. cognitive, emotional, linguistic).

The second, or operational, role of the prefrontal cortex is based on the neural transactions within and between cortical memory networks – of prefrontal cortex and elsewhere – in goal-directed

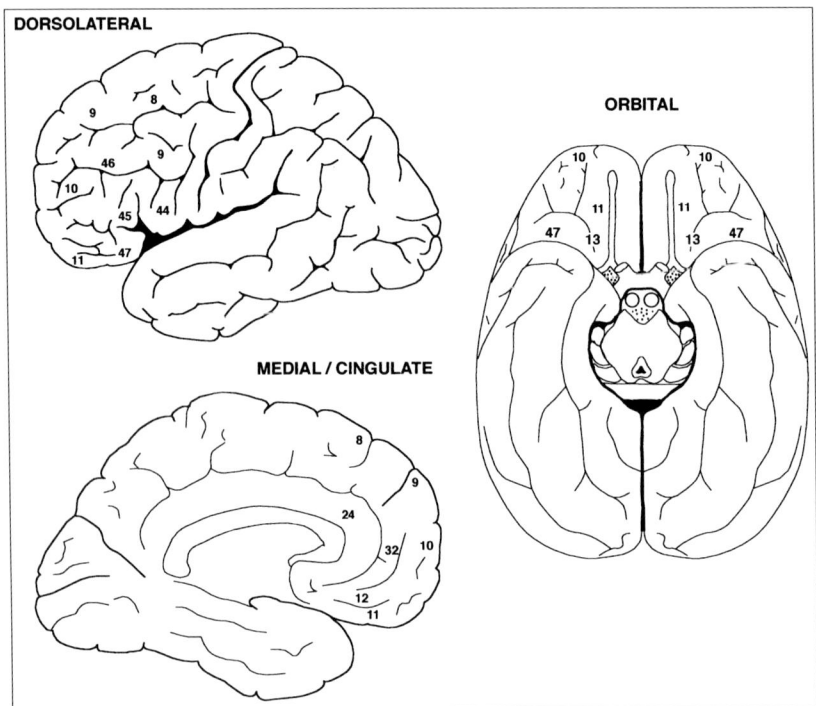

Fig. 1. The three principal regions of the frontal lobe of the human. Prefrontal areas are numbered in accord with the cytoarchitectonic map of Brodmann (1909).

actions. For the lateral prefrontal cortex, that role consists broadly in the temporal organization of behaviour, reasoning and language. This paper presents a brief review of the functions of the lateral prefrontal cortex in the temporal organization of behaviour.

Temporal integration

The lateral prefrontal cortex, which is the association cortex of the convexity of the frontal lobe, is the latest cortex to develop, phylogenetically as well as ontogenetically. In the human and non-human primate, its neuronal and connective substrate does not reach full maturity until adolescence. Some of its structure (e.g. the full myelination of intrinsic and extrinsic fibers) may take longer. It is profusely connected with many other neural structures, notably the medial and orbital prefrontal cortices, the mesencephalon, the dorsal thalamus, the basal ganglia, the limbic formations, and the cortex of the posterior regions of the cerebral hemispheres. By adaptive experience and through its connections with limbic structures (hippocampus and amygdala), the lateral prefrontal cortex can be assumed to become the store of executive memories, in other words, the substrate for cognitive networks representing schemas of goal-directed action. Those representations include old schemas with uncertainties or ambiguities that can only be resolved by temporal integration of environmental signals. This is the case in delay tasks (e.g. delayed response, delayed matching). The highest categories of prefrontal representation include the rules and contingencies for the execution of plans and schemas of behaviour. When activated, those cognitive representations, which include memories as well as plans of action, serve the organism to initiate and enact sequences of goal-directed behaviour.

Chapter 1 Functional anatomy of the prefrontal cortex

It is now well established, on the basis of neuropsychological studies, that the lateral prefrontal cortex plays a crucial role in the temporal organization of behaviour (Luria, 1966; Fuster, 1997). Human subjects with lesions of this cortex have difficulties in executing plans of behaviour, as well as sequences of propositional language and complex mental operations. These deficits are attributable to impairments in the representation and execution of goal-directed action sequences. In the past three decades, functional studies in the monkey and the human have helped us to understand the physiological functions and mechanisms supporting that role of the lateral prefrontal cortex in temporal organization. The available evidence from these studies allows us to postulate that temporal order in behaviour is essentially based on the mediation of cross-temporal contingencies, which is a core function of the prefrontal cortex. We further postulate that this function of temporal integration is supported by four cognitive functions in which that cortex crucially intervenes: (i) attention, (ii) working memory, (iii) preparatory set and (iv) monitoring. We review them successively below. Temporal order derives directly from the mediation of cross-temporal contingencies of behaviour, that is, from the integration of temporally separate fragments of perception, action and cognition into a sequence toward a goal (Fig. 2). Since temporal integration is essential to all goal-directed tasks (e.g. delay tasks), the lateral prefrontal cortex is necessary for their performance. Further, neuroimaging studies show that a large number of tasks activate in common a vast region of this cortex (Duncan & Owen, 2000). All those tasks can be shown to require some degree of temporal integration.

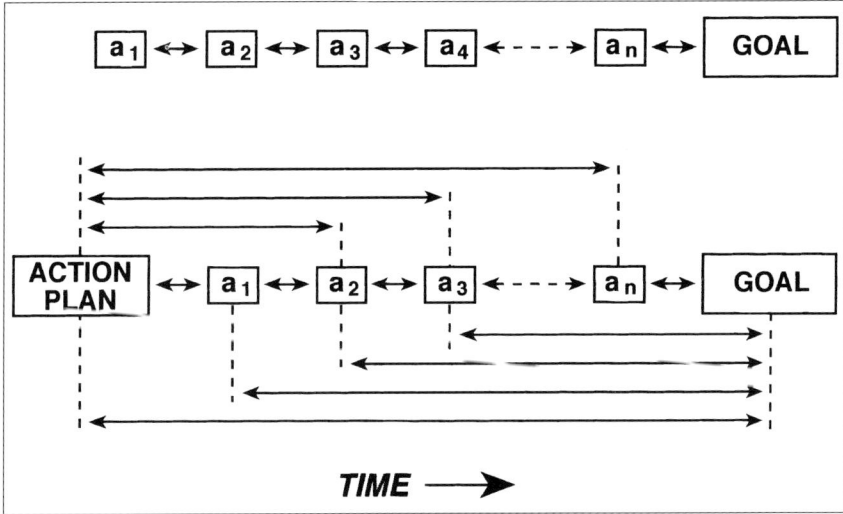

Fig. 2. Schema of the sequencing of actions toward a goal. Top: A routine sequence of acts (a_1... a_n), each leading to the next, in chain-like fashion, with contingencies (two-way arrows) only between successive acts. Bottom: A new sequence, where the acts are contingent across time on the plan, on the goal, and on other acts; the lateral prefrontal cortex mediates cross-temporal contingencies, and thereby organizes the sequence for achievement of the goal.

The mediation of cross-temporal contingencies results from the functional cooperation of the lateral prefrontal cortex with subcortical structures and, in addition, with other regions of the neocortex, such as the association cortices of parietal, occipital and temporal regions. This cooperation subserves the postulated four cognitive functions essential for temporal integration. All four are under prefrontal control. There is no conclusive evidence for the segregation of these functions by cortical area. The four are intimately entwined and operate in all lateral prefrontal areas. There is, however, evidence (reviewed in Fuster, 1997) for the topographical segregation of the contents of those cognitive functions, that is, of the material in long-term memory with which they operate. There seem to be separate frontal areas for different sectors of executive representation – e.g. locomotor, oculomotor, linguistic.

Attention

The temporal integration of information in the structuring of behaviour requires the selective and orderly activation of cortical networks that are highly specific with regard to information content, inputs and outputs. Such selective and orderly activation is essential for any novel and complex goal-directed behaviour. It takes place within a cortex-wide system of intersecting and overlapping networks that profusely share neurons and pathways. The prefrontal cortex ensures both selectivity and order in the recruitment of cortical networks for temporal integration, and thus for temporal organization. This role of the prefrontal has been called 'supervisory attentional control' (Shallice, 1988). It is supported by evidence from neurophysiology and neuroimaging. Humans with prefrontal damage have difficulty holding and shifting attention on sensory material. Thus they show a loss of attention-related modulation of sensory evoked potentials in posterior cortex (Knight, 1984; Daffner et al., 2000).

Functional imaging (Posner & Petersen, 1990; Pardo et al., 1990; Corbetta et al., 1993; Kastner et al., 1999) shows that cognitive tasks with heavy attention requirements activate three regions of the prefrontal cortex: the anterior cingulate, the orbital and the lateral. Each of those activations reflects a different aspect of attention. The cingulate activation reflects drive and motivation (the anterior cingulate cortex receives many afferents from limbic and brainstem structures). The orbital activation reflects mainly the inhibitory control and suppression of material unrelated to the current task. The lateral activation is related to the focus of attention on sensory as well as motor aspects of the task. Most relevant in this respect is the activation of area 8, which plays an important role in gaze and orientation.

Working memory

Working memory is attention focused on an internal representation. It was the first cognitive function of the prefrontal cortex to be supported by neuronal data (Fuster & Alexander, 1971; Fuster, 1973). Neurons engaged in working memory, or 'memory cells', were first found in the prefrontal cortex of monkeys performing delayed-response tasks. Those cells showed sustained elevated discharge during the memory period (delay) of delayed-response tasks. The discharge was higher during the delay than during inter-trial baseline periods. That delay discharge has the following relevant properties: (i) it occurs only when the stimulus before the delay calls for a motor act; (ii) it does not occur by simple expectation of reward; (iii) it is correlated with the animal's performance; and (iv) it can be disrupted by distraction.

Neuroimaging has substantiated the activation of prefrontal regions in working memory for visual information (Jonides et al., 1993; Cohen et al., 1994; Swartz et al., 1995) and for verbal information (Grasby et al., 1993; Smith et al., 1996). In the human, as in the non-human primate, the lateral prefrontal areas are most consistently activated in working memory. Imaging studies do not support the segregation of prefrontal areas in terms of the information that the subject retains in memory.

Those studies, however, substantiate the activation of lateral prefrontal areas in many tasks, not just delay tasks. Temporal integration seems to be the common element in all of them (Duncan & Owen, 2000).

Preparatory set

Preparatory set complements working memory in the temporal integration of behaviour. Whereas working memory is a temporally retrospective function that serves the retention of recent sensory information, preparatory set is a prospective function that serves the preparation of the organism for anticipated signals or actions. Both are functions of the lateral prefrontal cortex. The most direct neuropsychological evidence of the role of this cortex in preparatory set is the deficit that patients with lateral lesions have in predicting and preparing for actions. This deficit is closely related to the well-known planning deficit of such patients (Ackerly & Benton, 1947; Lhermitte *et al.*, 1972; Eslinger & Damasio, 1985). They are incapable of formulating and carrying out complex plans of future behaviour. At the root of the deficit there appears to be the difficulty in mediating contingencies between present events and their anticipated consequences. Included among those contingencies are those between a conceived goal and the acts that will lead to it. In general terms, the deficit can be characterized as a failure of prospective memory or 'memory of the future' (Ingvar, 1985). Neuroimaging confirms the activation of lateral prefrontal cortex in prospective preparation and planning (Partiot *et al.*, 1995; Baker *et al.*, 1996).

In the lateral prefrontal cortex of monkeys performing a delay task with double contingencies across time, Quintana & Fuster (1999) obtained cellular evidence of working memory and preparatory set. In that task, the animal had to first attend to a colour in the center of a panel. After 12 seconds of delay, a second visual signal appeared in the panel. Depending on the combination of the colour and the second signal, the animal had to touch a lighted disk on the right or on the left. Both the colour and the second signal were changed at random from trial to trial. Consequently, the choice of location at the end of each trial was based on the double contingency between the two visual stimuli separated by the delay. After the animal had been fully trained in performance of the task, the first signal (colour) predicted the second signal and the location of the correct choice with a given probability. Some colours predicted location with 100 per cent probability and others 75 per cent. Under those conditions, some cells responded specifically to the colour. Their discharge decreased gradually in the course of the delay (Fig. 3). Such cells could be characterized as working memory cells. Other cells, however, increased their firing in the delay period, and after it they reacted differentially to the side of the behavioural response – right or left. Moreover, the magnitude of acceleration of their discharge in the delay was proportional to the probability with which the monkey could anticipate the direction of the hand movement that the second stimulus would call for. Therefore, the cells of this second group were direction-coupled. They appeared to anticipate the manual response and participate in its preparation. The two kinds of cells were found intermingled in the cortex of the upper lateral convexity of the frontal lobe. Both working-memory cells and set cells were found intermingled in the lateral prefrontal cortex (upper bank of the sulcus principalis, areas 9 and 46). Both appeared to participate in the temporal integration of visual information with prospective action.

Monitoring

It would be reasonable to put all the three prefrontal functions of temporal integration just discussed under the heading of the first – attention: attention to sensory information, attention to the internal

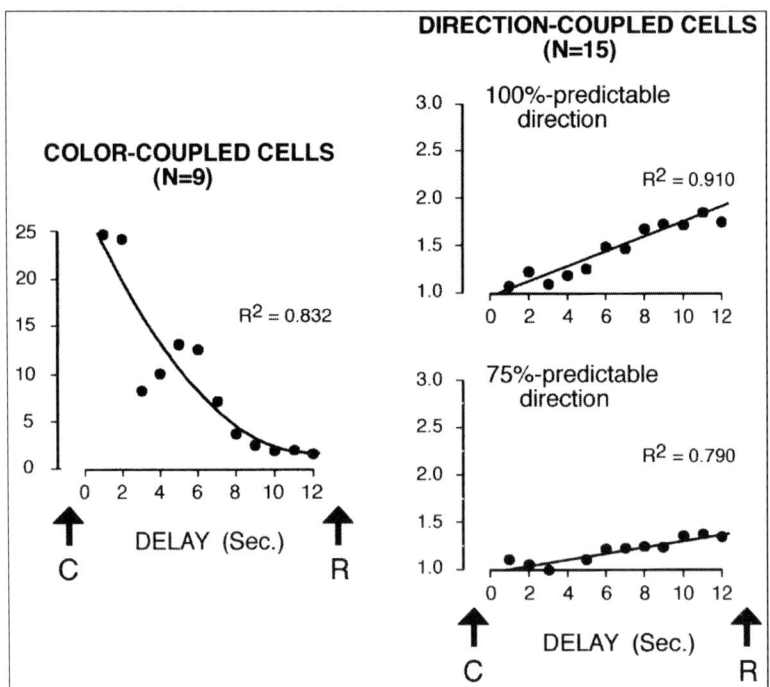

Fig. 3. Firing activity of prefrontal units during the delay period of a double-contingency task. Left: Working memory cells for colour (colour-coupled). Right: Preparatory-set cells (direction-coupled). Note the opposite temporal firing trends of the two cell types; in set cells, note also the relation between the slope of the accelerating trend of firing and the predictability of the direction of behavioural response. C, cue (first signal); R, behavioural response.

representation of that information (working memory) and attention to a forthcoming action (preparatory set). A fourth aspect of attention, monitoring, could be also considered as a prefrontal function serving temporal integration.

All goal-directed sequences of behaviour are performed within the broad physiological context of the perception-action cycle (Fuster, 1997), a process which is grounded on basic biological principles. This process is the circular cybernetic flow of cognitive information that links the organism to its environment. In the course of a sequence of behaviour, sensory inputs are processed in sensory structures. The result of that sensory processing leads to adaptive actions, which induce changes in the environment. These, in turn, generate new sensory signals, which feed back into the cycle and help control new action. That feedback control has been termed monitoring, and takes place at all levels of the hierarchy of sensory and motor structures of the central nervous system. Fig. 4 illustrates schematically the interactions in the cortical stages of the perception-action cycle.

The idea of a role of the prefrontal cortex in the monitoring of actions originated with the earlier concept of 'corollary discharge' (Teuber, 1972). Based on neuropsychological observations in the human, it was inferred that the prefrontal cortex was essential for the integration of information that stemmed from the organism's own actions. That information derived, in part, from efferent copies of executive actions and in part from sensory inputs (including proprioceptive) resulting from them.

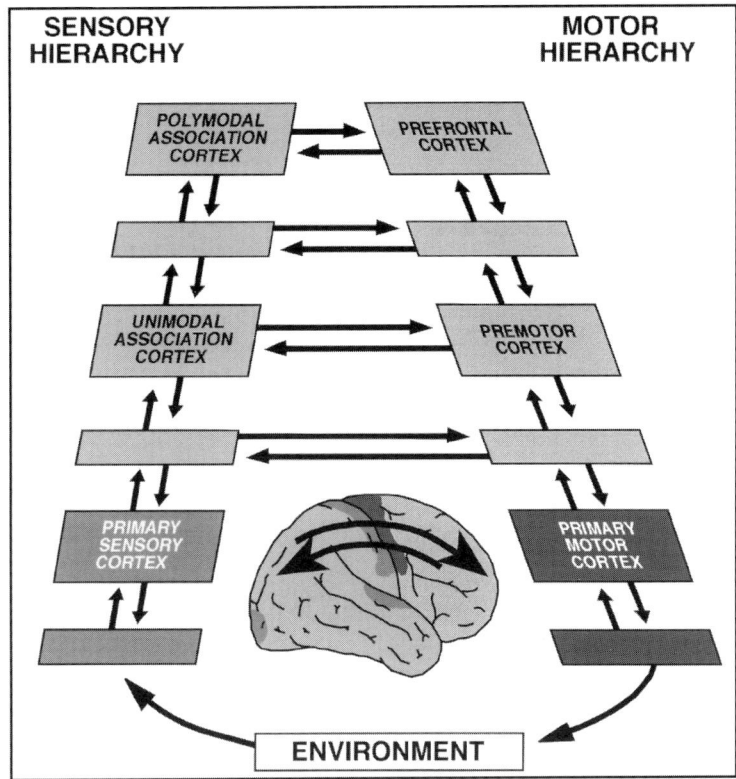

Fig. 4. Diagram of cortical interactions in the perception-action cycle (unlabeled rectangles signify intermediate areas or subareas in the sensory or motor hierarchy). All arrows signify general pathways identified anatomically in the brain of the monkey. The diagram of the human brain – inset in the centre – emphasizes the reciprocal interactions between posterior and frontal cortex.

Based on that information, the prefrontal cortex would generate corollary discharge, which would flow upon motor and sensory systems and prepare them for further actions. Lesion experiments in the monkey (Petrides, 1991) support the monitoring role of the prefrontal cortex and provide it with some topography in the lateral region. Neuroimaging in the human further supports that role of the lateral cortex (Petrides *et al.*, 1993; Fletcher *et al.*, 1998). To sum up, the lateral prefrontal cortex, with its temporal integrative functions of attention, working memory, set, and monitoring, sits at the top of the perception-action cycle. In that position, the prefrontal cortex helps the animal to organize novel and complex sequences of goal-directed behaviour.

Mechanisms of temporal integration

The neural mechanisms of temporal integration are only sketchily understood. Thus far, working memory is the temporal integrative function most intensely explored in this respect. As a result of microelectrode studies, we are coming to the conclusion that working memory is essentially the temporary activation of a neocortical network for the execution of prospective actions, and that both working memory and execution are under prefrontal control, especially the control of the dorsolateral prefrontal cortex. As the actions in a sequence are contingent on recent sensory events, the activation of the network allows the memory retention of those events and thus their integration with subsequent actions. Consequently, the network activation has the effect of mediating cross-temporal contingencies. It is reasonable to conclude, therefore, that prefrontal memory cells 'remember for action', in other words, for integrating actions in time.

It is now clear that the prefrontal cortex is not the only part of the neocortex involved in working memory. It is also clear that working memory is not the only function of the prefrontal cortex. Visual working memory activates inferotemporal units (Fuster & Jervey, 1982; Miller et al., 1993) as well as frontal units. Tactile working memory activates somatosensory units (Zhou & Fuster, 1996) as well as frontal units (Romo et al., 1999). Therefore, any working memory network appears to span both posterior and frontal regions, and includes neural representations of perceptual memory as well as of executive memory. Based on microelectrode and imaging studies it seems that a working memory network is an active network of long-term memory with perceptual as well as executive components. These components may include new percepts or new actions, which can be incorporated into active networks of long-term memory by categorization, similarity and other processes of perceptual or executive 'constancy'.

A recent microelectrode study (Fuster et al., 2000) supports the concept of the structural identity of working and long-term memory. We trained monkeys to perform a cross-modal delayed matching task. In it, the animal had to listen to a brief tone to choose a colour 12 seconds later. A high-pitched tone required a red choice and a low-pitched tone a green choice. Prefrontal cells reacted with different firing rates to the two tones and then again to the two colours. The cell reactions to tones and colours were correlated in accord with the rule of the task: some neurons responded more to low pitch and green than to high pitch and red, whereas others did the reverse. Those correlations between tones and colours disappeared when the monkey made errors in performing the task. In the course of correct performance, the correlations persisted through the period of delay or working memory. We concluded that prefrontal neurons integrate information across time and across two sensory modalities (sound and vision). Their discharge in working memory is not only related to a tone and to a colour, but to the association between the two, which is in long-term memory. The most plausible explanation for our observation is that prefrontal neurons are part of networks of long-term memory which, for working memory, are temporarily activated to integrate information of the two sensory modalities across time. The results of our study also imply that the prefrontal neurons of a working-memory network, that is of an active long-term memory network, receive task-related sensory inputs from posterior association cortex. Moreover, prefrontal memory cells are attuned to those inputs during the working-memory period.

There is empirical and computational evidence that working memory is maintained by recurrent excitation through reentrant neuronal circuits of the cerebral cortex. In working memory as well as in other executive functions of the frontal lobe, the prefrontal cortex cooperates with other brain structures, some of them subcortical, such as the thalamus and the basal ganglia. In addition, it cooperates with regions of posterior – i.e. post-central or post-Rolandic – cortex (Hasegawa et al., 1998; Kastner et al., 1999; Tomita et al., 1999; Daffner et al., 2000). In monkeys performing a visual delayed matching task, the reversible inactivation of prefrontal or inferotemporal cortex by local cooling induced the following effects (Fuster et al., 1985): (i) a deficit in working memory for colour and (ii) a decrease in the ability of neurons of either cortex to discriminate colours in the working-memory period. These observations indicate that the inactivation of either cortex, prefrontal or inferotemporal, interrupts neuronal loops of reverberating activity between them which are engaged in working memory and are critical for its retention. This concept is further supported by computational modeling. In a fully recurrent network trained to perform working memory, 'cells' have been found that behave like real cortical neurons engaged in working memory (Zipser *et al.*, 1993). Consequently, working memory seems to be a cognitive function that serves the temporal integration of behaviour by recurrent activation of cell assemblies in cortical networks of long-term memory.

Conclusions

Neuropsychological studies support the concept of a fundamental role of the prefrontal cortex in the representation and execution of plans and schemas of behaviour. Also from those studies derives the idea of a critical involvement of the lateral prefrontal cortex in the temporal organization of speech and behaviour. That organizing function of the lateral prefrontal cortex is based on its capacity to integrate information in the temporal domain; in other words, on its capacity to mediate contingencies across time. At least four prefrontal functions serve temporal integration: attention, working memory, preparatory set and monitoring. In all four, the lateral prefrontal cortex cooperates with subcortical structures and with posterior association cortex. Working memory seems essentially based on the activation of cortical networks of long-term memory, and sustained by reverberating activity between the neuron assemblies that constitute those networks.

References

Ackerly, S.S. & Benton, A.L. (1947): Report of case of bilateral frontal lobe defect. *Res. Publ. Ass. Nerv. Ment. Dis.* **27**, 479–504.

Baker, S.C., Rogers, R.D., Owen, A.M., Frith, C.D., Dolan, R.J., Frackowiak, R.S.J. & Robbins, T.W. (1996): Neural systems engaged by planning: a PET study of the Tower of London task. *Neuropsychologia* **34**, 515–526.

Brodmann, K. (1909): *Vergleichende Lokalisationslehre der Grosshirnrinde in ihren Prinzipien dargestellt auf Grund des Zellenbaues*. Leipzig: Barth.

Cohen, J.D., Forman, S.D., Braver, T.S., Casey, B.J., Servan-Schreiber, D. & Noll, D.C. (1994): Activation of the prefrontal cortex in a nonspatial working memory task with functional MRI. *Human Brain Map.* **1**, 293–304.

Corbetta, M., Miezin, F.M., Shulman, G.L. & Petersen, S.E. (1993): A PET study of visuospatial attention. *J. Neurosci.* **13**, 1202–1226.

Daffner, K.R., Mesulam, M.M., Scinto, L.F.M., Acar, D., Calvo, V., Faust, R., Chabrerie, A., Kennedy, B. & Holcomb, P. (2000). The central role of the prefrontal cortex in directing attention to novel events. *Brain* **123**, 927–939.

Duncan, J. & Owen, A.M. (2000): Common regions of the human frontal lobe recruited by diverse cognitive demands. *Trends NeuroSci.* **23**, 475–483.

Eslinger, P.J. & Damasio, A.R. (1985): Severe disturbance of higher cognition after bilateral frontal lobe ablation: patient EVR. *Neurology* **35**, 1731–1741.

Fletcher, P.C., Shallice, T., Frith, C.D., Frackowiak, R.S.J. & Dolan, R.J. (1998): The functional roles of prefrontal cortex in episodic memory. II. Retrieval. *Brain* **121**, 1249–1256.

Fuster, J.M. (1973): Unit activity in prefrontal cortex during delayed-response performance: neuronal correlates of transient memory. *J. Neurophysiol.* **36**, 61–78.

Fuster, J.M. (1997): *The prefrontal cortex: anatomy, physiology and neuropsychology of the frontal lobe*. Philadelphia: Lippincott-Raven.

Fuster, J.M. & Alexander, G.E. (1971): Neuron activity related to short-term memory. *Science* **173**, 652–654.

Fuster, J.M. & Jervey, J.P. (1982): Neuronal firing in the inferotemporal cortex of the monkey in a visual memory task. *J. Neurosci.* **2**, 361–375.

Fuster, J.M., Bauer, R.H. & Jervey, J.P. (1985): Functional interactions between inferotemporal and prefrontal cortex in a cognitive task. *Brain Res.* **330**, 299–307.

Fuster, J.M., Bodner, M. & Kroger, J. (2000): Cross-modal and cross-temporal association in neurons of frontal cortex. *Nature* **405**, 347–351.

Grasby, P.M., Frith, C.D., Friston, K.J., Bench, C., Frackowiak, R.S.J. & Dolan, R.J. (1993): Functional mapping of brain areas implicated in auditory-verbal memory function. *Brain* **116**, 1–20.

Hasegawa, I., Fukushima, T., Ihara, T. & Miyashita, Y. (1998): Callosal window between prefrontal cortices: cognitive interaction to retrieve long-term memory. *Science* **281**, 814–818.

Ingvar, D.H. (1985): 'Memory of the future': an essay on the temporal organization of conscious awareness. *Hum. Neurobiology* **4**, 127–136.

Jonides, J., Smith, E.E., Koeppe, R.A., Awh, E., Minoshima, S. & Mintun, M.A. (1993): Spatial working memory in humans as revealed by PET. *Nature* **363**, 623–625.

Kastner, S., Pinsk, M.A., De Weerd, P., Desimone, R. & Ungerleider, L.G. (1999): Increased activity in human visual cortex during directed attention in the absence of visual stimulation. *Neuron* **22**, 751–761.

Knight, R.T. (1984): Decreased response to novel stimuli after prefrontal lesions in man. *Electroencephalogr. Clin. Neurophysiol.* **59**, 9–20.

Lhermitte, F., Deroulsne, J. & Signoret, J.L. (1972): Analyse neuropsychologique du syndrome frontal. *Rev. Neurol.* **127**, 415–440.

Luria, A.R. (1966): *Higher cortical functions in man.* New York: Basic Books.

Miller, E.K., Li, L. & Desimone, R. (1993): Activity of neurons in anterior inferior temporal cortex during a short-term memory task. *J. Neurosci.* **13**, 1460–1478.

Pardo, J.V., Pardo, P.J., Janer, K.W. & Raichle, M.E. (1990): The anterior cingulate cortex mediates processing selection in the Stroop attentional conflict paradigm. *Proc. Natl. Acad. Sci. USA* **87**, 256–259.

Partiot, A., Grafman, J., Sadato, N., Wachs, J. & Hallett, M. (1995): Brain activation during the generation of non-emotional and emotional plans. *NeuroReport* **6**, 1269–1272.

Petrides, M. (1991): Monitoring of selections of visual stimuli and the primate frontal cortex. *Proc. R. Soc. Lond. B* **246**, 293–306.

Petrides, M., Alivisatos, B., Evans, A.C. & Meyer, E. (1993): Dissociation of human mid-dorsolateral from posterior dorsolateral frontal cortex in memory processing. *Proc. Natl. Acad. Sci. USA* **90**, 873–877.

Posner, M.I. & Petersen, S.E. (1990): The attention system of the human brain. *Ann. Rev. Neurosci.* **13**, 25–42.

Quintana, J. & Fuster, J.M. (1999): From perception to action: temporal integrative functions of prefrontal and parietal neurons. *Cerebral Cortex* **9**, 213–221.

Romo, R., Brody, C.D., Hernández, A. & Lemus, L. (1999): Neuronal correlates of parametric working memory in the prefrontal cortex. *Nature* **399**, 470–473.

Shallice, T. (1988): *From neuropsychology to mental structure.* New York: Cambridge University Press.

Smith, E.E., Jonides, J. & Koeppe, R.A. (1996): Dissociating verbal and spatial working memory using PET. *Cerebral Cortex* **6**, 11–20.

Swartz, B.E., Halgren, E., Fuster, J.M., Simpkins, F., Gee, M. & Mandelkern, M. (1995): Cortical metabolic activation in humans during a visual memory task. *Cerebral Cortex* **3**, 205–214.

Teuber, H.L. (1972): Unity and diversity of frontal lobe functions. *Acta Neurobiol. Exp.* **32**, 625–656.

Tomita, H., Ohbayashi, M., Nakahara, K., Hasegawa, I. & Miyashita, Y. (1999): Top-down signal from prefrontal cortex in executive control of memory retrieval. *Nature* **401**, 699–703.

Zhou, Y. & Fuster, J.M. (1996): Mnemonic neuronal activity in somatosensory cortex. *Proc. Natl. Acad. Sci. USA* **93**, 10533–10537.

Zipser, D., Kehoe, B., Littlewort, G. & Fuster, J. (1993): A spiking network model of short-term active memory. *J. Neurosci.* **13**, 3406–3420.

Chapter 2

Cognitive development and the frontal lobe

Federica Lucchelli

*Department of Neurology, Azienda Ospedaliera, Ospedale Niguarda Ca' Granda,
Piazza Ospedale Maggiore 3, 20162 Milan, Italy*
flucch@libero.it

Summary

The study of the development of cognitive functions attributed to the frontal lobe is still largely modelled on findings obtained in adults. Apart from work on the effects of early frontal lesions in non-human primates, two basic approaches have been followed. First, the application of neuropsychological tests originally devised for adults has yielded data on the emergence of frontal functions in children, showing that the maturation of these functions extends well beyond infancy and, for some functions, reaches into adolescence. Second, studies of children with focal frontal lesions or with disorders supposedly involving frontal dysfunction (e.g. phenylketonuria) have suggested clinical models of the frontal lobe syndrome in childhood. Despite considerable progress, contradictory results, and methodological biases and weaknesses, still hinder insight into the nature and the mechanisms of frontal lobe function in children.

Most information on the role of the frontal lobe in behaviour has been derived from the study of normal adults and those with frontal lobe lesions. Interest in developmental aspects of frontal lobe function is comparatively recent. Although the relative lack of knowledge of the development of frontal lobe functions may be due in part to the difficulty in finding children with well-documented frontal lobe lesions, it is also clear that a major difficulty in studying frontal lobe development is the lack of an accepted definition of what to study.

The frontal lobes include many cytoarchitectonic areas which differ in their links to other cortical and subcortical areas (Fuster, 1989), and functional diversification and heterogeneity have been demonstrated in the frontal lobe. A satisfactory comprehensive theory or conceptualization of frontal lobe function is understandably still lacking (Faglioni, 1999).

Attempts to identify a unitary function for the entire lobe have been so far largely unsuccessful. Perhaps the most accepted conceptualization of frontal lobe functions characterizes them as 'executive functions', i.e. capacities which enable a person to engage successfully in independent, purposeful, self-serving behaviour. They include the ability to plan and to organize behaviour across time and space in order to fulfil goals and intentions; they enable shifting of strategies and adaptation to changing circumstances. These capacities include planning, decision making, goal selection and monitoring of action (Shallice, 1982; Stuss & Benson, 1986).

The prefrontal cortex has a unique position in the cerebral economy, in that there is no cognitive function to which it is extraneous, or that is unaffected by damage to it. However, there is no function that it accomplishes alone and that cannot occur in its absence. It appears to have the special property of providing all cognitive and behavioural activity with rules and strategies that enable the subject to make coherent choices and fruitful decisions, avoiding harmful or useless ones. Therefore, the frontal lobe appears to be at the core of personality, endowing it with individual cognitive and emotional qualities.

It must be emphasized that since the brain is an integrated functioning unit, a strict localizationist approach is inappropriate. Terms such as 'executive functions', 'supervisory system' (Shallice, 1982) or 'dysexecutive syndrome' (Baddeley & Wilson, 1988), now widely used in neuropsychological parlance, relate more to psychological constructs than to anatomically localized functions. In the developmental literature this distinction is particularly relevant since the development of 'frontal functions' may relate not only to anatomical and biochemical maturation of the frontal lobes, but also to the integrative demands of tasks on multiple brain regions.

Table 1 shows a descriptive summary of functions found to be impaired by frontal lobe damage based on empirical data from the adult literature. Some of the most common tasks employed to tap these functional aspects are also listed. This summary does not imply any theoretical interpretation or unitary conceptualization of frontal lobe function. Moreover, overlap and interactions between functions are possible and even frequent.

Table 1. Frontal lobe functions

Functions	Standardized tasks	Behavioural abnormalities
Memory and temporal organization of experiences	Self-ordered pointing	Confabulations
Learning and learning strategies	Maze tests List learning	Rule-breaking
Productivity and creativity – spontaneous flexibility	Verbal fluency	Perseverations
Category discovering and abstract thinking	Wisconsin card sorting test	
Judgement and rationality	Cognitive estimates	
Planning and farsightedness	Tower of Hanoi/London	
Inhibition and self-control	Stroop test	Environmental dependency, utilization behaviour (Lhermitte, 1983, 1986)
Personality	Quantitative assessment not possible	

Several approaches have been taken to study the emergence of behaviours assumed to be controlled by the frontal lobes, and the changes that occur as the child gets older (reviewed in Smith et al., 1992; Temple, 1997).

The first is that of comparing the performance of non-human infant primates to human infants on tasks that have been proven to be effective in assessing frontal lobe functioning in monkeys, such as delayed response and delayed alternation tasks. The second approach involves applying to children the knowledge of frontal lobe function obtained from adults. Third, clinical models of frontal lobe dysfunction, such as the effects of focal frontal damage and the study of disorders supposed to involve frontal dysfunction, have been investigated in children.

The latter two points will be reviewed in some detail.

Adult models of frontal lobe functions

Frontal lobe development has been studied in normal children by applying models derived from the study of adults. Standard psychological tests of presumed frontal functions developed for adults, on which performance has been found to be sensitive to frontal damage, are administered to children of different ages. The idea is to outline a developmental pattern across a variety of ages to provide insight into the development rate of functions attributed to the frontal lobe.

These tasks include some traditional frontal tests, such as the Wisconsin card sorting test (Grant & Berg, 1948; Milner, 1963), fluency tasks, Tower of Hanoi/London (Anzai & Simon, 1979; Shallice, 1982), Self-ordered pointing (Petrides & Milner, 1982) and Stroop test (Stroop, 1935). It is important to point out that their frontal characterization has been claimed on the basis of specific disruption after frontal damage, in comparison with unimpaired performance by normal subjects or subjects with damage to other areas of the brain. This assumption has been challenged, at least for some of the tests (Anderson *et al.*, 1991). Therefore, it is important to keep in mind that the designation of a task as frontal does not necessarily mean that it is a consistent measure of frontal lobe function. In such studies it is assumed that the age at which children can perform the task as well as adults corresponds to the age at which the frontal lobes have reached maturity for the function in question.

Two different procedures have been applied, using tasks devised for adults in their original form, or tasks adapted to children usually by simplifying them. Several studies investigated children's performance in the Wisconsin card sorting test. Chelune & Baer (1986) administered this test to 105 children between the ages of 6 and 12 years and found that the performance of children was indistinguishable from that of adults by 10 years of age. This finding has been replicated in other studies (Chelune & Thompson, 1987; Levin *et al.*, 1991; Welsh *et al.*, 1991), but more recently has been challenged by data from a study of 685 children aged 9 to 14 years (Paniak *et al.*, 1996). Though showing improvement with increasing age, even the oldest children did not reach adult levels of performance. This is in line with results of studies of other cognitive aspects of frontal lobe function such as verbal fluency (Benton & Hamsher, 1976; Levin *et al.*, 1991; Yeudall *et al.*, 1986), motor sequencing and complex planning (Levin *et al.*, 1991; Welsh *et al.*, 1991), which found that adult levels are attained only later in adolescence.

The interpretation of these results is not straightforward. It must be pointed out that the criterion of attainment of adult levels as a measure of maturation of frontal functions may be inappropriate (Smith *et al.*, 1992); by focusing on adult-like performance we do not investigate the processes of development, but rather target its end stage. Moreover, early emergence of frontal abilities may be masked if adult tasks are too difficult for children for reasons unrelated to frontal functions, for example, because they are too long and fatiguing or because they require other abilities such as language and memory that are not as well-developed in children.

To overcome these difficulties some investigators have used simplified versions of adult tasks, for example in the case of the Wisconsin card sorting test, by reducing the number of categories, the number of intermediate category dimensions or the number of consecutive correct placements before shift (Diamond & Boyer, 1989); or, in the case of the Tower of Hanoi test, by reducing the number of disks (Welsh *et al.*, 1991). Adopting simplified versions, a developmental trend was observed, showing better performance with increasing age. However, the interpretation of these results is unclear; the requirements of the task have been changed, and therefore it is no longer certain that the task is still sensitive to frontal dysfunction unless independent validation of the new task is obtained. Perhaps the most interesting finding of these studies is the reported emergence of some executive skills even in pre-school children 3 and 4 years old (Diamond & Boyer, 1989), when the adult version of the task is inadequate.

A different line of research acknowledges the diversity of functions mediated by the frontal lobes, and studies developmental patterns of different behaviours in the same children, examining several different components in the same subject to assess differential developmental trends (Becker *et al.*, 1987; Fiducia & O'Leary, 1990; Welsh *et al.*, 1991). The basic hypothesis is that cognitive and behavioural skills that may tap different areas within the frontal lobe show developmental expression at different times and at different rates.

The best example of these studies is Welsh *et al.* (1991). They performed several tests of executive function in subjects aged from 3 to 28 years. By applying factor analysis, they argued for sequential development of skills, in that adult levels of performance seemed to be reached in three stages:

(1) simple planning and organized visual search by 6 years;
(2) set maintenance, hypothesis testing and impulsive responding control by 10 years (Wisconsin card sorting test);
(3) motor sequencing, complex planning (Tower of Hanoi) and verbal fluency later in adolescence (later than 12 years).

They also found that executive function was relatively independent of IQ. This confirms the common notion that measures generally used to assess intelligence, such as the Wechsler intelligence scale, are rather poor indicators of executive skills.

These studies suggest that frontal lobe behaviours do in fact follow a multi-stage process of development, and that developmental differences manifest themselves at different ages depending on the specific task. Each task may show its own developmental course. These findings may be interpreted in different ways. One possible interpretation is that behaviours or functions mediated by different areas of the frontal lobe emerge at different rates depending on the maturation of that particular region. However, different developmental trends may also be the expression of task differences related to degree of difficulty or dependence on other cognitive functions. Since many different abilities develop simultaneously in a child, it is likely that the structure of those abilities as well as their interactions change with age in complex ways. Again, it is important to emphasize that the most striking peculiarity of the prefrontal cortex relates to the fact that it exerts its influence on all cognitive abilities but at the same time, in order to perform its modulating function, it needs their valid contributions, with extremely complex multiple-way interactions.

Thus it is not clear whether the emergence of behaviours in children that resemble prefrontal behaviours in adults really reflects maturation of the prefrontal region alone. Any particular task could be measuring the development of a multitude of abilities, not necessarily exclusively nor directly related to the frontal lobe.

Some studies have approached this problem by administering both tasks assumed to involve prefrontal functions, and tasks assumed not to involve them. Kates & Moscovitch (1989) compared frontal tasks of temporal sequencing (recency judgement and temporal order tasks) to non-frontal tasks (digit span and visual block span). They found that adult levels of performance in temporal ordering tasks were attained quite early, by 7 years of age, but in the span tasks, performance did not reach adult levels until 11 years of age. The different developmental timetables for frontal and non-frontal tasks lend some support to the assumption that the cognitive abilities underlying these tasks and the brain regions mediating their performance are not the same. Simple conclusions about the relationship between cortical maturation and cognitive tests performance are however unwarranted.

The application of adult models to children may be difficult for several reasons (Smith *et al.*, 1992; Temple, 1997). Behaviour of adults with prefrontal lesions may differ from that of developing children in important ways, thus invalidating the comparison of their performance on the same or similar tasks. In adults, lesions occur in a fully developed brain and in a person with fully developed abilities. The loss of a previously established skill in the adult may not manifest itself in the same way as the interruption of a partially-developed or emerging skill in the child. For instance, the loss of planning ability in an adult results in a grossly distorted plan of action which little resembles the child's simplistic plan, effective but limited to simple courses of action. It is also possible that in the developing child some of the behaviours that emerge at a young age subsequently become redundant or useless, and disappear. Thus, the prefrontal lobe may mediate a particular behaviour in a young child that is no longer present when the child becomes older. The exclusive use of adult models may therefore result in ignoring or excluding from study certain behaviours that are indeed mediated by the prefrontal cortex in children.

Clinical models of frontal lobe functioning in children

The study of the effects of frontal lobes focal lesions represents the classical neuropsychological approach to the investigation of cognitive functions. In this perspective two lines of research have been followed: first, single case studies of children with focal frontal damage, and second, behavioural and neuropsychological investigations of clinical syndromes in which executive dysfunction is supposedly implicated, for instance phenylketonuria and disorders subsumed under the label of attention deficit hyperactivity disorder.

Single case studies

Well-documented reports of children with frontal lesions are still uncommon. The age at time of assessment and the range of neuropsychological procedures vary greatly and comparison of data is therefore hardly feasible. Earlier reports described the subjects as adults rather than at the time of the lesion and emphasized the long-term consequences of early frontal lesions. One of the most famous cases of frontal syndrome, patient J.P., first described by Ackerly & Benton (1947) and Ackerly (1964) and more recently re-evaluated by Benton (1992), represents a good example of this approach. The patient, with presumably congenital bilateral atrophy of both frontal lobes, was first assessed at the age of 20 years when cognitive and social impairment had been present for a long time. Cognitive difficulties typical of the frontal syndrome were documented, but the authors emphasized emotional changes and behavioural problems leading to major social impairment. A similar case (patient D.T.) was reported by Eslinger et al. (1989, 1990, 1992; Grattan & Eslinger, 1992), and it is noteworthy that the description of these subjects as adults is almost identical to the historical descriptions of patients, such as Phineas Gage, who sustained frontal lobe lesions in their adult years (Harlow, 1868).

A few, more recent reports described patients evaluated soon after the acute event. Williams & Mateer (1992) reported two young patients, D.R. and S.N., who were studied 1 month and 2 months respectively after traumatic frontal damage, left frontal contusion in the first case and bilateral contusions in the other. Marlowe (1992) described the effects of a right prefrontal lesion in a 4-year-old boy examined about 1 year after the trauma.

In these studies, neuropsychological assessment was carried out with traditional psychometric tests such as the Wechsler intelligence scale. The authors emphasize the difficulty in assessing changes in cognitive abilities immediately after the acute phase, when scores suggested good initial recovery of function. It was only after some time that formal tests began to reflect problems, which appeared to be related mainly to information and situations requiring new learning. The most affected areas of function were, once again, those associated with social and emotional development. Though significant executive deficits were found, none of these studies specifically investigated the level or the nature of the executive impairment or the specific cognitive processes disrupted by frontal damage.

On the whole, clinical studies indicate that long-term cognitive and behavioural effects of childhood frontal lesions are frequent and significant. Therefore, prolonged follow-up is needed for comprehensive assessment. The final outcome, however, is virtually indistinguishable from the adult presentation of the frontal syndrome. This can be true even for lesions acquired in early childhood, as in case P.L. reported by Marlowe (1992), who sustained frontal lobe injury at the age of about 4 years.

Clinical models of the frontal syndrome in children

Among medical disorders of childhood that have been proposed to involve frontal lobe dysfunction, phenylketonuria and attention deficit disorders have received special attention.

Phenylketonuria (PKU) is an autosomal recessive disorder in which there is inability to metabolize phenylalanine (Folling, 1994). The disorder affects myelination, with later-myelinating areas such as the frontal lobe thought to be particularly vulnerable. Children with PKU have specific behavioural and cognitive deficits that are not accounted for by their lower intelligence (Smith *et al.*, 1988).

A characteristic personality is also documented, with temper tantrums, irritability, hyperactivity, inattentiveness and impulsiveness. Cognitive deficits have been found in several domains including attention, concept formation, problem solving and visuo-motor integration (Crowie, 1971; Brunner *et al.*, 1983; Pennington *et al.*, 1985). Pennington *et al.* (1985) suggested that these deficits were not generalized but that the pattern was particularly suggestive of prefrontal dysfunction. They also hypothesized that cessation of dietary treatment around 6 years of age may contribute to the observed pattern since at that age dietary termination exerts its adverse effects only on later-developing systems such as the prefrontal areas, leaving language skills at least partially unaffected.

Welsh *et al.* (1990) used tasks presumed to measure executive functions (visual search, verbal fluency, motor planning and Tower of Hanoi) together with a discriminant control task (recognition memory), and supported the hypothesis that the PKU group had specific executive deficits, compared to a control group matched for age and IQ. The findings therefore suggested that PKU may provide a model for studying the effects of frontal impairment in childhood.

With respect to attention disorders, it should be remembered that, in child neuropsychology, there has been variation in diagnostic criteria for attention deficit hyperactivity disorder (ADHD) and within the clinical entity itself. Children with ADHD are often restless and easily distracted. A number of researchers have speculated that frontal lobe dysfunction underlies ADHD, accounting for the similarity between the characteristics of hyperactive children and the behavioural symptoms of adults with frontal damage. This similarity has been investigated by administering tasks known to be sensitive to frontal lobe dysfunction in adults. In several studies, the Wisconsin card sorting test, Trail making, the Stroop test, verbal fluency test and others were found to differentiate ADHD children from normal children (Pennington & Ozonoff, 1996). However, results have not been consistent (Loge *et al.*, 1990; McGee *et al.*, 1989) and have been criticized because of small sample sizes and variations in diagnostic criteria. For now, the evidence for frontal lobe dysfunction in ADHD is therefore rather weak.

Conclusions

Work on normal and brain-damaged subjects has produced a wealth of information on frontal lobe function in adults. Studies in children have also yielded significant knowledge about the development of frontal skills and the consequences of early frontal damage. However, many issues have not been addressed and many questions are still unanswered. Methodological biases represent a major problem.

It must be acknowledged that the principles of adult neuropsychology may be limited in their application to children. So far, most studies of the development of frontal lobe functions have been guided by concepts learned from the study of adults. Better or more fine-grained definitions are needed for frontal and executive functions in children, since they may be different from what we usually consider as frontal functions in adults. Behaviour that appears to be similar in adults and children may be the outcome of different processes or be regulated by different neural networks. Consequently, tests of frontal functions specifically devised for children are needed. Well-designed longitudinal studies of the development of normal children and of both cognitive and behavioural changes in brain-damaged children are especially important, but are still lacking. Until these goals are achieved, at least partially, we are left with good descriptions of frontal lobe phenomenology, but little insight into the nature and the mechanisms of frontal lobe function in childhood.

References

Ackerly, S.S. (1964): A case of paranatal bilateral frontal lobe defect observed for thirty years. In: *The frontal granular cortex and behaviour*, eds. J.M. Warren & K. Akert, pp. 192–218. New York: McGraw-Hill.

Ackerly, S.S. & Benton, A.L. (1947): Report of a case of bilateral frontal lobe defect. *Assoc. Res. Nerv. Ment. Dis.* **27**, 479–504.

Anderson, S.W., Damasio, H., Jones, R.D. & Tranel D. (1991): Wisconsin card sorting test performance as a measure of frontal lobe damage. *J. Clin. Exp. Neuropsychol.* **13**, 909–922.

Anzai, Y. & Simon, H.A. (1979): The theory of learning by doing. *Psychol. Rev.* **86**, 124–140.

Baddeley, A.D. & Wilson, B.A. (1988): Frontal amnesia and the dysexecutive syndrome. *Brain Cogn.* **7**, 212–230.

Becker, M.G., Isaac, W. & Hynd, G. (1987): Neuropsychological development of non-verbal behaviours attributed to 'frontal lobe' functioning. *Dev. Neuropsychol.* **3**, 275–298.

Benton, A.L. (1992): Prefrontal injury and behaviour in children. *Dev. Neuropsychol.* **7**, 275–281.

Benton, A.L. & Hamsher, K. de S. (1976): *Multilingual aphasia examination*. Iowa City: University of Iowa.

Brunner, R.L., Jordan, M.K. & Berry, H.K. (1983): Early-treated phenylketonuria: neuropsychologic consequences. *J. Pediatr.* **102**, 831–835.

Chelune, G.J. & Baer, R.A. (1986): Developmental norms for the Wisconsin Card Sorting Test. *J. Clin. Exp. Neuropsychol.* **8**, 219–228.

Chelune, G.J. & Thompson, L.L. (1987): Evaluation of the general sensitivity of the Wisconsin Card Sorting Test among younger and older children. *Dev. Neuropsychol.* **3**, 81–89.

Crowie, V.A. (1971): Neurological and psychiatric aspects of phenylketonuria. In: *Phenylketonuria and some inborn errors of aminoacid metabolism*, eds. H. Bickel, H. Hudson & L. Woolf, pp. 29–39. Stuttgart: Springer.

Diamond, A. & Boyer, K. (1989): A version of the Wisconsin Card Sort Test for use with preschool children and an explanation of their source of errors. Meeting of the International Neuropsychological Society, Vancouver, Canada (cited by Smith *et al.*, 1992).

Eslinger, P., Damasio, A.R., Damasio, H., & Grattan, L.M. (1989): Developmental consequences of early frontal-lobe damage. *J. Clin. Exp. Neuropsychol.* **11**, 51.

Eslinger, P., Grattan, L.M., Damasio, A.R. & Damasio, H. (1990): Childhood frontal lobe lesion and psychosocial development: patient DT. *J. Clin. Exp. Neuropsychol.* **12**, 95.

Eslinger, P.J., Grattan, L.M., Damasio, H. & Damasio A. (1992): Developmental consequences of childhood frontal lobe damage. *Arch. Neurol.* **49**, 764–769.

Faglioni, P. (1999): The frontal lobe. In: *Handbook of clinical and experimental neuropsychology*, eds. G. Denes & L. Pizzamiglio, pp. 525–569. Hove: Psychology Press.

Fiducia, D. & O'Leary, D.S. (1990): Development of behaviour attributed to the frontal lobes and the relationship to other cognitive functions. *Dev. Neuropsychol.* **6**, 85–94.

Folling, I. (1994): The discovery of phenylketonuria. *Acta Pediatr.* **407** (Suppl.), 4–10.

Fuster, J.M. (1989): *The prefrontal cortex: anatomy, physiology and neuropsychology of the frontal lobe.* New York: Raven Press.

Grant, D.A. & Berg, E.A. (1948): A behavioural analysis of degree of reinforcement and ease of shifting to new responses in Weigl-type card sorting problems. *J. Exp. Psychol.* **38**, 404–411.

Grattan, L.M. & Eslinger, P.J. (1992): Long-term psychological consequences of childhood frontal lobe lesions in patient DT. *Brain Cogn.* **20**, 185–195.

Harlow, J.M. (1868): Recovery after severe injury to the head. *Publ. Massachusetts Med. Soc.* **2**, 327–346.

Kates, M. & Moscovitch, M. (1989): Development of frontal-lobe functioning in children. Unpublished manuscript (cited by Smith *et al.*, 1992).

Levin, H.S., Culhane, K.A., Hartmann, J., Evankovic, K., Mattson, A.J., Harward, H., Righolz, G., Ewing-Cobbs, L. & Fletcher, J.M. (1991): Developmental changes in performance on tests of purported frontal lobe functioning. *Dev. Neuropsychol.* **7**, 377–395.

Lhermitte, F. (1983): 'Utilization behaviour' and its relation to lesions of the frontal lobes. *Brain* **106**, 237–255.

Lhermitte, F. (1986): Human autonomy and the frontal lobes. II. Patient behaviour in complex and social situations: the 'environmental dependency syndrome'. *Ann. Neurol.* **19**, 335–343.

Loge, D.V., Stanton, D. & Beatty, W.W. (1990): Performance of children with ADHD on tests sensitive to frontal lobe dysfunction. *J. Am. Acad. Child Adolesc. Psychiatr.* **29**, 540–545.

Marlowe, W.B. (1992): The impact of a right prefrontal lesion on the developing brain. *Brain Cogn.* **20**, 205–213.

McGee, R., Williams, S., Moffitt, T. & Anderson, J. (1989): A comparison of 13-year-old boys with attention deficit and reading disorder on neuropsychological measures. *J. Abn. Child Psychol.* **17**, 37–53.

Paniak, C., Miller H.B., Murphy, D., Patterson, L. & Keizer, J. (1996): Canadian developmental norms for 9- to 14-year-olds on the Wisconsin Card Sorting Test. *Can. J. Rehab.* **9**, 233–237.

Pennington, B.F. & Ozonoff, S. (1996): Executive functions and developmental psychopathology. *J. Child Psychol. Psychiatr.* **37**, 51–88.

Pennington, B.F., Van Doorminck, W.J., McCabe, L.L. & McCabe, E.R.B. (1985): Neuropsychologic deficits in early treated phenylketonuric children. *Am. J. Ment. Defic.* **89**, 467–474.

Petrides, M. & Milner, B. (1982): Deficits in subject-ordered tasks after frontal- and temporal-lobe lesions in man. *Neuropsychologia* **20**, 249–262.

Shallice, T. (1982): Specific impairments of planning. *Phil. Trans. Royal Soc. London* **B298**, 199–209.

Smith, I., Beasley, M.G., Wolff, O.H. & Ades, A.E. (1988): Behaviour disturbance in eight-year-old children with early treated phenylketonuria (PKU). *J. Pediatr.* **112**, 403–408.

Smith, M.L., Kates, M.H. & Vriezen, E.R. (1992): The development of frontal-lobe functions. In: *Handbook of neuropsychology*, vol. 7, pp. 309–330, eds. S.J. Segalowitz & I. Rapin. Amsterdam: Elsevier.

Stroop, J.R. (1935): Studies of interference in serial verbal reactions. *J. Exp. Psychol.* **18**, 643–662.

Stuss, D.T. & Benson, D.F. (1986): *The frontal lobes.* New York: Raven Press.

Temple, C. (1997): *Developmental cognitive neuropsychology*, pp. 287–316. Hove: Psychology Press.

Welsh, M.C., Pennington, B.F., Ozonoff, S., Rouse, B. & McCabe, E.R.B. (1990): Neuropsychology of early-treated phenylketonuria: specific executive function deficits. *Child Dev.* **61**, 1697–1713.

Welsh, M., Pennington, B.F. & Groisser, D.B. (1991): A normative-developmental study of executive function: a window on prefrontal function in children. *Dev. Neuropsychol.* **7**, 131–149.

Williams, D. & Mateer, C.A. (1992): Developmental impact of frontal lobe injury in middle childhood. *Brain Cogn.* **20**, 196–204.

Yeudall, L.T., Fromm, D., Reddon, F.R. & Stefanyk, W.O. (1986): Normative data stratified by age and sex for 12 neuropsychological tests. *J. Clin. Psychol.* **42**, 918–946.

Chapter 3

Epileptogenesis in the frontal lobe

Giuliano Avanzini

*Department of Experimental Research and Diagnostics, Istituto Nazionale Neurologico 'C. Besta',
via Celoria 11, 20133 Milan, Italy*
avanzini@istituto-besta.it

Summary

The complex integratory activity within the frontal lobe accounts for the complexity of frontal lobe seizures, which present with different combinations of motor, autonomic, emotional, and cognitive signs and symptoms. Knowledge of the cellular and local circuit properties and connectivity of different frontal areas is necessary to understand their susceptibility to epileptogenic agents and the patterns of discharge propagation.

The high concentration of N-methyl-D-aspartate (NMDA) receptors in the outer layers of the frontal cortex makes it prone to epileptogenesis especially in early infancy, when these receptors are not yet fully sensitive to voltage-dependent block by magnesium ions.

Stimulus-sensitive epileptic phenomena such as reflex seizures, some types of myoclonus elicited by somatosensory stimulation, and photosensitive seizures are related to the organization of afferent systems. These mechanisms appear particularly relevant to some age-related idiopathic partial epilepsies. In addition, thalamic afferents from mediodorsal nucleus may account for the sleep-related occurrence of partial seizures of frontal origin.

The rapid contralateral projection of epileptic discharge through the frontal callosal system is the basis for secondary bilateral synchrony which may produce bilaterally synchronous spike and wave discharges mimicking those of primary generalized epilepsy.

The biological bases of the cortical dysfunction underlying epileptic discharges are to be found in cellular and circuitry mechanisms leading to the generation of excessive and highly synchronized discharges and to their propagation along axonal pathways originating from the epileptogenic areas. Cortical susceptibility to epileptogenic agents and the clinical expression of epileptic discharges depend on the functional organization of different cortical areas and on maturational changes of nerve cell excitability and conduction. The influence of such variables is particularly difficult to evaluate when dealing with cerebral regions endowed with a complex anatomo-functional organization, such as the frontal lobe. The frontal lobe is a large region of isocortex (i.e. cerebral cortex with a basic six-layered structure) lying anterior to the central sulcus and its prolongation on the mesial surface. A number of cortical areas are located within these boundaries, heterogeneous both in structure and in function. Different classification schemes have been proposed according to differences in microscopic structure and connectivity; for the present chapter we will follow Karl Zilles' account (Fig. 1; Zilles, 1990), based mainly on Sanides (1962) and including two main divisions: the motor zone, comprising primary and non-primary motor areas; and the prefrontal associational region.

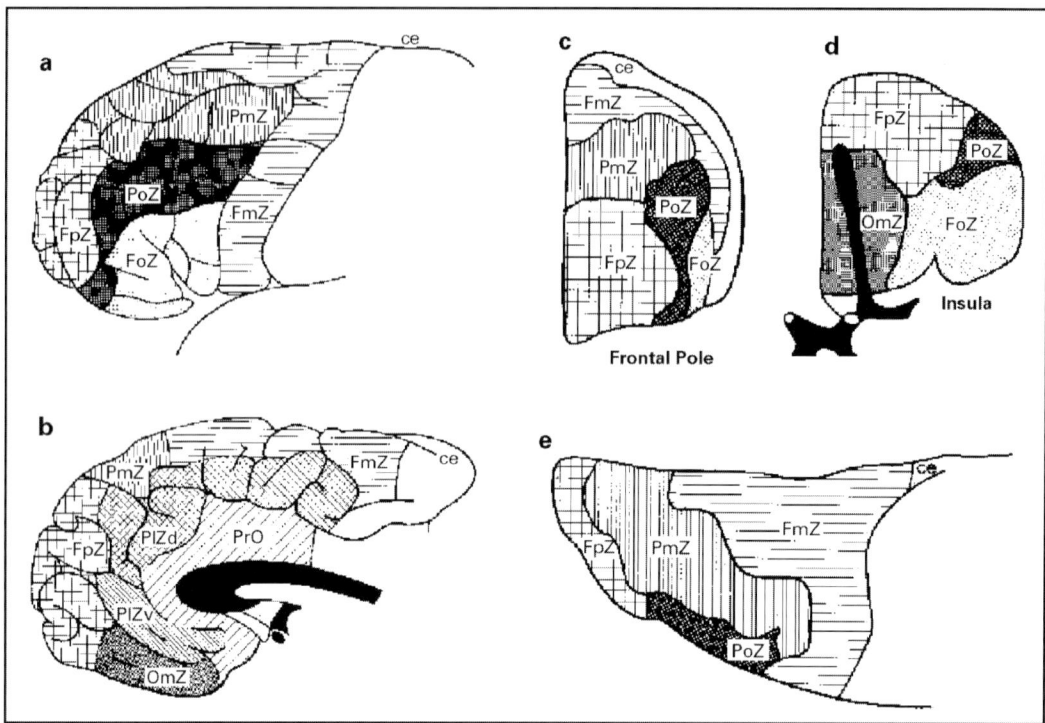

Fig. 1. Map of the frontal lobe. a: lateral; b: medial; c: frontal; d: basal; e: dorsal views. ce: central sulcus; FmZ: frontal motor zone; FoZ: fronto-opercular zone; FpZ: frontopolar zone; OmZ: orbitomedian zone; PlZd: dorsal paralimbic zone; PlZv: ventral paralimbic zone; PmZ: paramotor zone; PoZ: para-opercular zone; PrO: pro-isocortex. [From Zilles (1990), modified from Sanides (1962).]

Topography of the frontal lobe

Frontal motor zone (FmZ in Fig. 1): In the original Brodmann cytoarchitectonic classification (Brodmann, 1909) the frontal motor zone was defined as the agranular frontal cortex including primary (area 4) and nonprimary (area 6) motor regions (Fig. 2), the distinction being based on the presence of giant Betz cells in layer V of area 4 but not of area 6. This criterion however is no longer considered acceptable, nor is the identification of area 4 as the only source for pyramidal tract fibres. Additional sources for the pyramidal tract have been found in nonprimary motor, and primary and secondary somatosensory cortices (Brodal, 1969; Kuypers, 1958). Functional studies indicate that the nonprimary motor cortex is composed of two major areas, the premotor and the supplementary motor cortices, that are crucially involved in preparation, inhibition and sensory guidance of movement. The FmZ zone in Fig. 1 includes motor, premotor and supplementary motor cortices, but not the oculomotor field (Brodmann's area 8) which is indicated as paramotor zone (PmZ). The primary and nonprimary motor areas are widely interconnected with cortical and subcortical regions. The thalamic projections from the ventrolateral (VL) nucleus are particularly important; the rostral part of this nucleus, which is connected with the globus pallidus and substantia nigra, projects to the supplementary motor area, whereas the premotor area receives projections from a distinct part of VL (the nucleus X of Wise & Strick, 1984). The primary motor area receives its afferents from the caudal part of VL which is the thalamic relay for the cerebellar projection, and from the

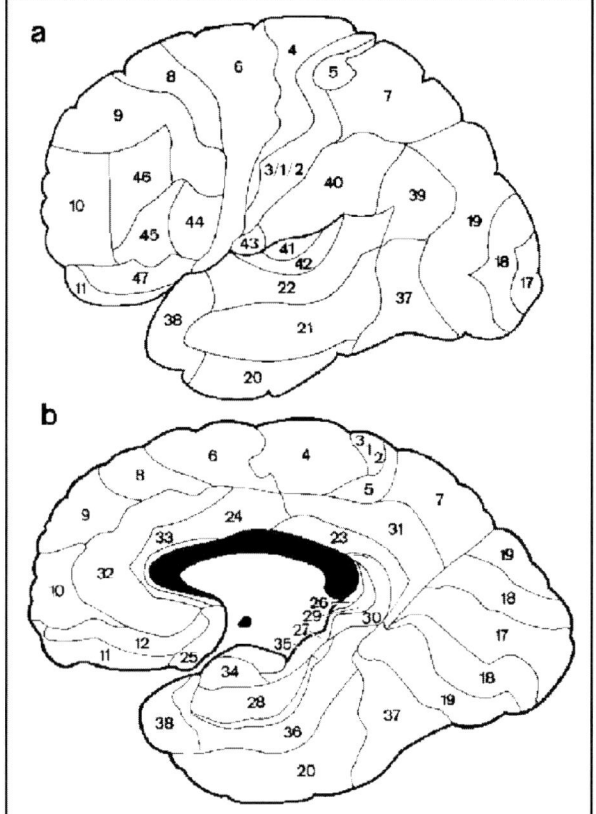

Fig. 2. Architectonic areal map in lateral (a) and medial (b) views after Brodmann (1909). [From Zilles (1990).]

ventroposterolateral (VPL) nucleus, which is the thalamic relay for the lemniscal system. Efferent projections from the supplementary and primary motor areas go directly to the spinal cord, whereas the premotor area projects indirectly to the spinal cord *via* the medullary reticular formation.

Information on the functional significance of the motor cortices has been obtained from animal experiments, and from clinical observations in humans with localized cortical lesions and the results of cortical stimulation during surgery. The primary motor area is activated during voluntary movements with a strict somatotopic organization as Penfield & Rasmussen (1950) impressively demonstrated by drawing their famous homunculus, whereas non-primary motor cortex is involved in preparation and inhibition; the premotor area is involved in the sensory guidance of movement. In contrast with the primary motor cortex, the non-primary motor areas are always activated bilaterally.

Prefrontal associational regions include the functionally heterogeneous zones PmZ, FoZ, PrO, PIZd, PIZv, FpZ and OmZ (Fig. 1) with a more or less visible inner granular layer, which is clearly recognizable in Brodmann's areas 8-12 and 44-47 (Fig. 2), less developed in dysgranular area 32 and least developed in area 24. The prefrontal cortex is reciprocally connected with the parietal, temporal, and visual association areas of the ipsi- and contralateral hemisphere and is the main target of the topographically organized cortical projection of the thalamic mediodorsal nucleus (MD). The mesial magnocellular MD division projects mainly to orbital and medial prefrontal cortices, whereas the lateral parvocellular division sends its afferents to the dorsolateral prefrontal cortex

(Goldman-Rakic & Porrino, 1985); a lateral crescent-like paralamellaris segment projects to PmZ (Fig. 1) corresponding to Brodmann's area 8 (Fig. 2). In addition, area 8 receives afferents from the pulvinar (Goldman-Rakic & Porrino, 1985; Barbas et al., 1991; Macchi et al., 1996).

Prefrontal associative functions are essential for social behaviour and cognitive processing. Disorders of prefrontal areas affect functions which substantially contribute to human personality such as motivational drive and planning of activities, emotional status and memory functions. Specific information can be drawn from experimental studies although important species differences make it difficult to extrapolate to humans the results obtained even in non-human primates. More direct insight is provided by observation in humans with spontaneous or surgical frontal lesions, including the aberrant practice of leucotomy, popularized by Moniz (1936) for the cure of various mental disorders, which leads to profound changes in personality and which should be remembered as an example of how brutal medical intervention can become when its ethical principles are disregarded. Very little has indeed been learned from the results of the shocking number of leucotomies performed with different techniques in many countries. The results of focal cortical stimulation protocols aimed at optimizing epilepsy surgery have been much more informative. Functional imaging is another important source of information and makes it possible to investigate the functional anatomy of the cerebral cortex in normal subjects and patients. Although detailed analysis of ictal phenomenology could also contribute to define the functional significance of the area involved in the epileptic discharge, difficulties arise because of the tendency of the discharge to spread to other cortical regions in more or less complex patterns. This is extensively discussed in other chapters.

Paramotor (PmZ) and fronto-opercular zones (FoZ) subserve special higher-order motor functions: control of eye movements (PmZ, mainly corresponding to Brodmann's area 8 and part of area 9), and motor speech (FoZ, mainly corresponding to areas 44, 45, and 47).

PmZ receives projections from cortical visual areas and contains cells responsive to visual stimuli which discharge before saccadic eye movements (Bruce & Goldberg, 1984), with directional selectivity. In humans, metabolic activation of area 8 is seen during ocular fixation, pursuit eye movements and various discrimination tasks (Roland, 1984).

FoZ, including Broca's motor speech region, receives its main afferents from Wernicke's area of the temporal lobe and from visual and auditory brain regions. Its metabolic rate is high during the analysis of visual or auditory information. As originally described by Broca (1863), a lesion of FoZ results in expressive aphasia, most probably due to a loss of the complex motor program for structured activation of neurons in the face region of area 4, whereas its stimulation evokes vocalizations (Penfield & Rasmussen, 1950). Functional magnetic resonance can define the localization of the speech area and analyse its function in individual subjects (McGraw et al., 2001; Demonet & Thierry, 2001).

Proisocortex (PrO) and dorsal and ventral paralimbic zones (PlZd and PlZv) correspond to Brodmann's areas 24 and 32. Brodmann (1909) included areas 24 and 32 in his anterior cingulate region together with areas 33 and 25 which belong properly to the periarchicortical region of the anterior cingulate gyrus, and together with areas 23 and 31 which have a clear isocortical structure but which belong to the posterior cingulate gyrus. These areas, however, are interconnected and are sometimes considered part of the limbic system the extent of which is still disputed. PrO and PlZ dorsal and ventral regions cooperate with PmZ in recruiting and controlling other cortical areas involved in actions which require prior instructions or analysis or which depend on comparison and decision about sensory discrimination followed by cues for voluntary movements. Ablation of PrO and PlZ in animals leads to increased tameness and reduction of social contacts, together with a reduced performance in delayed alternating tasks (Divac, 1971; Glees et al., 1950). This high-level integratory activity takes into account sensory information: PmZ is activated during tasks depending on patterned sensory information and its most basal and caudal parts are activated with PoZ during discrimination of auditory signals.

The frontopolar zone (FpZ) of Sanides (1962) is comparable to Brodmann's area 10 and has been shown to play an important role in cognition. Its dorsal part has its highest metabolic rate and blood flow in alert subjects; blood flow and metabolism drop to their lowest levels during sleep. The basal part of FpZ is significantly activated during discrimination of tone sequences, mental calculation and object categorization.

The orbitomedian zone (OmZ), including Brodmann's areas 11, 12, 13, and 14, is thought to integrate autonomic and emotional functions. Early reports documented 'sham rage' in monkeys after ablation of its most medial portion (area 14). A detailed analysis of OmZ is difficult because of its inaccessibility.

Interactions between different prefrontal areas for performing the temporal integration of emotional, social and visceral aspects of information are comprehensively discussed by Fuster (2003), whose work has greatly contributed to our understanding of the role of the prefrontal cortex in the temporal organization of behaviour (Fuster, 1997).

Biological bases of epileptogenesis

Epileptic seizures are the result of highly synchronized discharges arising in a population of hyperexcitable neurons in which intrinsic mechanisms of excitability and neurotransmitter-mediated cell-to-cell communication are significantly altered (Fig. 3). Experiments (reviewed in Avanzini, 2002) have shown that imbalance between excitatory aminoacid (EAA) neurotransmitters and the inhibitory neurotransmitter gamma-aminobutyric acid (GABA), and dysfunction of depolarizing Na^+ and Ca^{2+} transmembrane currents and repolarizing K^+ currents flowing through voltage-gated channels are the most relevant determinants of cortical epileptogenesis. Such changes can lead cortical neurons to fire robust burst discharges (Fig. 4), first described by Matsumoto & Ajmone Marsan (1964a; 1964b) as paroxysmal depolarization shifts (PDSs). The tendency of epileptogenic neuronal aggregates to fire with a high probability of highly synchronized PDSs is facilitated by a special subpopulation of cortical pyramidal neurons in layer V that are physiologically endowed with an intrinsic Na^+-dependent bursting property (Fig. 5). Such intrinsically bursting (IB) neurons are associated with a well-developed system of neuronal collaterals that extends widely tangentially to the cortical surface and that can thus synchronize large populations of pyramidal neurons (Chagnac-Amitai & Connors, 1989).

To what extent can the specific anatomical and functional organization of the frontal lobe be correlated with the biological bases of frontal epileptogenesis? One way to address this question is to analyse the influence of functional topographic representation within the frontal cortex on the clinical patterns of frontal seizures. This issue is extensively discussed in chapters analysing the different types of frontal seizures.

In this section, some cellular and circuit properties that may account for discharge propagation and for a special susceptibility to epileptogenic agents will be highlighted.

Morrisett *et al.* (1987) have shown that the concentration of N-methyl-D-aspartate (NMDA) receptors in the outer layers of rat frontal cortex is remarkably high. NMDA receptors are a subtype of EAA receptors coupled with a Na^+- and Ca^{2+}- permeable ionophore and thus are particularly effective in depolarizing the postsynaptic neuron. At resting membrane potential, EAA binding to NMDA receptors does not depolarize the membrane because the NMDA-associated ionophore is blocked

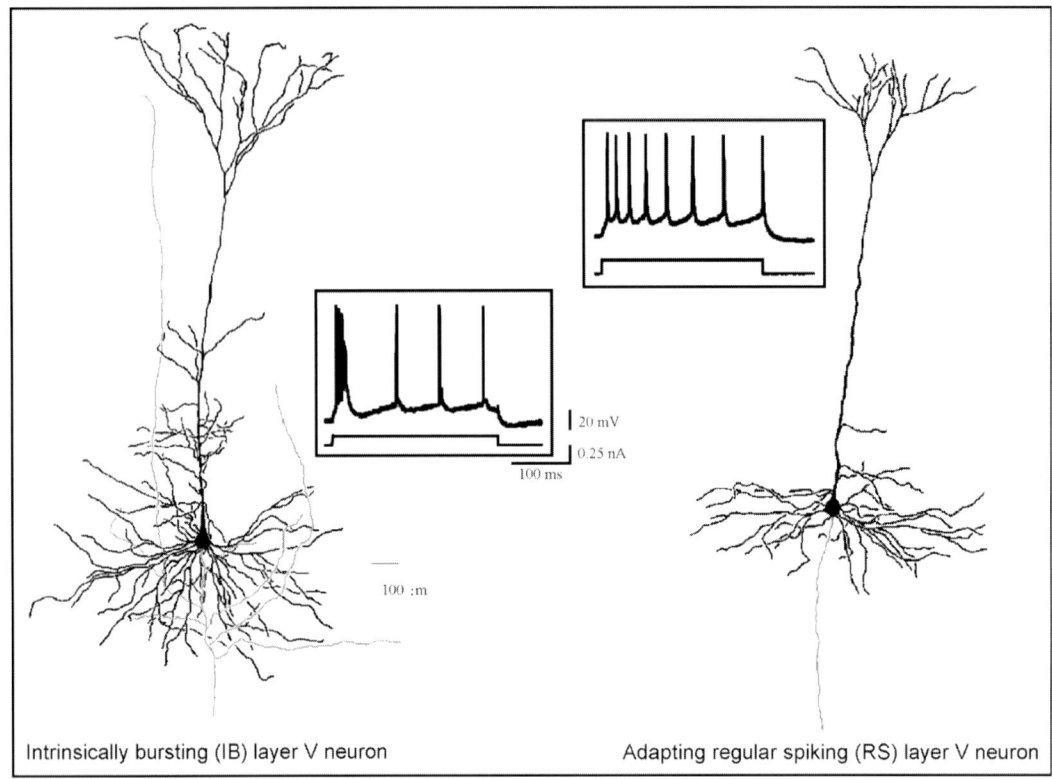

Fig. 3. Synaptic (top) and intrinsic (bottom) excitable cellular mechanisms whose alteration can lead to epileptogenic discharges here shown (right side) by PDS. Top left: cortical local circuit made by a GABAergic interneuron receiving a collateral of the axon of a pyramidal neuron and projecting back to it. The postsynaptic $GABA_A$ and $GABA_B$ receptors are coupled respectively to chloride- (Cl^-) and potassium- (K^+) permeable ionophores. Top middle: EAA receptors of subtype AMPA (left), permeable to sodium (Na^+) ions and NMDA (right) permeable to both Na^+ and Ca^{2+} ions whose flow however at resting potential is prevented by a magnesium (Mg^{2+}) ion which is removed by membrane depolarization. Top right: transformation from a physiological excitatory-inhibitory postsynaptic discharge (bottom line) into a PDS (top line) due to an imbalance between excitatory and inhibitory synaptic influences. Bottom left: voltage-dependent Na^+, Ca^{2+} and K^+ channels which are the main determinants of intrinsic neuronal excitability. Bottom right: dysfunction of voltage-dependent channels can lead to transformation of regular firing (top line) into an excessive high-frequency discharge (bottom line) constituted by repeated PDSs (better shown on the right by expanding the time axis).

by a magnesium ion. Membrane depolarization relieves this voltage-dependent block by removing the magnesium ion from the channel pore, thus further depolarizing the membrane towards the spike generation level (Fig. 3). The high concentration of NMDA receptors in the frontal lobe would be expected to make this region particularly prone to the effect of agents affecting the balance between excitatory and inhibitory neurotransmission. A systematic analysis of topographic differences in receptor and channel distribution and in other determinants of neuronal excitability relevant to epileptogenesis in different zones of the frontal lobe has not been carried out.

Another aspect of frontal cortical organization relevant to epileptogenesis is related to its connectivity, with ascending associative and commissural systems which account for stimulus sensitivity, relationship to vigilance, and bihemispheric synchronization of epileptic manifestations arising from the frontal lobe.

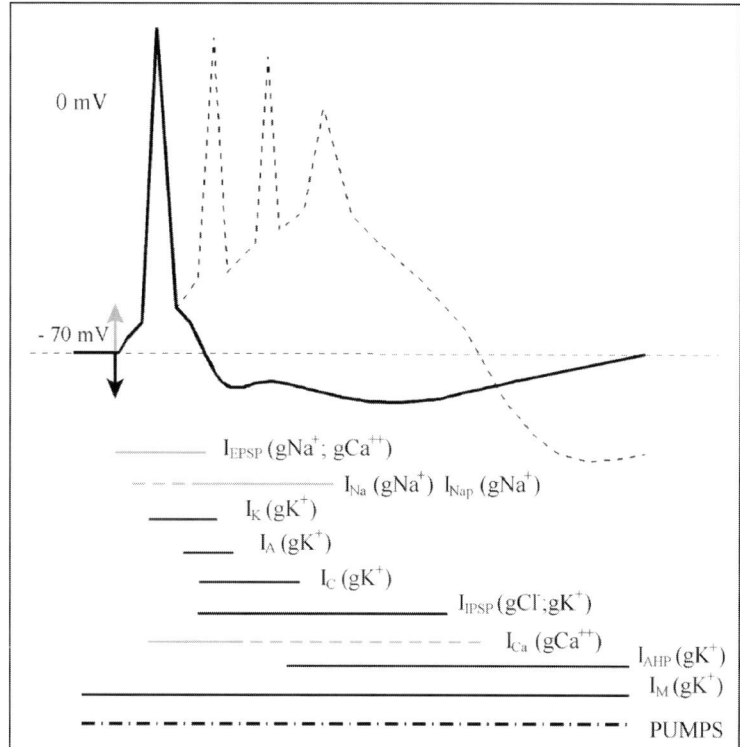

Fig. 4. Time course of different neurotransmitter and voltage-activated ionic conductances which are activated in sequence during a single spike cell discharge (black line, top). I_{EPSP} and I_{IPSP} refer respectively to excitatory and inhibitory postsynaptic potential currents. Each line indicates the activation and inactivation time of the ionic currents with respect to the cell response. Broken lines indicate slowly- or non-inactivating currents which have a primary role in prolonging membrane depolarization thus promoting the transformation of a simple spike discharge (black line, top) into a PDS (broken line, top).

Stimulus-sensitive seizures have their pathophysiological basis in transcortical reflexes. The afferent arm of the transcortical reflex arc is provided by sensory systems reaching the frontal lobe through primary or non-primary afferents. Typical examples of the first case are the somatosensory afferents, i.e. lemniscal fibres terminating not only in the parietal areas 1, 2 and 3, but also in the primary motor area 4 (Wiesendanger, 1973; Wong et al., 1974) where a subset of thalamocortical fibres, originating in the lemniscal relay nucleus ventro-postero-lateral (VPL), terminate. Non-primary visual and auditory afferents reach the frontal cortex through multisynaptic pathways, usually involving cortico-cortical fibres, and eventually end in several frontal areas as described in the previous section.

Studies of stimulus-sensitive myoclonus have shown that cortical reflex myoclonus is due to a transcortical reflex mechanism involving somatosensory afferent pathways, the motor cortex and its efferent corticospinal and corticobulbar fibres (Hallett et al., 1979). Hyperexcitability of this transcortical loop can account for some other types of motor seizures. De Marco (1980) described an unusual form of idiopathic partial epilepsy with extreme somatosensory evoked potentials (ESEPs) and in collaboration with Tassinari (De Marco & Tassinari, 1981) was able to show that ESEPs can be recorded before the onset of seizures in subjects that subsequently developed the complete syndrome and also in some subjects who never had seizures thereafter. The conclusion was

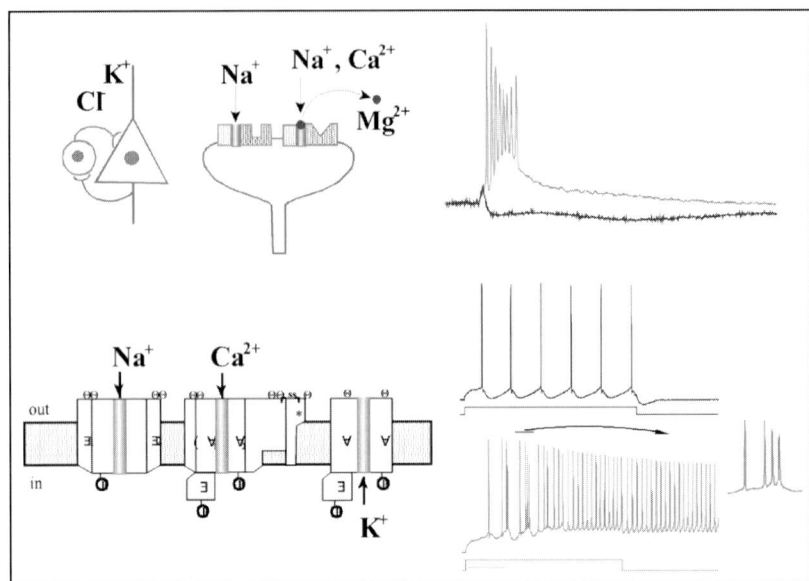

Fig. 5. Camera lucida reconstruction of layer V. Intrinsically bursting (IB, left) and regular spiking (RS, right) cortical neurons are depicted with examples of their typical firing patterns. Note the tangential arborization of the IB axon.

that between 4 and 6 years of age, somatosensory evoked activities are enhanced in some subjects and that this can predispose them to an age-related idiopathic partial epilepsy that usually subsides before 9 years of age.

The frontal cortex has been proven to be involved in another type of stimulus-sensitive epilepsy, the photosensitive epilepsy occurring spontaneously in the baboon *Papio papio* first reported by Killam *et al.* (1966) and intensively studied by Naquet and his group (Naquet & Meldrum, 1972). In this animal, intermittent light stimulation induces EEG discharges which appear as bilaterally synchronous spike and wave or polyspike and wave discharges invariably beginning in the fronto-Rolandic region, and which consistently correlate with burst discharges of frontal, but not parietal or occipital neurons. Since most of the visual input reaching the frontal cortex is thought to be relayed by the occipital visual cortex (see above), the photosensitive discharges of *Papio papio* are triggered by non-primary visual afferents; and, unlike stimulus-sensitive motor discharges, are not linked to a local evoked potential which is generated elsewhere. Whether similar pathophysiology applies to human photosensitive epilepsies, and what mechanism is responsible for simian frontal hyperexcitability and thus responsible for these visually-triggered epileptic discharges, are still open questions.

The interconnection between the thalamic nucleus MD (see above) and the prefrontal cortex is involved in facilitating the occurrence of frontal seizures during sleep. MD implication in sleep mechanisms was first suggested by the observation of an Italian family with familial fatal insomnia, transmitted as an autosomal dominant trait and associated with a selective atrophy of anterior and MD thalamic nuclei (Lugaresi *et al.*, 1986; Marini *et al.*, 1989). Experimental lesions of MD in cats confirmed the role played by this thalamic nucleus in transferring synchronized sleep patterns to the frontal cortex (Marini *et al.*, 1989). The precipitating effect of synchronized sleep on frontal lobe seizures is well illustrated by the syndrome autosomal dominant nocturnal frontal lobe epilepsy (ADNFLE), due to a mutation of acetylcholine receptor genes, in which explosive partial seizures of frontal origin occur predominantly or exclusively during slow wave sleep (Steinlein *et al.*, 1995).

Finally the role of frontal callosal projections in interhemispheric synchronization of epileptic discharges deserves mention. Marcus & Watson (1968) reported that bilateral frontal homotopic epileptogenic foci in the rhesus monkey produced bilaterally synchronous and symmetrical spike and wave discharges, but that symmetrical foci located in other parts of the cortex usually remained independent. Marcus & Watson were able to obtain fairly typical bisynchronous spike and wave activity associated with short staring spells resembling childhood absence with PmZ lesions and polyspike and wave complexes associated with interruption of motor activities and prominent myoclonus involving the muscle of the face and forelimbs with lesions of the anterior part of FmZ, mainly corresponding to Brodmann's area 6. The more posterior the foci along FmZ, towards area 4, the more pronounced the motor component which tended eventually to generalize. Bilateral anterior foci in the FpZ produced prolonged localized polyspike discharges, but no definite alteration of behaviour.

Development

The frontal cortex gains its final configuration after complex changes during foetal life. During early foetal development, the telencephalic ventricular zone (VZ) provides glial and neuronal stem cells that eventually form the mature layered cortex through an 'inside-out' sequence of neuronal layer formation. That is, the neurons of the deepest cortical layers migrate first, followed by the neuroblasts that are committed to the more superficial cortical layers (Sidman & Rakic, 1973). Postmitotic neuroblasts migrate by climbing the radial glial fibres from the VZ to the pial surface to form the cortical plate (CP) around the 10th week of gestation (Rakic, 1990; Schmechel & Rakic, 1979). While layer I derives from the primordial plexiform layer (PPL) which is thought to provide a framework for successive migration (Marin-Padilla, 1988, 1990; Rakic & Goldman-Rakic, 1982) the cortical layers II-VI originate from the CP.

Disturbances of prenatal maturational processes may result in different types of dysplasia, usually highly epileptogenic, and beyond the topic of this chapter.

In the mammalian neocortex, however, major maturational processes continue after birth and have both morphological and physiological aspects. Most of the available data are drawn from experimental data on rats; it is therefore important to establish some relationship between human and rat postnatal developmental stages. At birth the rat neocortex is less mature than the human neocortex and reaches a stage around postnatal day 5 corresponding to about 1 month of human postnatal life. From this point, developmental rates in rat and human diverge so that the third human postnatal month corresponds to days 13–15 in the rat. In the rat sensorimotor cortex, neocortical layering is still incomplete at birth; on the second postnatal day (P2), layer V appears completely separate from the cortical plate, and during the next few days, layers II, III and IV further differentiate from the cortical plate and gradually increase in thickness. Most of the morphogenetic processes affecting cell bodies, dendrites and axons also occur after birth. Cell bodies progressively enlarge and attain their final size by the end of the first month, while the volume of neuropil increases, principally due to the growth of dendritic arborization (Eayers & Goodhead, 1959). Axonal proliferation and synapse formation occur at different rates in pyramidal and local circuit neurons, so that the axons of projection neurons begin to extend and form synapses a week before the axons of local circuit neurons (Miller, 1988).

Substantial changes in physiological properties occur in connection with morphological development and involve both synaptic transmission and intrinsic membrane excitability (McCormick & Prince, 1987; Kriegstein *et al.*, 1987; Avanzini *et al.*, 1992; Franceschetti *et al.*, 1998). Rat neocortical neurons undergo significant maturational changes in passive membrane properties and active mechanisms, which determine their mature firing properties. The substantial increase in ion channel density and the significant changes in the different ionic currents contributing to the membrane potential are crucial in bringing about the changes in membrane excitability that occur during this time. Concurrently, immature synaptic transmission, characterized by facilitation of EAA-mediated transmission due to an incomplete sensitivity to voltage-dependent magnesium block of NMDA receptors (see previous section and Fig. 3), and by a reduced GABA-induced hyperpolarization, evolves towards the adult state. Low ion channel density in axons may be a limiting factor for synaptic transmission in immature neocortex neurons. The ionic currents which are activated close to the resting membrane potentials may contribute significantly to shaping both excitatory and inhibitory post-synaptic potentials evoked by different inputs. For example, the inward current persisting during burst discharge, which is easily activated by threshold depolarizing events, can lead the neuron to respond to an excitatory input with a strong repetitive discharge of action potentials in mature animals, amplifying the effect of the input, while this amplification does not occur in immature animals during the first two weeks of life.

These developmental processes would also be expected to have a major influence on the response of the immature brain to pathological events in early life. Analysis of the age-dependent changes to intrinsic neuronal properties may therefore help to understand the development of epilepsy in childhood. More than two-thirds of human epilepsies begin during childhood and adolescence, when the anatomical and functional maturation of the brain is still incomplete; furthermore the clinical presentation of such epilepsies is also age-dependent (ILAE Commission on classification, 1989).

As shown in Table 1a, immature synaptic features, passive properties and voltage-dependent current characteristics on which neuronal firing depends, suggest that the immature brain is hyperexcitable

Table 1.

a) Physiological properties suggesting increased propensity to excitability in the immature brain		
Characteristic	**Effect**	
• Reduced sensitivity of NMDA receptors to voltage-dependent magnesium block	Enhanced NMDA-mediated neurotransmission	Weeks I-II
• Reduced GABA-induced hyperpolarization	Less effective inhibitory neurotransmission	Weeks I-II
• Less negative resting membrane potential	Neurons closer to depolarization threshold	Weeks I-II
• Higher input resistance	Amplification of depolarizing inputs	Weeks I-II
• Shorter electrotonic length	Increased gain of inputs	Weeks I-II
• Slower repolarization following action potential	Less effective fast hyperpolarization	Weeks I-II
• Lower efficiency of spike frequency adaptation in regular spiking neurons	Less effective control of firing	Week II
b) Physiological properties consistent with asynchronous and 'fragmentary' expression of neuronal hyperexcitability in the immature brain		
Characteristic	**Effect**	
• Slow rising phase of action potential	Reduced ability to generate fast, high-frequency action potentials	Weeks I-II
• Inability to discharge during long lasting depolarizing pulses	Inability to generate long-lasting high-frequency firing leading to sustained epileptic discharges	Week I
• Absence of intrinsically generated bursts, characterizing intrinsically bursting neurons	Less effective neocortical synchronization	Weeks I-II

compared to the mature brain. Experimental evidence (Table 1b) also indicates that many factors restrain membrane excitability, thereby decreasing the probability of developing long-lasting, high-frequency discharges, on which the mature expression of seizure activity depends.

The relatively depolarized resting potential present in immature animals holds the neuron close to the threshold for action potential generation; furthermore, the higher membrane resistance to input may act in conjunction with the rather short electrotonic length to amplify incoming depolarizing signals, so that immature neurons would seem to be predisposed to hyperexcitability. This tendency is further enhanced by the relative predominance of excitatory over inhibitory synaptic transmission and by the immaturity of firing properties, i.e. the less effective repolarization following an action potential and the delayed maturation of firing frequency adaptation.

In contrast however, the inability of more immature neurons to sustain fast, high-frequency action potentials would inhibit the generation of epileptic discharges. The delayed maturation of IB pyramidal neurons may serve to counteract intracortical synchronizing mechanisms, developing in layer V. These factors may partially explain the fragmentary and asynchronous expression of seizures in the immature brain (Mares, 1991) and suggest a physiological basis for the chaotic EEG expression of epileptic discharges in human epileptic encephalopathies.

Conclusions

The complex anatomo-functional organization of the frontal lobe accounts for the complex manifestations of frontal lobe seizures which can include different combinations of motor, vegetative, and emotional signs and symptoms, depending on the site of origin and the propagation of the epileptic discharge. Results of clinical and experimental studies provide evidence for cellular and circuit mechanisms which may make the frontal cortex susceptible to epileptogenesis and apt to recruit cellular populations of both hemispheres in synchronized activities.

The high concentration of NMDA receptors in outer layers of the frontal cortex may facilitate an imbalance between excitatory and inhibitory synaptic systems, thus enhancing the effect of epileptogenic agents. This factor can be particularly important in the early stages of postnatal life when the voltage-dependent sensitivity of NMDA receptors to magnesium is physiologically incomplete and therefore the contribution of NMDA receptors to excitatory synaptic transmission is particularly prominent.

The motor and premotor areas of the frontal lobe are richly provided with multisensory afferents which can trigger abnormal activities and sustain cortical excitability. Lemniscal afferents are responsible for somatosensory-evoked cortical reflex myoclonus and other stimulus-sensitive epileptic phenomena, whereas non-primary visual afferents are responsible for some types of frontally-generated photosensitive seizures. A special facilitation of the cortical evoked activity occurs in some children between 4 and 6 years old and is considered a predisposing factor for an age-dependent idiopathic partial epilepsy with extreme somatosensory evoked potentials. Non-specific afferents reaching the prefrontal region through the thalamic MD nucleus may account for the sleep-related occurrence of seizures in partial epilepsies of frontal origin such as ADNFLE.

Callosal transfer of frontal epileptic activity from one hemisphere to the other is particularly rapid. This explains the tendency of frontal epileptic discharges to occur bilaterally, often synchronously and sometimes symmetrically, thus mimicking genuine generalized epilepsies.

References

Avanzini, G. (in press): Mechanisms of epileptogenesis. In: *The treatment of epilepsy*, 2nd ed., eds. S. Shorvon, D.R. Fish, E. Perucca, W.E. Dodson & A. Olivier. Boston: Blackwell Science.

Avanzini, G., Franceschetti, S., Panzica, F., & Buzio, S. (1992): Age-dependent changes in excitability of rat neocortical neurons studied in vitro. In: *Molecular neurobiology of epilepsy (Epilepsy Rev.* Suppl. 9), eds. J. Engel Jr., C. Wasterlain, E.A. Cavalheiro, U. Heinemann & G. Avanzini, pp. 95–105. Amsterdam: Elsevier Science Publishers.

Barbas, H., Haswell-Henion, T.H. & Dermon, C.R. (1991): Diverse thalamic projections to the prefrontal cortex in the rhesus monkey. *J. Comp. Neurol.* 313: 65–94.

Broca, P.P. (1863): Localisation des fonctions cérébrales. Siège du langage articulé. *Bull. Soc. Anthropol. (Paris)* 4, 200–204.

Brodal, A. (1969): Neurological anatomy in relation to clinical medicine. 2nd ed. London and New York: Oxford University Press.

Brodmann, K. (1909): *Vergleichende Lokalisationslehre der Grosshirnrinde*. Leipzig: Barth.

Bruce, C.J. & Goldberg, M.E. (1984): Physiology of the frontal eye fields. *Trends Neurosci.* 7, 436–441.

Chagnac-Amitai, Y. & Connors, B.V. (1982): Synchronized excitation and inhibition driven by intrinsically bursting neurons in neocortex. *J. Neurophysiol.* 48, 1302–1320.

Commission on Classification and Terminology of the International League Against Epilepsy (1989): Proposal for revised classification of epilepsy and epileptic syndromes. *Epilepsia* 30, 389–399.

De Marco, P. (1980): Possibilities of a temporal relationship between the morphology and frequency of parietal somatosensory evoked spikes and the occurrence of epileptic manifestations. *Clin. Electroencephal.* 11, 132–135.

De Marco, P. & Tassinari, C.A. (1981): Extreme somatosensory evoked potential (ESEP): an EEG sign forecasting the possible occurrence of seizures in children. *Epilepsia* 22, 569–575.

Demonet, J.F. & Thierry, G. (2001): Language and brain: what is up? What is coming up? *J. Clin. Exp. Neuropsychol.* 23, 49–73.

Divac, I. (1971): Frontal lobe system and spatial reversal in the rat. *Neuropsychologica* 9, 175–183.

Eayers, J.T. & Goodhead, B. (1959): Postnatal development of the cerebral cortex of the rat. *J. Anat.* 93, 385–402.

Franceschetti, S., Sancini, G., Panzica, F., Radici, C. & Avanzini, G. (1998): Postnatal differentiation of firing properties and morphological characteristics in layer V pyramidal neurons of the sensorimotor cortex. *Neurosciences* 83, 1013–1024.

Fuster, J.M. (1997): *The prefrontal cortex: anatomy, physiology and neuropsychology of the frontal lobe*. Philadelphia: Lippincott-Raven.

Fuster, J.M. (2003): Functional anatomy of the prefrontal cortex. In: *Frontal seizures and epilepsies in children*, eds. A. Beaumanoir, F. Andermann, P. Chauvel, L. Mira & B. Zifkin, pp. 1–10. Mariani Foundation Paediatric Neurology Series, vol. 11. Paris, London: John Libbey Eurotext.

Glees, P., Cole, J., Whitty, C.W.M. & Cairns, H. (1950): The effects of lesions in the cingulate gyrus and adjacent areas in monkeys. *J. Neurol. Neurosurg. Psychiatry* 13, 178–190.

Goldman-Rakic, P.S. & Porrino, L.J. (1985): The primate medio-dorsal (MD) nucleus and its projection to the frontal lobe. *J. Comp. Neurol.* 242, 535–560.

Hallett, M., Chadwick, D., Adam, J. & Marsden, C.D. (1979): Cortical reflex myoclonus. *Neurology* 29, 1107–1125.

Killam, K.F., Killam, E.K. & Naquet R. (1966): Mise en évidence chez certains singes d'un syndrome myoclonique. *C.R. Acad. Sci. (Paris)* 262, 1010–1012.

Kriegstein, A.R., Suppes, T. & Prince D.A. (1987): Cellular and synaptic physiology and epileptogenesis of developing rat neocortical neurons *in vitro*. *Dev. Brain Res.* 34, 161–171.

Kuypers, H.J.M. (1958): Cortico-bulbar connections to the pons and lower brain stem in man. *Brain* 81, 364–388.

Lugaresi, E., Medori, R., Montagna, P., Baruzzi, A., Cortelli, P., Lugaresi, A., Tinuper, P., Zucconi, M. & Gambetti, P. (1986): Fatal familial insomnia and dysautonomia with selective degeneration of thalamic nuclei. *N. Engl. J. Med.* 315, 997–1003.

Macchi, G., Bentivoglio, M., Minciacchi, D. & Molinari, M. (1996): Trends in the anatomical organization and functional significance of the mammalian thalamus. *Ital. J. Neurol. Sci.* 17, 105–129.

McCormick, D.A. & Prince, D.A. (1987): Post-natal development of electrophysiological properties of rat cerebral cortical pyramidal neurons *J. Physiol.* 393, 743–762.

McGraw, P., Mathews, V.P., Wang, Y. & Phillips, M.D. (2001): Approach to functional magnetic resonance imaging of language based on models of language organization. *Neuroimaging Clin. North Am.* 11, 343–353.

Marcus, E.M. & Watson, C.W. (1968): Symmetrical epileptogenic foci in monkey cerebral cortex: mechanisms of interaction and regional variations in capacity for synchronous discharges. *Arch. Neurol.* 18, 99–116.

Mares, P. (1991): Epileptic phenomena in the immature brain. *Physiol. Res.* **40**, 577–584.

Marin-Padilla, M. (1988): Early ontogenesis of the human cerebral cortex. In: *Development and maturation of cerebral cortex*, vol. 7, eds. A. Peters & E.G. Jones, pp. 1–34. New York: Plenum Press.

Marin-Padilla, M. (1990): Three-dimensional structural organization of layer I of the human cerebral cortex. A Golgi study. *J. Comp. Neurol.* **229**, 89–105.

Marini, G., Gritti, I. & Mancia, M. (1989): Changes in EEG spindle activity induced by ibotenic acid lesions of medialis dorsalis thalamic nuclei in the cat. *Brain Res.* **500**, 395–399.

Matsumoto, H. & Ajmone Marsan, C. (1964a): Cortical cellular phenomena in experimental epilepsy. Interictal manifestations. *Exp. Neurol.* **9**, 286–304.

Matsumoto, H. & Ajmone Marsan, C. (1964b): Cortical cellular phenomena in experimental epilepsy. Ictal manifestations. *Exp. Neurol.* **9**, 305–326.

Miller, M.W. (1988): Development of projection and local circuit neurons in neocortex. In: *Cerebral cortex. Development and maturation of cerebral cortex*, vol 7. eds. A. Peters & E.G. Jones, pp. 133–175. New York: Plenum Press.

Moniz, E. (1936): Tentatives opératoires dans le traitement de certaines psychoses. Paris: Masson.

Morrisset, R.A., Nadler, J.V. & McNamara, J.O. (1987): Evidence for enhanced N-methyl-D-aspartate receptor mediated inhibition of carbachol-stimulated phosphoinositide hydrolysis in kindled rats. *Neurosci. Abstr.* **13**, 946.

Naquet, R. & Meldrum, B.S. (1972): Photogenic seizures in baboon. In: *Experimental models of epilepsy*, eds. D.P. Purpura, J.K. Penry, D. Tower, D.M. Woodbury & R. Walter, pp. 374–406. New York: Raven Press

Penfield, W. & Rasmussen, T. (1950): *The cerebral cortex of man*. New York: Macmillan.

Rakic, P. (1990): Principles of neuronal cell migration. *Experientia* **46**, 882–891.

Rakic, P. & Goldman-Rakic, P.S. (1982): The development and morphology of the cerebral cortex: overview. *Neurosci. Program. Bull.* **20**, 439–451.

Roland, P.E. (1984): Metabolic measurement of the working frontal cortex in man. *Trends Neurosci.* **7**, 430–435.

Sanides, F. (1962): *Die Architektonik des menschlichen Stirnhirns*. Berlin and New York: Springer-Verlag.

Schmechel, D.E. & Rakic, P. (1979): A Golgi study of radial glial cells in developing monkey telencephalon: morphogenesis and transformation into astrocytes. *Anat. Embryol.* **156**, 115–152.

Sidman R.L. & Rakic P. (1973): Neuronal migration disorders, with special reference to developing human brain: a review. *Brain Res.* **62**, 1–35.

Steinlein, O.K., Mulley, J.C., Propping, P., Wallace, R.H., Phillips, H.A., Sutherland, G.R., Scheffer, I.E. & Berkovic, S.F. (1995): A missense mutation in the neuronal nicotinic acetylcholine receptor α4 subunit is associated with autosomal dominant nocturnal frontal lobe epilepsy. *Nat. Genet.* **11**, 201–203.

Wiesendanger, M. (1973): Input from muscle and cutaneous nerves of the hand and forearm to neurons of the precentral gyrus of baboons and monkeys. *J. Physiol.* **228**, 203–219.

Wise, S.P & Strick, P.L. (1984): Anatomical and physiological organization of the non-primary motor cortex. *Trends Neurosci.* **7**, 442–446.

Wong, Y.C., Kwan, H.C. & Murphy, J.T. (1974): Projection of primary muscle spindle afferents to motor sensory cortex. *Can. J. Physiol Pharmacol.* **52**, 349–351.

Zilles, K. (1990): Codistribution of receptors in the human cerebral cortex. In: *Receptors in the human nervous system*, eds. G. Paxinos & F.A.O. Mendelsohn. San Diego: Academic Press.

Chapter 4

Cognitive evoked potentials in the study of frontal lobe executive functions and their maturation

Luis García-Larrea

Inserm E342 and University of Lyon-I, Human Neurophysiology Laboratory, CERMEP,
59, boulevard Pinel, 69003 Lyon, France
larrea@univ-lyon1.fr

Summary

Cognitive evoked potentials are electrophysiological counterparts of sensory integration processes, i.e. processes whereby the information contained in a stimulus is progressively incorporated into the subject's internal world and can generate adequate behavioural responses. The cortical potentials that follow a task-relevant stimulus may be classified into several functional modules reflecting stimulus evaluation, perceptual decision and cognitive closure stages, which we shall describe and discuss. To these post-stimulus stages we should add the pre-stimulus negativities reflecting stimulus anticipation and preparation to react.

Executive functions are reflected in event-related potentials (ERPs) by pre-stimulus slow negative potentials (indicating anticipation and preparatory processes), and by post-stimulus P3 amplitude (reflecting the amount of processing capacities allocated to the stimulus). The *executive cost* of dual task situations, typically challenging the frontal executive system, may be estimated by attenuation of such pre- and post-stimulus components.

Maturation of a number of executive capacities may be studied by coupling ERPs to performance measures during the Posner attention-shifting paradigm. In this test, subjects respond to left and right visual targets by pressing the corresponding left or right button of a computer mouse. In most of the trials the targets are preceded by a spatial cue appearing before target onset. Under these conditions, cortical responses may be separated into *cue-related* ERPs, developing during the cue-to-target period, and *target-related* ERPs which emerge upon target presentation. Performance, reaction times and ERPs were studied during performance of this test in 7–9 years old children, and in 18–30 years old adults. While the morphology of responses to visual targets was very similar in the two groups, we found striking differences between children and adults in ERPs evoked by the cue stimuli that preceded target presentation. In children, cue stimuli evoked a series of sensory (P1) and cognitive potentials (N2-P3 complex), whereas in adults these potentials were surmounted by a long-lasting, high-amplitude negative wave consistent with a pre-stimulus preparation ERP (readiness potential or RP). Response times in adults were very significantly shorter than in children, and these differences could not be explained by differences in target detection times. Thus, children processed the cues as if they were relevant as such, while adults appeared to use the information contained in the cue mainly to prepare a response. Using external information to anticipate a forthcoming stimulus and prepare a response pertains to frontal executive functions, the ERP concomitants of which were absent in 7–10 years old children in this study. The higher speed of adults in responding to targets was therefore related to their superior capacities for stimulus anticipation and motor preparation, rather than to a superior ability for attention orienting or target detection.

Cognitive electrophysiology is a powerful tool to assess maturational cognitive changes. Brain mechanisms can be accessed with millisecond accuracy and disclose activity changes that would not be detected by behavioural analysis alone. Such techniques are being applied to study children with disorders involving frontal dysmaturation such as attention deficit hyperactivity disorder. Combined with neuropsychological testing, they should be helpful to assess possible cognitive delays and responses to therapy in children with frontal epilepsies.

Introduction to cognitive evoked potentials

Cognitive evoked potentials are electrophysiological counterparts of sensory integration processes, whereby the information contained in a stimulus is progressively incorporated into the subject's internal world and may then give rise to adequate behavioural responses. The cortical responses that follow a task-relevant stimulus may be classified into several functional modules each reflecting different aspects of sensory integration, which we shall describe as the evaluative, decisional and closure stages.

The evaluative stage

Activities during this period reflect progressive extraction of the stimulus features (intensity, location, modality), and their comparison with memory templates. Such sensory-cognitive analysis is needed to decide whether or not the stimulus is behaviourally relevant, i.e. whether it needs a response or not. This evaluative period is reflected in event-related potentials (ERPs) by two different effects: first, by amplitude modulation of early responses in primary sensory areas, either auditory (Picton & Hillard, 1974), visual (Rugg et al., 1987; Luck & Hillyard, 1994) or somatosensory (Desmedt et al., 1983; García-Larrea et al., 1991); and second by changes in the so-called N1 potential (Hillyard et al., 1973). Of particular importance are changes in the 'processing negativity', a subcomponent of the N1 described by Näätänen (1978, 1982), the amplitude of which is directly proportional to the concordance between the incoming and the expected stimulus.

The decision stage

The conscious or unconscious decision that the incoming stimulus has possible behavioural relevance is reflected by the N2 family of responses, which follow the N1 and typically appear within 150-250 ms after the eliciting stimulus. Among members of the N2 family we emphasize the *mismatch negativity* (MMN), appearing whenever an auditory stimulus deviates from a series of monotonous inputs presented previously (Sams et al., 1985; Näätänen, 1990); the N2b response, which reflects the classification of a given stimulus into an expected category (Ritter et al., 1979); and the N400 potential, developing in response to words semantically incongruent within a given context (Kutas & Hillyard, 1981). The presence of an activity of the N2 type is a signal that the eliciting stimulus has been identified by the brain as being potentially relevant for behaviour whatever the reason for it. It is believed that the time of occurrence of the N2 after a given stimulus is the closest ERP indication of stimulus identification (Ritter et al., 1979; Kekoni et al., 1995). Therefore, the N2 latency time can be used to estimate the stimulus evaluation time (Starr et al., 1995).

The post-decision, or 'cognitive closure' stage

This is reflected by a high-amplitude positive response labelled P300 or P3. The P3 appears in response to stimuli that are both selectively expected and unpredictable in time (reviewed in Picton, 1992), and is almost always preceded by an N2. Although initially the P3 response was considered to reflect detection of the expected stimulus (it was called the 'aha!' wave), it was soon demonstrated that the P3 usually follows, rather than precedes, the motor response (Ritter et al., 1972; Goodin & Aminoff, 1984), thus making unlikely that it would reflect the sensory decision itself. Rather, it is generally accepted that the P3 reflects cognitive processes operating immediately after stimulus classification has been completed.

The specific operations reflected by the P3 wave are still a subject of debate and it is impossible in this chapter to discuss all the proposed theories in detail. In brief, the P3 has been considered to index working memory updating processes (Donchin, 1979), phasic deactivation of the ascending reticular formation (Desmedt & Debecker, 1979) or of polymodal association cortex (Verleger, 1988), and conscious encoding of the stimulus in intermediate/long-term memory (Picton, 1992). Regarding this latter hypothesis, recent data have shown that a well synchronized P3 is necessary to ensure stimulus retrieval, and that replacement of P3 by other activities, notably of opposite polarity, precludes this retrieval (García-Larrea et al., 2000). These different views converge in seeing the P3 as reflecting closure, a post-perceptual process triggered by stimulus identification. The preservation of such a mechanism appears crucial to ensure accurate encoding of the stimulus in memory structures.

The amplitude of P3 appears to reflect the amount of attentional resources allotted to the processing of the eliciting stimulus (reviews in Picton, 1992; Kok, 1997), while the latency of the P3 may be viewed as a reflection of stimulus evaluation time (Kutas et al., 1977). However, being a post-decisional response, the P3 latency reflects such evaluation time less accurately than the N2 (Ritter et al., 1979; Starr et al., 1995). In general terms (Kok, 1997), N2 and P3 latencies reflect computational aspects of stimulus processing (i.e. the time needed to perform these processes), while their amplitude (notably that of P3) reflects the amount of processing capacities allocated to the eliciting stimulus.

Event-related potentials and frontal executive functions

The term *executive functions* refers to a domain of cognitive abilities that allow mental flexibility and the planning of behaviour. This is a vast domain and a precise yet comprehensive definition of executive functions is difficult to provide; instead, neuropsychologists have often preferred to enumerate the major brain abilities requiring executive control. Among the most frequently cited (Rabbitt, 1997) are novelty management (dealing with novel, goal-oriented tasks), deliberate memory search, sequence initiation while interrupting ongoing activity, control of inappropriate responses, coordination in dual task situations, error correction, stimulus and response anticipation, and long-lasting sustained attention. Abundant evidence in normal subjects, and in patients with cerebral lesions, suggests that executive capacities are mediated by prefrontal regions and their various interconnecting structures (see reviews in Rabbitt, 1997; Van der Linden et al., 1999; Fuster, 2000).

Because the central executive system is thought to be crucial for coordinating concurrent processing, it has commonly been investigated by using dual-task paradigms, in which two behavioural tasks are performed concurrently (Baddeley, 1986; Hegarty et al., 2000; Adcock et al., 2000). Dual tasks have also been applied to ERP paradigms and have provided rather consistent results. Typical dual-task ERP experiments have included a combination of a sensory detection and a motor task (e.g. Wickens et al., 1984; Schubert et al., 1998), and more recently of two tasks free of any motor response (García-Larrea & Cézanne-Bert, 1998).

ERP experiments in dual-task settings have helped identify some of the mechanisms underlying the alterations in performance, notably increases in reaction times, observed when executive functions are challenged by simultaneous task demands. The effects of dual-task paradigms on ERPs are mainly reflected in the N2-P3 responses and in pre-stimulus negativities (see above for description), and may be summarized in three points (see also Fig. 1):

(a) The amplitude of the P3 response evoked by one class of stimuli (task n° 1) decreases when the load of a second task increases (Israel et al., 1980; Wickens et al., 1983). In accordance with the notion that P3 amplitude reflects the capacity for processing task-relevant stimuli (Picton, 1992; Kok, 1997), P3 attenuation in dual tasks is thought to reflect a decrease in the processing resources allocated to the detection task when a concurrent activity must be simultaneously performed (Wickens et al., 1983; Ragazzoni et al., 1996; García-Larrea & Cézanne-Bert, 1998).

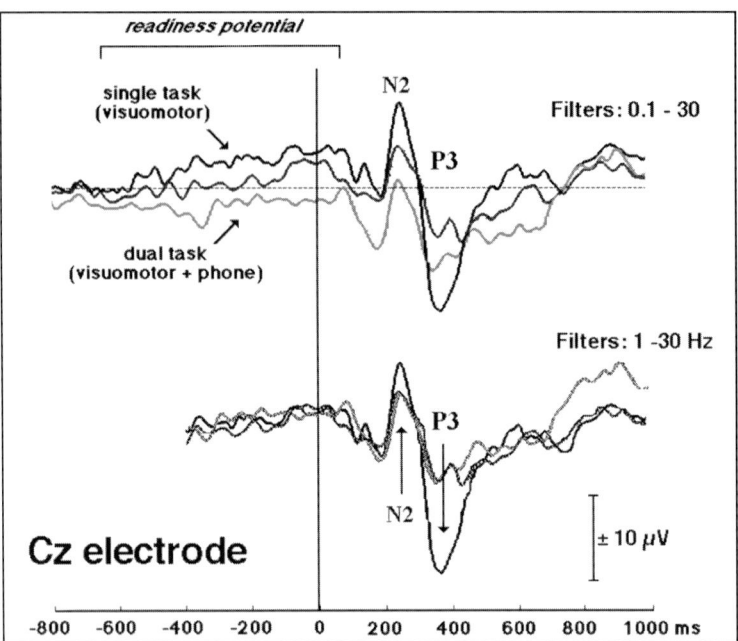

Fig. 1. ERP effects of a dual task situation combining a visuomotor task (pushing a button upon detection of a visual target) and a conversation on a mobile telephone. ERP traces correspond to the responses to visual targets; responses obtained in the single task (visuomotor alone) have been superimposed on those recorded in dual-task situations (conversation with the telephone in the hand or in 'hands-free' mode). A: In the first row (filters 0.1-30Hz), the slow negative potential reflecting preparation to respond to the target (readiness potential) decreases or disappears when the task is performed concurrently with the telephone conversation. B: In the lower row the low frequencies have been filtered out to eliminate the effect on pre-stimulus negativities. This brings out significant attenuation of the P3 wave in dual-task situations relative to the control condition. Note that the latencies of the N2 and P3 potentials do not vary within conditions, indicating that the longer reaction times during dual tasks (see arrows) were not due to a delay in stimulus evaluation, but rather to increased transfer time from stimulus identification to response production. (Negative potentials up; arrows on time axis indicate reaction times.) [Data from García-Larrea et al., 2001.]

(b) The peak latencies of the N2 and P3 responses to one class of stimuli typically do not vary in spite of a second task being performed concurrently (Israel et al., 1980; Sirevaag et al., 1989; Ragazzoni et al., 1996; Schubert et al., 1998). This suggests that the time needed for discrimination and identification of target stimuli is short or not increased in dual tasks.

(c) Slow negativities preceding an imperative stimulus decrease when a second task must be performed concurrently, and especially so when the concurrent task includes a motor component (García-Larrea et al., 2001). Pre-stimulus slow negativities reflect anticipation of the incoming stimulus and preparation of the response; their attenuation suggests therefore that the cognitive cost of adding a second task is reflected in a weakening of anticipatory processes.

These ERP results provide a framework to understand the altered performance observed in dual tasks, notably the increase in reaction times (RTs). RT slowing does not appear to depend on a delay in stimulus identification, since the brain events reflecting this stage (N2 and P3) are typically not delayed in dual tasks. Conversely, ERP results indicate disturbance of anticipatory processes (attenuation of pre-stimulus negativities) leading to decreased attention allocated to sensory targets (attenuation of P3 responses). Loss of anticipatory processes prolongs RTs by increasing the time to access and select motor programs (review in Brunia, 1993). Thus, delayed motor reactions in multi-task settings are most probably explained by a selective disturbance in cognitive stages that use the information conveyed by the stimulus to activate a motor response (Fig. 1). We shall denote these as transfer stages, as they correspond to the transfer of sensory information to modules involved with the access, selection and mobilisation of motor programs.

Apart from their theoretical implications, these changes in cognitive evoked potentials may be used in clinical practice to quantify the executive cost, as the supplementary burden imposed upon executive functions when resources must be shared among several tasks. For example, decrease of anticipatory response activation in dual settings has been shown to be more pronounced if the secondary task requires motor control (García-Larrea et al., 2001). Also, Parkinsonian patients confronted with a dual-task paradigm show significantly greater P3 attenuation than age-matched controls even in tasks not requiring any motor response (García-Larrea et al., 1997; García-Larrea & Cézannne-Bert, 1998), suggesting that the executive cost imposed by the secondary task is pathologically increased in Parkinson's disease independently of motor impairment. The fact that this is detectable even when the two tasks are correctly performed underlines the importance of coupling electrophysiological measures to behavioural data.

Event-related potentials and maturation of executive functions

Dual tasks commonly used to assess executive cost on ERPs are hardly applicable to children, and are of little use for maturational studies. Cognitive ERP paradigms designed for maturational research must present lively and if possible, amusing tasks. Otherwise children are rarely compliant enough for useful recordings. Also, it is often advisable to use tests that incorporate a number of different cognitive axes within a single task, which may reveal differences in the maturation of different abilities. One test that meets these criteria is the Posner paradigm (Posner, 1984; 1987). In a variant form presented here (Fig. 2), subjects are asked to respond to a visual target stimulus (a red star) presented 5° to the left or to the right of a central fixation point. Eighty percent of targets are preceded by a cue stimulus occurring 500 ms prior to target onset. The cue consists of a bright yellow rectangle also appearing at 5° left or right of the screen centre, which remains on the screen until the target appears. The cue is said to be 'valid' when it correctly predicts the location of the target stimulus; in this case the target star appears within the yellow cue rectangle. Conversely, an 'invalid' cue is one that appears in the field opposite the subsequent target. Finally, in some trials the target appears without any preceding cue ('no cue' condition). It has been repeatedly shown that presentation of valid cues significantly decreases RTs to the ensuing targets, relative to either the invalid or to the no cue conditions (Posner, 1984; 1987; 1988).

By coupling this procedure with ERP recordings (Fig. 3), cortical responses may be separated into cue-related ERPs developing during the cue-to-target period, and target-related ERPs which emerge upon target presentation (Verleger et al., 1996; Perchet & García-Larrea, 2000). This opens the possibility of assessing the ERP concomitants of different cognitive operations or axes within a single recording session. In particular:

    (a) pre-stimulus negativities reflect anticipation of stimulus-response contingencies (Brunia, 1993; Starr et al., 1995) and therefore index executive mechanisms;

    (b) enhancement of early sensory responses (P1) reflects sensory priming of correctly cued stimuli (Heinze et al., 1990; 1994; Luck & Hillyard, 1994);

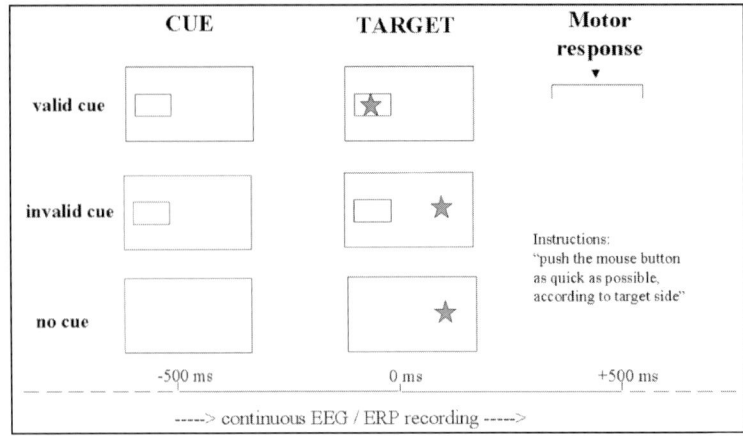

Fig. 2. Schematic representation of the Posner paradigm used in the reported study.

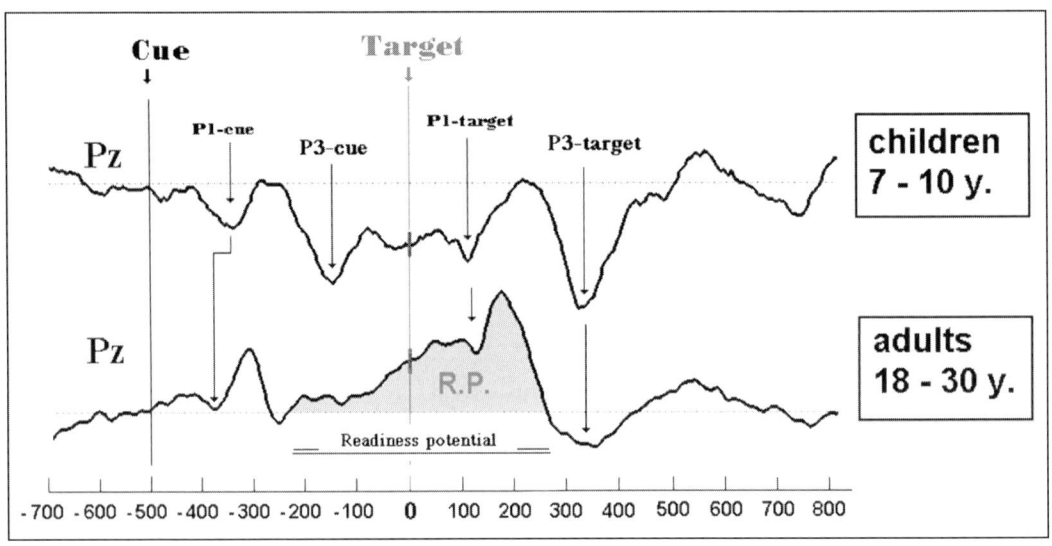

Fig. 3. Averaged responses to cue and target stimuli during the Posner paradigm (see text and Fig. 2) obtained in a sample of 12 children 7–9 years old, and in 12 young adults. Each trace is the average of all subjects in the corresponding group; only the responses obtained at the vertex electrode are presented. The main differences in both groups corresponded to responses to the cue stimuli; while children produced target-like responses to them, including a N2-P3 complex, adults mainly used the information contained in the cue to prepare their response, as reflected by the slow negative readiness potential. Maturation of executive responses is in this case reflected by the development of cognitive strategies that favour anticipation of upcoming information over immediate processing of all incoming inputs.

(c) N2 and P3 latency comparisons across conditions reflect changes in stimulus detection times as a result of attentional misallocation ('validity effect') (Perchet & García-Larrea, 2000);

(d) late positive components following P3 indicate response selection and/or motor reprogramming in case of invalid cues (Falkenstein *et al.*, 1994; Verleger *et al.*, 1996; Perchet & García-Larrea, 2000).

We recently attempted to study maturation of these cognitive abilities by assessing behavioural performances (error rates, error types, RTs) and event-related potentials in 7–9 years old children and 18–30 years old young adults while they performed a computerized variant of the Posner attention-shifting paradigm. All subjects were required to signal the detection of each target by pressing as quickly as possible the left or right button of a computer mouse according to the side of target presentation.

Surprisingly, very little differences were observed between children and adults in the three last axes described above (b, c and d), while striking dissimilarities between the groups appeared in ERPs to the cue stimuli. In children, cues evoked a series of stereotyped sensory and cognitive responses (P1-N2-P3), whereas in adults these were much smaller than a long-lasting, high-amplitude negative wave which was morphologically and topographically consistent with a readiness potential (RP). As shown in Fig. 3, the ERP responses to cue stimuli in children were virtually identical to those developed to the ensuing targets, indicating that children processed the cues as if they were relevant as such, while adults appeared to use the information contained in the cue mainly to prepare a response.

Frontal executive functions allow 'cross-temporal integration' between past and upcoming experience (see Fuster, 2000, 2003). Using external information to anticipate a forthcoming stimulus and prepare a response clearly pertains to this class of executive capabilities. Whereas the electrophysiological concomitants of such anticipatory activity (i.e. pre-stimulus negativities) were readily obtainable in young adults, they were absent in 7–10 years old children. This reflects a relative immaturity of executive frontal control over external inputs in children at this age, which contrasts with their more rapid achievement of adult values as assessed by ERPs for other cognitive axes such as attentional priming, re-orienting of attention and target detection. We may therefore contend that the faster motor responses of adults to targets (see arrows in Fig. 3) were mainly related to their superior capacities for response anticipation, rather than to superior attentional or perceptual abilities. As a corollary it may be proposed that development of baseline attentional and perceptual capabilities in children remains of limited behavioural use, in terms of performance, if the executive control over these functions is not fully developed.

We observed one exception to this lack of electrophysiological signs of anticipation in children; a slow negative wave preceding the target was observed in those trials without any preceding cue. Although we have no clear explanation why this ERP sign should appear in children only in this particular setting, it is interesting to note that even this limited sign of executive control disappeared in a group of children of similar age with attention deficit hyperactivity disorder (ADHD), who were otherwise comparable to normal control children for other ERP markers such as N2 and P3 (Perchet *et al.*, 2001).

Recent neuropsychological work has suggested that, rather than a sum of specific attentional deficits, ADHD children may suffer from a global dysfunction in attentional control (i.e. in the capacity to regulate attentional allocation in complex situations), linked to a frontal executive deficit (Boucugnani & Jones, 1989; Reader *et al.*, 1994; Oosterlaan & Sergeant, 1995). Our results, showing ERP signs consistent with frontal executive dysmaturation relative to age-matched children, lend objective support to this notion. In addition, the results in adults, healthy children and ADHD children help establish a gradient in the normal and abnormal development of electrophysiological signs of executive anticipatory control from childhood to adulthood.

Conclusions

These examples have shown that cognitive electrophysiology is a powerful tool to assess both established and maturational changes in cognitive strategies, especially when coupled to quantification of behavioural performance. Cerebral responses can be traced with millisecond accuracy and disclose activity changes that would be invisible to behavioural analysis alone. As compared with functional imaging, which mainly aims to localize cerebral functions, electrophysiology allows detailed assessment of their temporal course, the knowledge of which has been shown to be essential for the understanding of executive interaction between frontal lobes and other association areas (Fuster, 2000). Combined with neuropsychological testing, ERP techniques should become increasingly helpful to identify possible cognitive delays and response to therapy in children with frontal epilepsies.

References

Adcock, R.A., Constable, R.T., Gore, J.C. & Goldman-Rakic, P.S. (2000): Functional neuroanatomy of executive processes involved in dual-task performance. *Proc. Natl. Acad. Sci. USA* **97**, 3567–3572.

Baddeley, A.D. (1986): *Working Memory*. Oxford: Clarendon Press.

Boucugnani, L.L. & Jones, R.W. (1989): Behaviours analogous to frontal lobe dysfunction in children with attention deficit hyperactivity disorder. *Arch. Clin. Neuropsychol.* **4**, 161–173.

Desmedt, J.E. & Debecker, J. (1979): Wave form and neural mechanism of the decision P350 elicited without pre-stimulus CNV or readiness potential in random sequences of near-threshold auditory clicks and finger stimuli. *Electroencephalogr. Clin. Neurophysiol.* **47**, 648–670.

Desmedt, J.E., Nguyen, T.H., & Bourget, M. (1983): The cognitive P40, N60 and P100 components of the somatosensory evoked potentials and the earliest signs of sensory processing in man. *Electroencephalogr. Clin. Neurophysiol.* **56**, 272–282.

Donchin, E. (1979): Event-related potentials: a tool in the study of human information processing. In: *Evoked potentials and behaviour*, ed. H. Begleiter, pp. 13–88. New York: Plenum Press.

Fuster, J.M. (2000): Executive frontal functions. *Exp. Brain Res.* **133**, 66–70.

Fuster, J.M. (2003): Functional anatomy of the prefrontal cortex. In: *Frontal seizures and epilepsies in children*, eds. A. Beaumanoir, F. Andermann, P. Chauvel, L. Mira & B. Zifkin, pp. 1–10. Mariani Foundation Paediatric Neurology Series, vol. 11. Paris, London: John Libbey Eurotext.

García-Larrea, L. & Cezanne-Bert, G. (1998): P3, positive slow wave and working memory load: a study on the functional correlates of slow wave activity. *Electroencephalogr. Clin. Neurophysiol.* **108**, 260–73.

García-Larrea, L., Bastuji, H., & Mauguière, F. (1991): Mapping study of somatosensory evoked potentials during selective spatial attention. *Electroencephalogr. Clin. Neurophysiol.* **80**, 201–214.

García-Larrea, L., Broussolle, E., Cézanne-Bert, G. & Mauguière, F. (1997): P300 and 'frontal executive' functions: application of a dual-task paradigm in normal subjects and patients with Parkinson's disease and progressive supranuclear palsy. *Electroencephalogr. Clin. Neurophysiol.* **103**, 148.

García-Larrea, L., Perrin, F. & Bastuji, H. (2000): ERPs, memory encoding and stimulus awareness. Lessons from a forced awakening test. *Electroencephalogr. Clin. Neurophysiol.* **111** (Suppl. 1), S1–S2.

García-Larrea, L., Perchet, C., Perrin, F. & Amenedo, E. (2001): Interference of cellular phone conversations with visuomotor tasks: an ERP study. *J. Psychophysiol.* **15**, 14–21.

Goodin, D.S. & Aminoff, M.J. (1984): The relationship between the evoked potential and brain events in sensory discrimination and motor response. *Brain* **107**, 241–251.

Hegarty, M., Shah, P. & Miyake, A. (2000): Constraints on using the dual-task methodology to specify the degree of central executive involvement in cognitive tasks. *Mem. Cognit.* **28**, 376–385.

Heinze, H.J., Luck, S.J., Mangun, G.R. & Hillyard, S.A. (1990): Visual event-related potentials index of focused attention within bilateral stimulus arrays. I. Evidence for early selection. *Electroencephalogr. Clin. Neurophysiol.* **75**, 511–527.

Heinze, H.J., Mangun, G.R., Burchert, W., Hinrichs, H., Scholz, M., Munte, T.F., Gos, A., Scherg, M., Johannes, S., Hundeshagen, H., Gazzaniga, M.S. & Hillyard, S.A. (1994): Combined spatial and temporal imaging of brain activity during visual selective attention in humans. *Nature* **372**, 543–546.

Israel, J.B., Chesney, G.L., Wickens, C. & Donchin, E. (1980): P300 and tracking difficulty: evidence for multiple resources in dual-task performance. *Psychophysiology* **17**, 259–273.

Kekoni, J., Hamalainen, H., McCloud, V., Reinikainen, K. & Näätänen, R. (1995): Is the somatosensory N250 related to deviance discrimination or conscious target detection? *Electroencephalogr. Clin. Neurophysiol.* **100**, 115–125.

Kok, A. (1997): Event-related potential (ERP) reflections of mental resources: a review and synthesis. *Biol. Psychol.* **45**, 19–56.

Kutas, M., & Hillyard, S.A. (1981) Reading senseless sentences: brain potentials reflect semantic incongruity. *Science* **207**, 203–205.

Kutas, M., McCarthy, G., & Donchin, E. (1977): Augmenting mental chronometry: the P300 as a measure of stimulus evaluation time. *Science* **197**, 792–795.

Luck, S.J. & Hillyard, S.A. (1994): Electrophysiological correlates of feature analysis during visual search. *Psychophysiology* **31**, 291–308.

Näätänen, R. (1982): Processing negativity: an evoked-potential reflection of selective attention. *Psychol. Bull.* **92**, 605–640.

Näätänen, R. (1990): The role of attention in auditory information processing as revealed by event-related potentials and other brain measures of cognitive function. *Behav. Brain Sci.* **13**, 201–288.

Näätänen, R., Gaillard, A.W.K. & Mäntysalo, S. (1978): Early selective attention effect on evoked potential reinterpreted. *Acta Psychologica* **42**, 313–329.

Oosterlaan, J. & Sergeant, J.A. (1995): Response choice and inhibition in ADHD, anxious and aggressive children: the relationship between S-R compatibility and the stop signal task. In: *Eunethydis: European approaches to hyperkinetic disorder*, ed. J.A. Sergeant, pp. 225–240. Amsterdam: University of Amsterdam.

Perchet, C. & García-Larrea, L. (2000): Visuospatial attention in children: an electrophysiological study of the Posner paradigm. *Psychophysiology* **37**, 231–341.

Perchet, C., Revol, O., Fourneret, P., Mauguière, F. & Garcia-Larrea, L. (2001): Attention shifts and anticipatory mechanisms in hyperactive children: an ERP study using the Posner paradigm. *Biol. Psychiatry* **50**, 44–57.

Picton T.W. (1992): The P300 wave of the human event-related potential. *J. Clin. Neurophysiol.* **9**, 456–479.

Picton, T.W. & Hillyard, S.A. (1974): Human AEPs. II. Effects of attention. *Electroencephalogr. Clin. Neurophysiol.* **36**, 191–199.

Posner, M.I. & Cohen, Y. (1984): Components of visual orienting. In: *Attention and performance X*, eds H. Bouma & D. Bowhuis, pp. 531–556. Hillsdale, NJ: Erlbaum.

Posner, M.I., Inhoff, A.W., Friedrich, F.J. & Cohen, A. (1987): Isolating attentional systems: a cognitive-anatomical analysis. *Psychobiology* **15** (2), 107–121.

Posner, M.I., Petersen, S.E., Fox, P.T. & Raichle, M.E. (1988): Localization of cognitive operations in the brain. *Science* **240**, 1627–1631.

Rabbitt, P. (1997): Methodologies and models in the study of executive function. In: *Methodology of frontal and executive function*, ed. P. Rabbitt, pp. 1–38. Hove, East Sussex: Psychology Press.

Ragazzoni, A., Mata, S., Grippo, A. & Pinto, F. (1996): Dual-task performance: effects of increasing difficulty on auditory ERPs and RTs. In: *Functional Neuroscience* (EEG Suppl. 46), eds. C. Barber, G. Celesia, C. Comi & F. Mauguière, pp. 253–260. Amsterdam: Elsevier.

Reader, M., Harris, E., Schuerholz, L. & Denckla, M. (1994): Attention deficit hyperactivity disorder and executive dysfunction. *Dev. Neuropsychol.* **10**, 493–512.

Ritter, W., Simson, R. & Vaughan, H.G. Jr. (1972): Association of cortex potentials and reaction time in auditory discrimination. *Electroencephalogr. Clin. Neurophysiol.* **33**, 547–555.

Ritter, W., Simson, R., Vaughan, H.G. & Friedman, D.A. (1979): A brain event related to the making of sensory discrimination. *Science* **203**, 1358–1361.

Ritter, W., Simson, R., Vaughan, H.G. Jr. & Macht, M. (1982): Manipulation of event-related potential manifestations of information processing stages. *Science* **218**, 909–911.

Rugg, M.D., Milner, A.D., Lines, C.R. & Phalp, R. (1987): Modulation of visual event-related potentials by spatial and non-spatial visual selective attention. *Neuropsychologia* **25**, 85–96.

Sams, M., Paavilainen, P., Alho, K. & Näätänen, R. (1985): Auditory frequency discrimination and event-related potentials. *Electroencephalogr. Clin. Neurophysiol.* **62**, 437–448.

Schubert, M., Johannes, S., Koch, M., Wieringa, B.M., Dengler, R. & Munte, T.F. (1998): Differential effects of two motor tasks on ERPs in an auditory classification task: evidence of shared cognitive resources. *Neurosci. Res.* **30**, 125–134.

Sirevaag, E.J., Kramer, A.F., Coles, M.G. & Donchin, E. (1989): Resource reciprocity: an event-related brain potentials analysis. *Acta Psychol.* **70**, 77–97.

Starr, A., Sandroni, P. & Michalewski, H.J. (1995): Readiness to respond in a target detection task: pre- and post-stimulus event-related potentials in normal subjects. *Electroencephalogr. Clin. Neurophysiol.* **96**, 76–92.

Van der Linden, M., Seron, X., Le Gall, D. & Andrés, P. (1999): *Neuropsychologie des lobes frontaux*, pp. 379. Marseille: Solal Éditeur.

Verleger, R. (1988): Event-related potentials and cognition: a critique of the context updating hypothesis and an alternative interpretation of P3. *Behav. Brain Sci.* **11**, 343–427.

Verleger, R., Heide, W., Butt, C., Wascher, E. & Kompf, D. (1996): On-line brain potential correlates of right parietal patients' attentional deficit. *Electroencephalogr. Clin. Neurophysiol.* **99**, 444–457.

Wickens, C., Kramer, A., Vanasse, L. & Donchin, E. (1983): Performance of concurrent tasks: a psychophysiological analysis of the reciprocity of information-processing resources. *Science* **221**, 1080–1082.

Chapter 5

The neuroethological interpretation of motor behaviours in 'nocturnal-hyperkynetic-frontal seizures': emergence of 'innate' motor behaviours and role of central pattern generators

Carlo Alberto Tassinari, Elena Gardella, Stefano Meletti and Guido Rubboli

Department of Neurological Sciences, University of Bologna, Bellaria Hospital, via Altura n. 3, 40139 Bologna, Italy
carloalberto.tassinari@ausl.bologna.it

Summary

Nocturnal hyperkinetic frontal seizures are characterized by complex motor behaviours with the following peculiar features: arousal-orienting behaviour; grasping movements with upper limbs; vocalizations; bimanual and bipedal limb movements, with trunk and pelvis thrusting; dystonic posturing; fugue, with body pronation and attempt to escape. In our hypothesis, we suggest that these behaviours can be related to the activation of brainstem, bulbar or even spinal cord circuitries, where the 'central pattern generators' (CPGs) of these behaviours are located, far away from the cortex, where the epileptic discharge arises. CPGs subserve innate motor behaviours essential for survival (such as walking, swimming, sexual copulatory behaviour, and other forms of rhythmic motor sequences). The epileptic activity, originating from the epileptogenic zone, sets up a cascade of ictal and post-ictal modifications that render possible the emergence of innate motor behaviours, which then develop independently. Therefore, the seizure would act as 'trigger' for the excitation or, more likely, the release from cortical inhibitory influences, of CPGs. Similarities in semiology between these types of epileptic motor events and certain parasomnias (for instance, nocturnal wandering, jactatio capitis, tooth grinding) might suggest that the same CPGs can be called in action independently from the nature of the causative trigger, be it an epileptic phenomenon or a sleep-related dysfunction.

> '... These symptoms do not occur in, but after, the paroxysm; they are too coordinated movements to result directly from epileptic discharges; there is, I think, a duplex condition: 1) negatively, loss of control; 2) positively, increased activity of healthy lower centres. Nevertheless, the association, or sequence, is very significant.' (H. Jackson, 1876)

It should be firmly stated that when we refer to seizure types using common anatomical or functional terminology, such as 'fronto-mesial' (Williamson *et al.*, 1985; Wada *et al.*, 1989), we strictly imply the motor behaviour of which the semiological features suggest the involvement of fronto-mesial structures, not the seizure onset region or the epileptogenic zone.

From the final discussion it will be evident that we eventually suggest that the behaviours observed in a 'fronto-mesial' seizure could be better related to the activation of brainstem, bulbar or even spinal cord circuitries, where the 'central pattern generators' (CPGs) of these behaviours are located, far away from the cortex where the epileptic discharge arises. Further, when referring to a sequence of motor behaviours, as observed in 'fronto-mesial nocturnal seizures', we are fully aware that the seizure onset could be in other cortical areas, for instance temporal or parietal. Therefore, when a given sequence of motor behaviours is observed, we simply assume and accept the terminology of the literature suggesting an ictal fronto-mesial or fronto-orbital involvement.

Our hypothesis is based on data observed in a selected cohort of patients, who:
- (a) had a video polygraphic recording of at least one nocturnal epileptic seizure featuring the complete motor sequence of events as described by Wada in his article 'Predominantly nocturnal recurrence of intensely affective vocal and facial expression associated with powerful bimanual, bipedal, and axial activity as ictal manifestation of mesial frontal lobe epilepsy' (Wada, 1989). Here, we refer to these seizures as 'nocturnal-hypermotor-frontal seizures' with an exclusively descriptive meaning (Lüders et al., 1998) or, more appropriately, 'nocturnal hyperkinetic' as per ILAE Glossary (Blume et al., 2001);
- (b) had evidences of epileptic nature of ictal events. Some of these patients were reported in a previous paper (Fusco et al., 1990).

In a few patients, we video-polygraphically recorded 'nocturnal-hyperkinetic-frontal seizures' with an evident stereotypy, as observed at intervals from three to ten years. Moreover, in the same patients with the full-blown hyperkinetic seizure, we also recorded 'fragments' of seizures, as we will discuss further.

The full 'nocturnal-hyperkinetic-frontal seizure' is composed by a sequence of motor behaviours which have the following features:
- (1) at onset (first seconds), arousal-orienting behaviour (Wada, 1989) at times with a startle response; common features are: head lateral deviation, mouth grimacing (with depression of mouth corners), and elevation of the shoulders; a movement of one arm toward the head is also frequently observed;
- (2) grasping with reaching – as described by Gardella & Tassinari (2002) (Fig. 1a);
- (3) vocalizations;
- (4) 'wild' repetitive, more or less cyclic bimanual and bipedal limb movements, with trunk and pelvis thrusting of various duration and intensity (see Riggio & Harner, 1995);
- (5) dystonic posturing – 'hypnogenic paroxysmal dystonia', as described by Lugaresi & Cirignotta (1981);
- (6) fugue behaviour, with body pronation and attempt to escape;
- (7) end of the motor event, usually abrupt; then, can follow
- (8) affective behaviours (fear as in Fig. 1b, or sham aggressive behaviours) and finally
- (9) movements suggesting 'embarrassment', such as self-touching of body or face (Meletti et al., 2001), dress adjustments, smiles, downward or lateral gaze, a to and fro movement of the legs.

Chapter 5   The neuroethological interpretation of motor behaviours in 'nocturnal-hyperkynetic-frontal seizures'

This is the most frequent sequence, from onset to the end, of a 'nocturnal-hyperkynetic-frontal seizure', as evidenced by our recordings. During sleep, this behaviour could repeatedly occur many times, with variable intensity and duration. The full-blown nocturnal-hyperkynetic-frontal seizure can be viewed as a drama, a 'display' as in non human primates, composed of various sequential motor behaviours (schematically indicated from 1 to 9) that can be better understood with a *neuro-ethological* approach.

The arousal behaviour

Arousal, which occurs firstly during slow sleep, is an alerting response. It can be interpreted as an investigative behaviour, mainly depending on the activation of mesolimbic and striatal dopaminergic systems, without which the appropriate sensory-motor coordination does not take place (Iversen & Koob, 1977). As described by Mogenson *et al.* (1980), mesencephalic dopaminergic systems are unequivocally involved in the control of the neural interface between motivation and increased movement activity: there is a need to move, the shoulders contract, the head is pulled down, protected by the shoulder, the hands uplifted toward the head in a defensive reaction. These types of responses have received extensive video-documentation and occur universally as innate defensive reactions (Eibl-Eibesfeldt, 1984), observed in separate, small secluded human aggregates (in New Guinea, in Brasil, etc.). Interestingly, these motor behaviours can be associated with a startle reaction at the onset of the hyperkynetic seizures. The raising of the shoulders toward the head (the 'neck-shoulder reaction' described by Eibl-Eibesfeldt) is also the first muscular event at the onset of a tonic epileptic seizure.

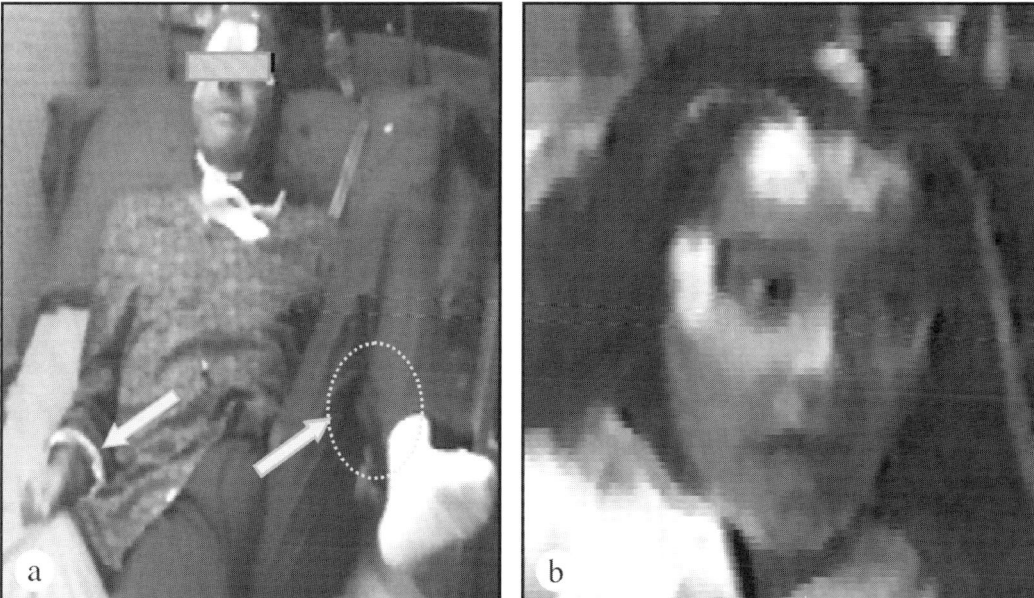

Fig. 1a: Ictal bilateral repetitive grasping in a patient with frontal nocturnal seizures. Arrows indicate grasping of the bed sheets with the right hand, and of the left thigh with the left hand. 1b: Ictal facial expression of fear (as confirmed by FACS, facial action coding system) in a patient with frontal nocturnal seizures. Fear facial expression is one of the five universal facial expressions of emotion, the others being happiness, disgust, anger and sadness. [Darwin, 1872.]

The grasping and the cyclic motor bimanual-bipedal patterns

Grasping of one hand toward an object is one of the innate behaviours present in mammals and is essential for survival in non-human and human primates. The occurrence of grasping in 'nocturnal-hyperkinetic-frontal seizures' has been emphasized for the first time by us (Gardella & Tassinari, 2002). In the phylogeny, grasping is a fragment of 'undulatory or tetrapod locomotion', subserved by CPGs. Such behaviour, however, was noted by Williamson et al. (1985).

Patients concomitantly exhibit coordinated limb-trunk flexion-extension movements, rhythmically repeated, which have the features of walking or running. Stimulation of mesencephalic areas in decerebrate cats (Sherrington, 1906) evokes rhythmic stepping, as well as rhythmic alternating walking movements such as can be observed in tetraplegic human subjects (Dimitrijevich et al., 1998). The patient during the 'nocturnal-hyperkinetic-frontal seizures' enacts a series of coordinated repetitive movements – the bimanual-bipedal pattern, as described by Wada (1989) – as during walking, or, if we refer to non-human primates, as during climbing a tree. In this respect, it is significant that the repetitive grasping is coordinated with upper and lower limbs alternating movements, such as to render the grasping a support to trunk and arms displacements (the brachiation, as during the evolutive process of arboreal progression in monkeys).

Despite all the intense laboring, with wild struggling, thrusting, moaning when the hyperkynetic sequence stops abruptly the patient usually can recall what he 'unwillingly' did. The patient indeed is the 'conscious' spectator of his own performance, i.e. of the fixed motor sequences imposed on him by the CPGs. When, and this is an hypothesis, the frontal more than the limbic structures are involved, he is surprisingly 'cool' as if not concerned: he had to do it (as it occurs in other involuntary movements), a 'consummatory' act such as other inborn motor sequences (as reproductive copulatory or predatory behaviours).

Vocalizations

After the arousal behaviour, and in correspondence of the first motor manifestations, the patients produce vocalizations, which can be of three types: (i) noises, brief and not repetitive; (ii) rapid repetition of words; (iii) repetitive sound emission, fixed and stereotyped in different hyperkynetic seizures, recorded over the years. Acoustic analysis of such stereotyped (type iii) vocalizations led to the hypothesis that they might represent 'encoded' acoustic behaviours (Esposito et al., 2000).

At the end of the hyperkynetic sequence there can be a fugue behaviour, which concludes the enacted motor drama.

Concluding remarks

Genes are responsible for producing the neural networks of a behaviour, as well as enzymes, hormones, and peptides, that regulate its expression. CPGs subserve innate motor behaviours essential for survival, such as swimming, and other forms of rhythmic motor sequences (Grillner & Wallen, 1985).

In our analysis of 'nocturnal-hyperkinetic-frontal seizures', behaviour is equated to movement, whose fixed motor sequence leads to the concept of instinctive behaviours, which are characterized by their stereotypy (Gardella et al., 2000). Fixed action patterns are generated by genetically determined central motor programs, i.e. the CPGs.

Chapter 5   The neuroethological interpretation of motor behaviours in 'nocturnal-hyperkynetic-frontal seizures'

The neuronal networks subserving instinctive movements are mainly located outside the cerebral cortex, from the brainstem down to the spinal cord. The epileptic 'cortical' discharge, arising from the epileptogenic zone, sets up a cascade of ictal and post-ictal modifications that enable the emergence of innate motor behaviours or fixed actions, which then develop independently (and far away from the ictal event) (Tassinari, 2000; Tassinari *et al.*, 2003). Therefore, a series of physiological sequences of muscular contractions, leading to 'normal' synergic movements (flexion, extension, grasping) appear. Indeed, the mesencephalic 'locomotion' region of the mammalian brainstem can be stimulated to induce exploratory (arousal) and locomotory behaviours (Jordan, 1998). The seizure could allow the excitation or, more likely, the release from cortical inhibitory influences, of CPGs: for instance, grasping is an example of a release phenomenon from frontal and parietal structures (Seyffarth & Denny-Brown, 1948). The ictal event – in our case the paroxysmal discharge, involving areas of frontal and limbic systems – acts as a trigger for 'innate releasing mechanisms', which then develops independently, like a music box playing its own fixed 'motor symphony'. The motor symphony can be complete from the onset (arousal) through the various fixed subsequent behaviours (see above, from 1 to 9), ultimately leading to fugue. However, in some instances, the music box can shut down after the first note, then we may have only fragments of the motor symphony, such as 'the arousal seizure', 'the dystonic seizure', 'the wandering seizures' (Tinuper *et al.*, 1990; Zucconi *et al.*, 1997; Oldani *et al.*, 1998; Provini *et al.*, 1999), each fragment related to its own specific innate CPGs. To what extent sleep mechanisms play a role in triggering the 'nocturnal seizures' and in reducing their electroclinical expressions (i.e. how many sequential CPGs participate to the event) is to be determined. In this respect, significant is also the 'confusion' that emerges from the debate in the literature (Oldani *et al.*, 1996; Plazzi *et al.*, 1997; Ambrosetto, 1997; Zucconi *et al.*, 1997) between parasomnias (of non-epileptic origin) and 'nocturnal frontal' epileptic seizures. Our hypothesis suggests that the semiology of parasomnias and certain epileptic motor events could be very similar if the same CPGs are called in action, independently from the nature of the causative trigger, be it an epileptic phenomenon (as it certainly is in our cases) or a sleep-related dysfunction.

Acknowledgments: We thank Mrs. Clementina Giardini for editorial assistance.

References

Ambrosetto, G. (1997): Autosomal dominant nocturnal frontal lobe epilepsy. *Epilepsia* **38**, 739–740.

Darwin, C. (1872): *The expression of emotions in man and animals*. London: Murray.

Dimitrijevich, M.R., Gerasimenko, Y. & Pinter, M. (1998): Evidence for a spinal central pattern generator in humans. In: *Neuronal mechanisms for generating locomotor activity*, eds. O. Kiehn *et al. Ann. N.Y. Acad. Sci.*, **860**, 360–376.

Eibl-Eibesfeld, I. (1984): *Die Biologie des menschlichen Verhaltens: Grundriss der Humanethologie*. Munchen: R. Piper Verlag.

Esposito, A., Gardella, E., Rubboli, G. *et al.* (2000): Acoustic analysis of vocalizations during 'hyperkynetic frontal' seizure: can they be interpreted as pre-encoded (instinctive) behaviours? [abstract]. *Epilepsia* **41** (Suppl. Florence), 101.

Fusco, L., Iani, C., Fredda, M.T. *et al.* (1990): Mesial frontal epilepsy: a clinical entity not sufficiently described. *J. Epilepsy* **3**, 123–135.

Gardella, E., Rubboli, G., Meletti, S. *et al.* (2000): Stereotypy of motor patterns during 'frontal hypermotor' epileptic seizures. *Epilepsia* **41** (Suppl. Florence), 172.

Gardella, E. & Tassinari, C.A. (2002): Grasping during 'frontal' 'hyperkynetic' seizures: a release of innate behaviour? *Epilepsia* **43** (Suppl. 7), 155.

Grillner, S. & Wallen, P. (1985): Central pattern generators for locomotion, with special reference to vertebrates. *Ann. Rev. Neurosci.* **8**, 233–261.

Iversen, S. & Koob, G. (1977): Behavioural implications of dopaminergic neurons in the mesolimbic system. *Adv. Biochem. Psychopharmacol.* **16**, 209–214.

Jordan, L. (1998): Initiation of locomotion in mammals. In: *Neuronal mechanisms for generating locomotor activity*, eds. O. Kiehn *et al. Ann. N.Y. Acad. Sci.*, **860**, 83–93.

Lüders, H., Acharya, J., Baumgartner, C. *et al.* (1998): Semiological seizure classification. *Epilepsia* **39** (9), 1006–1013.

Lugaresi, E. & Cirignotta, F. (1981): Hypnogenic paroxysmal dystonia: epileptic seizure or a new syndrome? *Sleep* **4**, 129–138.

Meletti, S., Rondelli, F., Volpi, L. *et al.* (2001): The face-wiping and the nose-wiping behaviour: periseizures time courses of a unique innate pattern of behaviour. *Epilepsia* **42** (7), 135.

Mogenson, G.J., Jones, D.L. & Yim, C.Y. (1980): From motivation to action: functional interface between limbic and motor systems. *Prog. Neurobiol.* **14**, 69–97.

Oldani, A., Zucconi, M., Ferini-Strambi, L. *et al.* (1996): Autosomal dominant nocturnal frontal lobe epilepsy: electroclinical picture. *Epilepsia* **37**, 964–976.

Oldani, A., Zucconi, M., Asselta, R. *et al.* (1998): Autosomal dominant nocturnal frontal lobe epilepsy. A video-polysomnographic and genetic appraisal of 40 patients and delineation of the epilepsy syndrome. *Brain* **121**, 205–223.

Plazzi, G., Montagna, P., Tinuper, P. *et al.* (1997): Autosomal nocturnal frontal lobe epilepsy. *Epilepsia* **38**, 738–740.

Provini, F., Plazzi, G., Tinuper, P., Vandi, S., Lugaresi, E. & Montagna, P. (1999): Nocturnal frontal lobe epilepsy. A clinical and polygraphic overview of 100 consecutive cases. *Brain* **122**, 1017–1031.

Riggio, S. & Harner, R.N. (1995): Repetitive motor activity in frontal lobe epilepsy. In: *Epilepsy and the functional anatomy of the frontal lobe*, eds. E.H. Jasper *et al. Adv. Neurol.* **66**, 153–166.

Seyffarth, H. & Denny-Brown, D. (1948): The grasp reflex and the instinctive grasp reaction. *Brain* **71**, 9–183.

Sherrington, C.S. (1906): *The integrative action of the nervous system*. New Haven: Yale University Press.

Tassinari, C.A. (2000): *A neuroethological approach to epileptic seizures*. Invited lecture presented at the 4th European congress on Epilepsy. Florence, October 7, 2000.

Tassinari, C.A., Gardella, E., Meletti, S. & Rubboli, G. (2003): Emergence of innate motor behaviours in human epileptic seizures. In: *Emotion inside out: 130 years after Darwin's The expression of the emotions in man and animals*, eds. P. Ekman, J. Campos, R. Davidson & F. De Waal. *Ann. N.Y. Acad. Sci.* (submitted).

Tinuper, P., Cerullo, A., Cirignotta, F., Cortelli, P., Lugaresi, E. & Montagna, P. (1990): Nocturnal paroxysmal dystonia with short-lasting attacks: three cases with evidence for an epileptic frontal lobe origin of seizures. *Epilepsia* **31** (5), 549–556.

Wada, J.A. (1989): Predominantly nocturnal recurrence of intensely affective vocal and facial expression associated with powerful bimanual, bipedal, and axial activity as ictal manifestations of mesial frontal lobe epilepsy. *Adv. Epileptol.* **17**, 261–267.

Williamson, P.D., Spencer, D.D., Spencer, S.S., Novelly, R.A. & Mattson, R.H. (1985): Complex partial seizures of frontal lobe origin. *Ann. Neurol.* **18**, 497–504.

Zucconi, M., Oldani, A., Ferini-Strambi, L., Bizzozero, D. & Smirne, S. (1997): Nocturnal paroxysmal arousals with motor behaviours during sleep: frontal lobe epilepsy or parasomnia? *J. Clin. Neurophysiol.* **14**, 513–522.

Chapter 6

Natural history of frontal lobe epilepsies

Fabienne Picard and Anne de Saint Martin*

*Clinical Epileptology and Electroencephalography Unit, Department of Neurology,
University Hospital of Geneva, 24, rue Micheli-du-Crest, 1211 Geneva, Switzerland
Fabienne.Picard@hcuge.ch
* Paediatric Department and INSERM U398, Neurologic Clinic,
University Hospitals of Strasbourg, Strasbourg, France*

Summary

The prognosis of a frontal lobe epilepsy depends on the type of epilepsy (symptomatic, cryptogenic, idiopathic). The frontal lobe is often involved in symptomatic epilepsies. Their response to antiepileptic drugs is similar to that of other symptomatic neocortical epilepsies (lateral temporal, parietal, occipital). Almost all cryptogenic epilepsies originating in the frontal lobe correspond to the syndrome described as nocturnal frontal lobe epilepsy (NFLE). This can be familial (autosomal dominant nocturnal frontal lobe epilepsy, ADNFLE) or sporadic. It had been described as nocturnal paroxysmal dystonia but has since been identified as a form of epilepsy. Some features are characteristic of NFLE: (i) each patient's seizures have a remarkably stereotyped motor pattern that does not change even in patients who have had the seizures for more than 30 years. NFLE seems to be non-progressive, with a fixed focus. This differs from symptomatic epilepsies and cryptogenic temporal or occipital lobe epilepsies in which progressive modification of seizures and secondary epileptogenesis are frequent; (ii) in familial cases, we reported a tendency of the seizures to disappear around the third or fourth decade but this seems more dubious in sporadic cases according to the report of a large Italian series; (iii) low doses of carbamazepine are remarkably effective in NFLE. After the discovery of nicotinic receptor mutations in some ADNFLE families, the recent demonstration of an increased sensitivity to carbamazepine of the nicotinic receptors carrying an ADNFLE mutation may help in understanding such a specific sensitivity.

Childhood epilepsy with frontal paroxysms may account for around 5 to 10 per cent of idiopathic age-related partial epilepsies. This differs from the classical benign childhood epilepsy with centro-temporal spikes and childhood epilepsy with occipital paroxysms in (i) the frequency of bilateral interictal discharges reflecting a facilitated spreading of electrical abnormalities, and (ii) an increased risk of abnormalities of behaviour and cognition during the active phase. Long-term outcome is, however, good with remission of the epilepsy at adolescence.

While the exact incidence of frontal lobe epilepsies is not known, reports from epilepsy surgery programs estimate that around 25 per cent of patients with localization-related epilepsy have an epileptogenic focus in the frontal lobe (Williamson, 1992). A similar rate was observed in a large sample of epileptic outpatients followed in a French epilepsy unit. However this unit received referrals of intractable patients and the study did not include patients under 16 years of age (Semah *et al.*, 1998). Frontal lobe epilepsies do not constitute a single entity with a single natural history. We will discuss in this chapter the natural history of frontal lobe epilepsies following the aetiological classification of the Commission on classification (1989). In symptomatic epilepsies, the localization, although related to a frontal lobe lesion, is of little consequence for the natural history of the epilepsy. A more specific frontal lobe epilepsy syndrome will be observed when the frontal localization is related to a particular pathophysiological mechanism. The only such syndrome now appears to be nocturnal frontal lobe epilepsy (NFLE), representing the majority of cryptogenic frontal lobe epilepsies. Sporadic cases of NFLE and familial forms (autosomal dominant nocturnal frontal lobe epilepsy, ADNFLE) show a homogeneous pattern. Lastly, the idiopathic frontal form of benign partial epilepsy of childhood, frequently misdiagnosed, seems to have a specific pattern and prognosis directly related to the localization of the epileptic activity.

Lesional partial epilepsies

Intractable epilepsy is more frequent in patients with MRI abnormalities than in patients without MRI-detected lesions, but the location of the epileptogenic zone is not a major prognostic factor and is associated with only slight differences between the lobar subgroups of lesional partial epilepsies. Semah et al. (1998) observed no significant differences in the rate of complete seizure control among the extra-temporal lobe epilepsy subgroups (parietal, occipital and frontal). Similarly, no significant difference was found between patients with temporal lobe epilepsy without hippocampal sclerosis and those with extra-temporal lobe epilepsy. Thus lesional frontal lobe epilepsies are as responsive to medication as are lesional epilepsies of other lobes, except for temporal lobe epilepsies associated with hippocampal sclerosis, which are known to have a less favourable outcome. The type of underlying brain abnormality was found to have great influence on the rate of intractability. Hippocampal sclerosis, dual pathology (hippocampal sclerosis with another lesion) and cerebral dysgenesis are associated with the worst outcome, whereas other lesions (stroke, vascular malformation, tumour) have a more favourable prognosis for seizure control. Thus the prognosis of a symptomatic epilepsy seems to be closely related to the causal lesion, and little influenced by its location. Nevertheless, it should be emphasized that localization of the epileptogenic zone is difficult in most cases of partial seizures, and is limited to a lobar classification which does not allow definite conclusions as to the organization of the epileptogenic zone and its relation to intractability (Semah et al., 1998).

Cryptogenic partial epilepsies

Most of the cryptogenic frontal lobe epilepsies correspond to NFLE, which has not yet been individualized in the International Classification. This form of epilepsy is often accompanied by a normal interictal and even ictal EEG, and has such specific clinical features and course that it had been described in the 1980's as a non-epileptic disorder, 'nocturnal paroxysmal dystonia' (Lugaresi & Cirignotta, 1981; Lugaresi et al., 1986). The nature of the disorder had long been debated before most authors came to consider it as a frontal epilepsy (Hirsch et al., 1994). Some of the arguments were that the ictal semiology was similar to that observed in some lesional frontal lobe epilepsies, and that some patients also had generalized tonic-clonic seizures (GTCSs) or epileptiform EEG abnormalities. Sporadic (non-familial) cases are more frequent, but large families with a monogenic autosomal dominant transmission of the disorder have been reported (ADNFLE, Scheffer et al., 1994, 1995). In about 20 per cent of ADNFLE families, different mutations have been identified in genes encoding subunits of the neuronal nicotinic receptor (alpha4 or beta2 subunit) (Steinlein et al., 1995, 1997; Saenz et al., 1999; Hirose et al., 1999; Fusco et al., 2000). This familial condition demonstrates that genetic factors may play a causal role in frontal lobe cryptogenic epilepsies. It is important to specify that the clinical and EEG features are identical in sporadic and in familial forms.

Clinical features and evolution of NFLE

The mean age at onset reported in NFLE is 8–12 years (Scheffer *et al.*, 1995; Oldani *et al.*, 1998; Picard *et al.*, 2000). Seizures last less than one minute and hyperkinetic, dystonic or tonic motor manifestations predominate. They occur at night, and frequently in clusters, with a mean of eight seizures per night (Scheffer *et al.*, 1995). Interictal or ictal EEG abnormalities have been identified in 12–65 per cent of cases in different studies. They remain lateralized to the same side throughout the course of the disease. The seizures of ADNFLE reportedly tend to disappear around the fourth decade without relapse after cessation of drug therapy. This tendency to spontaneous remission was not observed by Provini *et al.* (1999) in a group consisting mainly of sporadic cases of NFLE, but the mean age of patients at the time of evaluation (26 years) may have been too young for a decrease in seizures to be observed. Thirty per cent of NFLE patients are pharmacoresistant. The remainders are particularly responsive to low doses of carbamazepine of about 600 mg/d. This suggests pathophysiological mechanisms different from those of other epilepsies. The recent demonstration of an increased sensitivity to carbamazepine of the nicotinic receptors carrying an ADNFLE mutation (Picard *et al.*, 1999) may partly explain this specific drug sensitivity.

The stereotyped character of the seizures in a given patient is a striking feature of NFLE. An exception has to be made when the epilepsy begins in early childhood, since the seizures then occur as tonic postures and change within a few years to the classic NFLE seizures with dystonic or hyperkinetic components (Tinuper, 2003). However, the ictal semiology then remains unchanged throughout life in a given patient. This suggests a stability of the regions of initiation and propagation of epileptic discharges. Secondary epileptogenesis has never been observed in NFLE, although it has been described in symptomatic partial epilepsies and observed less often in cryptogenic partial epilepsies with other localizations. Morrell & de Toledo-Morrell (1999) reported a secondary focus, consisting of an independent mirror focus, in 40 per cent of patients with frontal lobe epilepsies associated with tumour after 5 years of evolution. The following elements associated with a greater likelihood of secondary epileptogenesis are all observed in NFLE: (i) age at seizure onset < 25 years; (ii) high frequency of attacks; and (iii) high density of direct excitatory interhemispheric connections of the cells of the primary focus (Morrell, 1989). The absence of progression of the epilepsy in NFLE is therefore surprising. We hypothesize a pathophysiological mechanism that is different from other epilepsies and consider that the epileptogenic network may involve part of the thalamocortical network generating sleep spindles.

Pathophysiological mechanisms of NFLE: hypothesis

Sleep spindles are physiological neuronal oscillations, consisting of waves at 11–15 Hz grouped in sequences of at least 0.5 seconds, that recur periodically during stage 2 non-REM sleep, usually every 5–10 seconds, with a maximum over the frontal regions. They are generated by a recurrent synaptic loop that links thalamic and cortical circuits and modulates arousal (see Fig. 1). Why do we think that the NFLE epileptic circuit uses this thalamocortical circuit? Two reasons are that (i) ictal EEGs exhibit seizures that apparently begin on a sleep spindle (see Fig. 2); and (ii) nicotinic receptors that have been implicated in ADNFLE are abundant in the thalamus and seem to play a role in the modulation of thalamocortical activity during the spindle stage of sleep. In the ferret, Lee & McCormick (1995) have shown that nicotinic activation of reticular thalamic cells by ACh may contribute to the cessation of spindle oscillations at the time of an arousal. It activates the inhibitory reciprocal connections between reticular thalamic nucleus (RTN) cells that normally serve to desynchronize thalamocortical activity (Huguenard, 2000) (Fig. 1). A computer model of the thalamic network also pointed out that the increase in $GABA_A$ in the RTN may be detrimental to the occurrence of synchrony (Thomas & Lytton, 1998). We can hypothesize that deficient nicotinic receptors would sometimes not allow an increase of intra-RTN GABAergic transmission sufficient to properly interrupt spindles. Spindles could then persist at the time of an arousal, and change into pathological oscillations. It is thus of interest that the mean number of seizures per night in ADNFLE is equivalent to the mean number of arousals per night in normal controls.

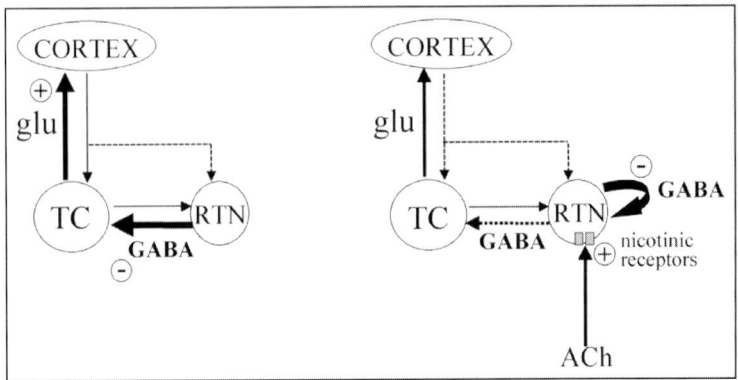

Fig. 1a: RTN is the 'pacemaker' of spindles and is composed of GABAergic neurons that each project to widespread regions of dorsal thalamus (divergence). The rhythmic activation of some reticular thalamic GABAergic cells triggers a synchronous inhibition in many thalamocortical cells, succeeded by a rebound activation, that transmits to the cortex (especially frontal and parietal), and initiates reverberant activity in the reticular thalamic cells. Several cycles of inhibition/activation in this circuit will give rise to a spindle (von Krosigk et al., 1993; McCormick & Bal, 1997). 1b: Through nicotinic receptors located on the GABAergic cells of the RTN, ACh activates the inhibitory reciprocal intra-RTN interconnections and thus desynchronizes thalamocortical activity. This could participate in the interruption of sleep spindles at the time of arousal. TC, thalamocortical cells; RTN, reticular thalamic nucleus; glu, glutamate; ACh, acetylcholine.

Transformation of the physiological oscillations generated by thalamocortical circuitry into generalized spike and wave activity (SW) has been proposed in absence epilepsy based on animal models. In feline generalized penicillin epilepsy, sleep spindles are gradually transformed into SW after parenteral penicillin because of a diffuse cortical hyperexcitability. The excitatory post-synaptic potentials that summate to form spindles are more likely after penicillin to reach the firing threshold of cortical neurons (Gloor & Fariello, 1988). The genetic model Genetic Absence Epilepsy Rats from Strasbourg (GAERS) also proved that the thalamocortical circuits involved in the genesis of the SW are those that normally sustain sleep spindles (Avanzini et al., 2000). However, in another feline model with injections of a GABA antagonist in cats under barbiturate anaesthesia, Steriade & Contreras (1998) found data in favour of a leading role of the neocortex in the generation of SW seizures.

In NFLE, we postulate (i) that the epileptic network uses a pre-existing, normal network corresponding to the part of the thalamocortical circuit generating spindles that is also involved in movement control; and (ii) that it involves a very small cortical region. The cortico-subcortical loop that allows the performance of an accurate voluntary movement and inhibits all other interfering movements comprises only a few thalamic nuclei, especially the lateral ventral and anterior ventral nuclei. The abnormal firing of this loop may not inhibit some additional movements. In conclusion, we postulate an unusual pathophysiological mechanism as the basis of NFLE compared with the other cryptogenic partial epilepsies. The proposed focal firing of a normal thalamocortical circuit could explain the frequent lack of ictal EEG abnormalities on scalp EEG and the non-progressive nature of this epilepsy.

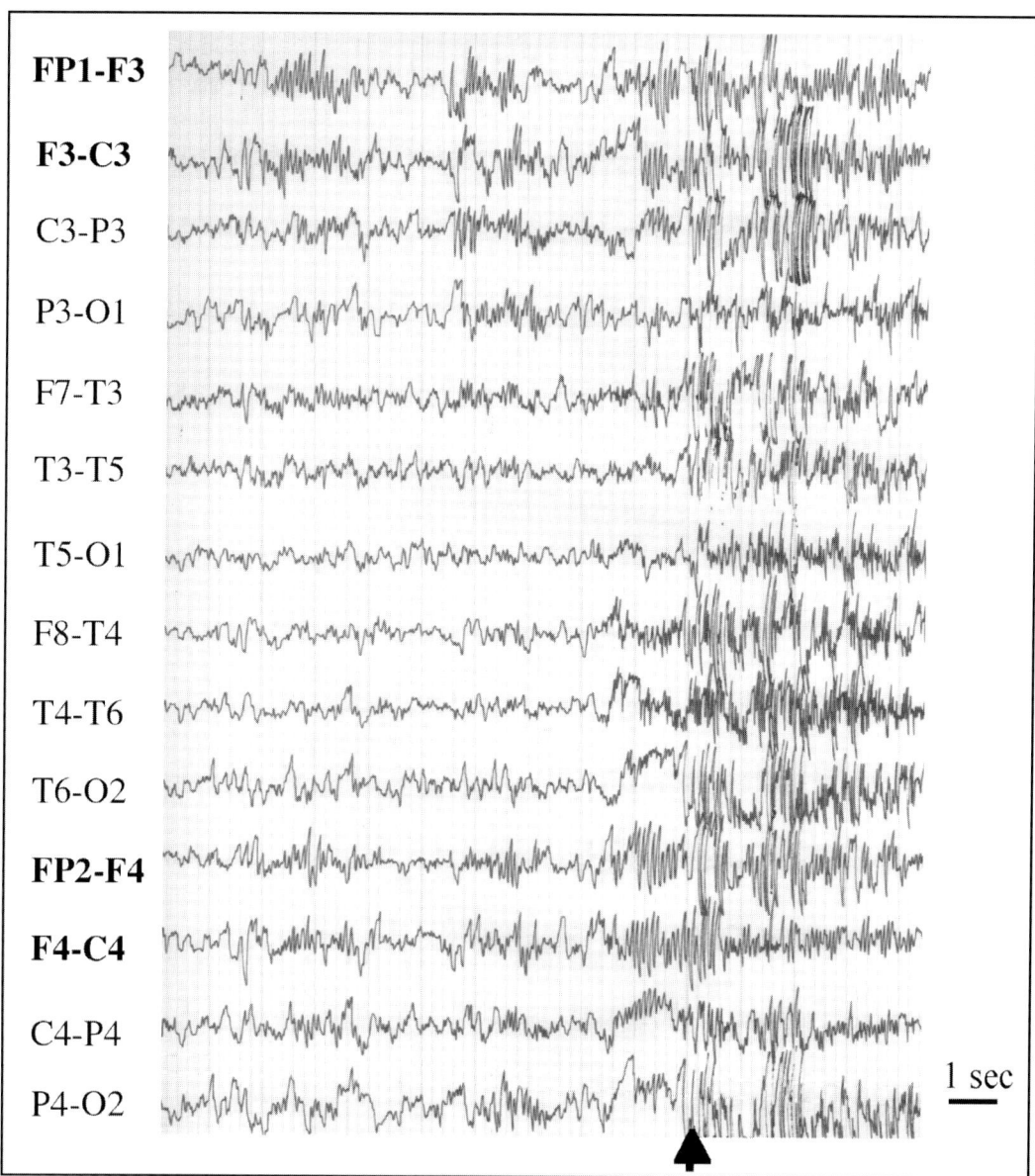

Fig. 2. Ictal EEG (first part) of a nocturnal seizure in a 12-year-old boy with ADNFLE. The seizure occurred in stage 2 of sleep. The EEG modification began 1 second before the first clinical manifestations (arrow) with sustained bifrontal rhythmic activity of the same frequency (12 Hz) and location as sleep spindles. This was followed a few seconds later by muscle artifacts without visible underlying EEG abnormalities. Clinical manifestations were tachypnoea related to a feeling of being 'out of breath', followed by forced, abrupt and irregular movements of the extremities and trunk for 20 seconds.

Idiopathic partial epilepsies with frontal spikes

Beaumanoir & Nahory (1983) described a frontal form of benign partial epilepsy of childhood based on a series of 11 children. These children had had at least two seizures. The clinical picture was polymorphic; most often, seizures consisted of alteration of consciousness, tonic head and possibly trunk deviation, more seldom amyotonia of an upper limb or of the head, and facial flushing. Interictal EEGs showed repetitive SW located in fronto-polar or frontal areas, becoming more widespread during sleep. Prognosis for seizure control was good, with disappearance of seizures before the age of 11 years and of EEG abnormalities before the age of 12 ½. Neuropsychological disorders were reported in three cases, with school difficulties in two and personality problems in one. No other case of benign partial epilepsy of childhood with frontal paroxysms has been reported since.

However, we recently found this disorder in the Department of Neurology of the University Hospital of Strasbourg in four girls and one boy identified in a cohort of children with idiopathic partial epilepsy. We present their electroclinical features.

Electroclinical features and evolution in our series

The age at onset of epilepsy was between 2 and 6 years. Clinical neurological examination and cerebral MRI were normal in all. Seizures mainly occurred during sleep, with heterogeneous symptoms. Loss of consciousness was common. Tonic postures (head and trunk rotation, or brief generalized tonic posture) were described in two patients. Hemiconvulsions, and more rarely facial clonic elements or forward falling of the head, were reported. Four children have also had brief episodes of loss of consciousness similar to absences. Active periods with frequent seizures sometimes occurred, particularly at the beginning of the epilepsy disorder.

EEG features were very homogeneous, with (i) normal EEG background activity; (ii) high-voltage fronto-polar SW, either unilateral or bilateral, synchronous or slightly asynchronous, and frequently occurring in clusters; (iii) intermittent slow waves in the same location (Fig. 3); (iv) brief bursts of generalized SW at 2.5-3 Hz (Fig. 4) since the first recording in all children, with concomitant cervical or shoulder myoclonia in one; (v) subsequent association with an independent spike focus: typical Rolandic spikes (Fig. 5) were observed in four out of five children, 2 to 8 years after seizure onset. In addition, one child had independent left and right frontal SW. The initial frontal focus, usually lateralized, remained so in follow-up EEGs, and was present in all patients when other foci appeared. However the Rolandic spikes sometimes persisted alone for a few months after the disappearance of the frontal focus.

During non-REM sleep recordings, frontal SW were activated and tended to diffuse (Fig. 6). On arousal, two patients had a transitory appearance of rhythmic focal delta slow waves, sometimes spreading, for 20 to 60 seconds.

The children have had no seizures for 1 to 9 years. EEG abnormalities have disappeared in only two of them at the time of the study, but the other three are less than 10 years of age. Thus, the long-term evolution was favourable. However, during the active phase of the epilepsy, neuropsychological problems occurred in all the patients.

The neuropsychological disturbances

All five children had cognitive deficits with impact on schooling and family life. Three had to repeat a year of primary school. Three had attention disorders, and two were treated with methylphenidate. Detailed neuropsychological assessment demonstrated impairments of executive functions in three, particularly in planning; mood disorders in three, consisting of inhibition/passivity in two patients and euphoria in one; and difficulties in short-term memory in three. These results suggest frontal lobe dysfunction.

Chapter 6 Natural history of frontal lobe epilepsies

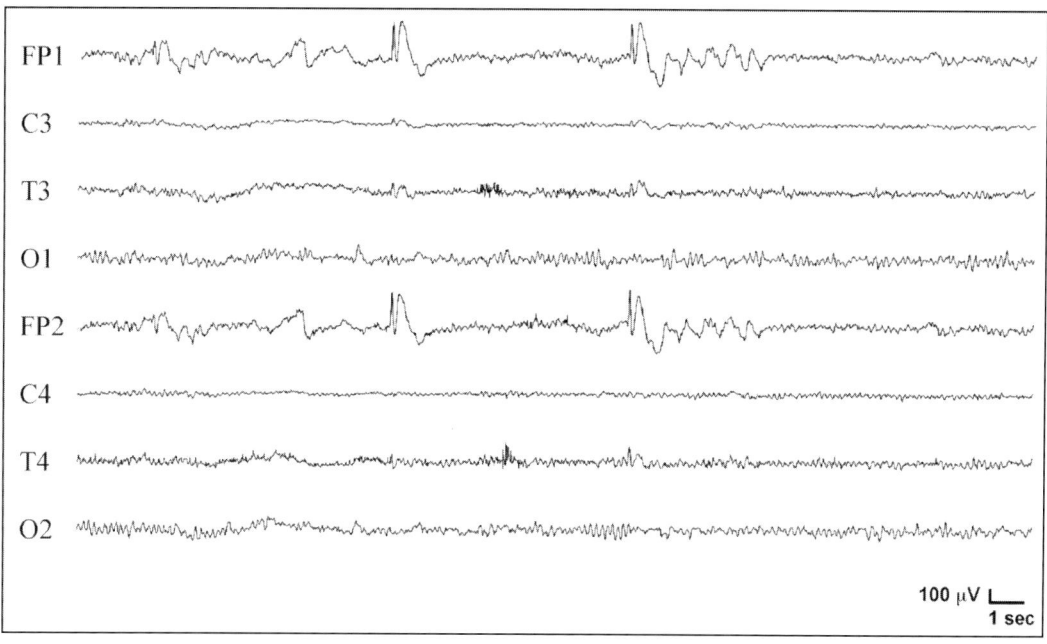

Fig. 3. Sporadic synchronous spike and wave activity in both fronto-polar regions in a 10-year-old girl (G.G.) with a frontal form of benign partial epilepsy of childhood. A train of slow waves is visible in the same locations after one of these spike-and-wave complexes. (Monopolar derivations recalculated against the average reference.)

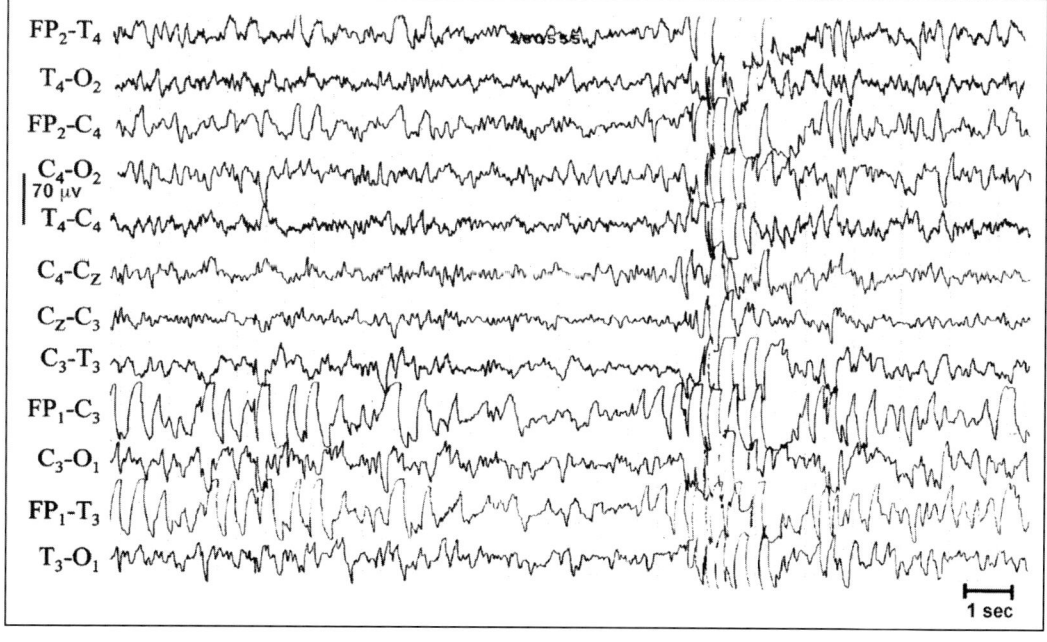

Fig. 4. Burst of generalized spike and wave activity at 2.5 Hz, in addition to focal spike and wave activity and slow waves in the left fronto-polar area, in a patient (N.M.) with a frontal benign partial epilepsy of childhood.

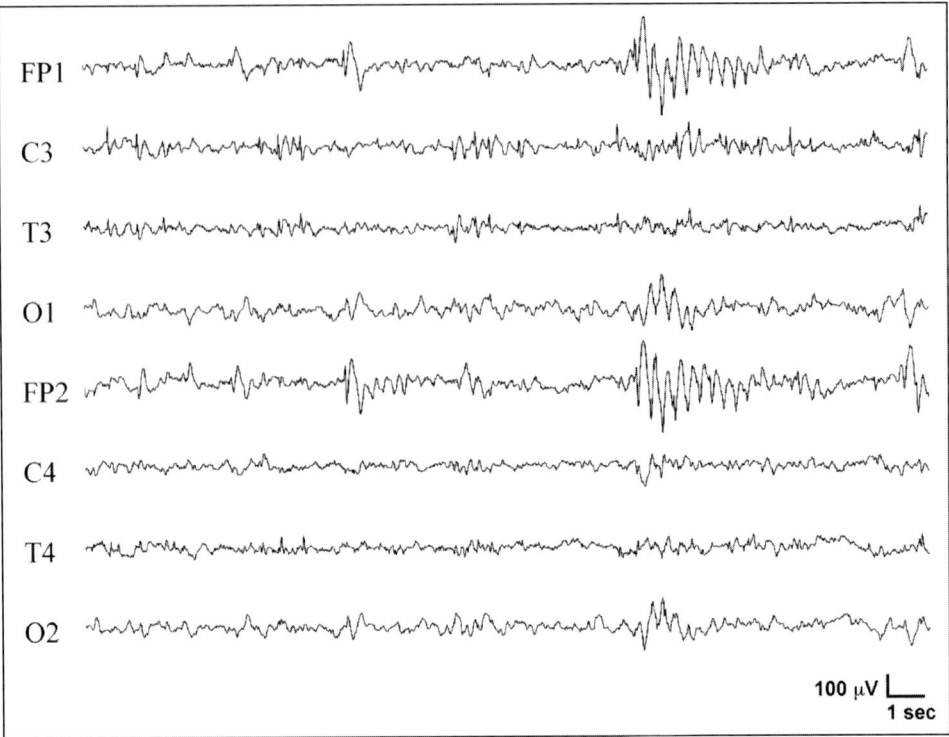

Fig. 5. Independent left centro-temporal spikes are observed in the same patient as in Fig. 3, aged 8 years. (Monopolar derivations recalculated against the average reference.)

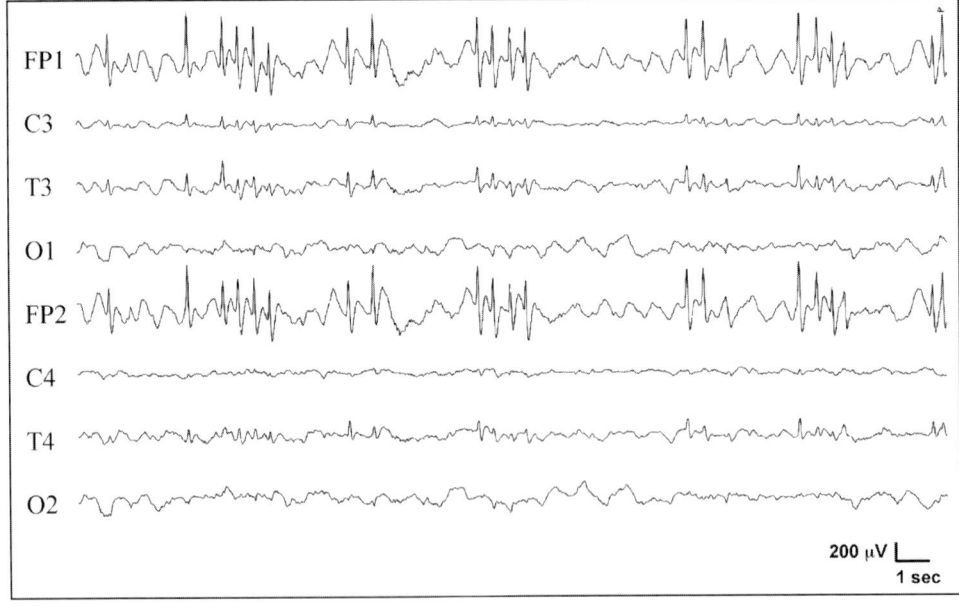

Fig. 6. Activation of the fronto-polar spike and wave activity and slow waves, and tendency to diffusion of the spike and wave activity during non-REM sleep in the same patient as in Fig. 3, aged 10 years. (Monopolar derivations recalculated against the average reference.)

Several elements may contribute to this frequent occurrence of disabling neuropsychological disorders. Firstly, EEGs consistently showed an intermittent slow focus consisting of sequences of rhythmic high-voltage slow waves. A succession of slow waves is considered more disruptive of cognitive functions than are spikes. Shewmon & Erwin (1988) showed that the after-coming slow wave within a spike and wave complex transiently disrupts cortical functioning. In addition, the electrical abnormalities in the frontal form of benign partial epilepsy of childhood often involve both frontal lobes because of secondary bilateral synchrony. This may prevent contralateral compensation for the frontal cognitive functions. Lastly, at the time the epilepsy develops, the frontal lobes are in the midst of maturation (Smith *et al.*, 1992). Luria (1966, 1973) suggested that the frontal lobes are not mature until the age of 7 years, in contrast to more posterior and subcortical areas that mature earlier.

Cognitive disturbances of a frontal nature have been reported in benign focal epilepsy of childhood with Rolandic spikes (Metz-Lutz *et al.*, 1999). They were ascribed to a distant effect of the epileptiform EEG abnormalities on functions that are maturing at the age when this epilepsy occurs, while other functions have already reached a high level of organization around 3–4 years. However, only a small subgroup of these patients had disturbances with consequences in daily life. The EEG focus was more active in this subgroup.

To conclude, idiopathic partial epilepsy of childhood with frontal spikes is probably less rare than was initially thought. It may correspond to about one-twelfth of idiopathic partial epilepsy cases in childhood and thus be at least as frequent as idiopathic partial epilepsy of childhood with occipital spikes. In our small series, some cases were long misdiagnosed as cryptogenic frontal lobe epilepsy resistant to carbamazepine or vigabatrin, or atypical absence epilepsy. The recognition of this form of idiopathic partial epilepsy of childhood is thus important for proper treatment and adequate neuropsychological follow-up.

Acknowledgments: We wish to thank R. Massa, R. Carcangiu, E. Raffo, C. Seegmuller, M.N. Metz-Lutz, E. Hirsch for their contribution to the study of the children with benign partial epilepsy of childhood with frontal paroxysms. In particular, we greatly appreciated the helpful discussion with C. Marescaux.

References

Avanzini, G., Panzica, F. & de Curtis, M. (2000): The role of the thalamus in vigilance and epileptogenic mechanisms. *Clin. Neurophysiol.* **111**, S19–S26.

Beaumanoir, A. & Nahory, A. (1983): Les épilepsies bénignes partielles: 11 cas d'épilepsie partielle frontale à évolution favorable. *Rev. E.E.G Neurophysiol.* **13**, 207–211.

Commission on Classification and Terminology of the International League Against Epilepsy (1989): Proposal for revised classification of epilepsies and epileptic syndromes. *Epilepsia* **30**, 389–399.

Fusco, M.D., Becchetti, A., Patrignani, A., Annesi, G., Gambardella, A., Quattrone, A., Ballabio, A., Wanke, E. & Casari, G. (2000): The nicotinic receptor beta2 subunit is mutant in nocturnal frontal lobe epilepsy. *Nat. Genet.* **26**, 275–276.

Gloor, P. & Fariello, R.G. (1988): Generalized epilepsy: some of its cellular mechanisms differ from those of focal epilepsy. *TINS* **11**, 63–68.

Hirose, S., Iwata, H., Akiyoshi, H., Kobayashi, K., Ito, M., Wada, K., Kaneko, S. & Mitsudome, A. (1999): A novel mutation of CHRNA4 responsible for autosomal dominant nocturnal frontal lobe epilepsy. *Neurology* **53**, 1749–1753.

Hirsch, E., Sellal, F., Maton, B., Rumbach, L. & Marescaux, C. (1994): Nocturnal paroxysmal dystonia: a clinical form of focal epilepsy. [Review]. *Neurophysiol. Clin.* **24**, 207–217.

Huguenard, J.R. (2000): Circuit mechanisms of spike-wave discharge: are there similar underpinnings for centrotemporal spikes? *Epilepsia* **41**, 1076–1077.

Lee, K.H. & McCormick, D.A. (1995): Acetylcholine excites GABAergic neurons of the ferret perigeniculate nucleus through nicotinic receptors. *J Neurophysiol* **73**, 2123–2128.

Lugaresi, E. & Cirignotta, F. (1981): Hypnogenic paroxysmal dystonia: epileptic seizure or a new syndrome? *Sleep* **4**, 129–138.

Lugaresi, E., Cirignotta, F. & Montagna, P. (1986): Nocturnal paroxysmal dystonia. *J. Neurol. Neurosurg. Psychiatry* **49**, 375–380.

Luria, A.R. (1966): *Higher cortical functions in man.* New York: Basic Books.

Luria A.R. (1973): *The working brain.* New York: Basic Books.

McCormick, D.A. & Bal, T. (1997): Sleep and arousal: thalamocortical mechanisms. *Annu. Rev. Neurosci.* **20**, 185–215.

Metz-Lutz, M.N., Kleitz, C., de Saint Martin, A., Massa, R., Hirsch, E. & Marescaux, C. (1999): Cognitive development in benign focal epilepsies of childhood. *Dev. Neurosci.* **21**, 182–190.

Morrell, F. (1989): Varieties of human secondary epileptogenesis. *J. Clin. Neurophysiol.* **6**, 227–275.

Morrell, F. & de Toledo-Morrell, L. (1999): From mirror focus to secondary epileptogenesis in man: an historical review. In: *Advances in neurology*, vol. 81, pp. 11–23, eds. H. Stefan, F. Andermann, P. Chauvel & S. Shorvon, Philadelphia: Lippincott Williams & Wilkins.

Oldani, A., Zucconi, M., Asselta, R., Modugno, M., Bonati, M.T., Dalprà, L., Malcovati, M., Tenchini, M.L., Smirne, S. & Ferini-Strambi, L. (1998): Autosomal dominant nocturnal frontal lobe epilepsy: a video-polysomnographic and genetic appraisal of 40 patients and delineation of the epileptic syndrome. *Brain* **121**, 205–223.

Picard, F., Bertrand, S., Steinlein, O.K. & Bertrand, D. (1999): Mutated nicotinic receptors responsible for autosomal dominant nocturnal frontal lobe epilepsy are highly sensitive to carbamazepine. *Epilepsia* **40**, 1198–1209.

Picard, F., Baulac, S., Kahane, P., Hirsch, E., Sebastianelli, R., Thomas, P., Vigevano, F., Genton, P., Guerrini, R., Gericke, C.A., An, I., Rudolf, G., Herman, A., Brice, A., Marescaux, C. & LeGuern, E. (2000): Dominant partial epilepsies: a clinical, electrophysiological and genetic study of 19 European families. *Brain* **123**, 1247–1262.

Provini, F., Plazzi, G., Tinuper, P., Vandi, S., Lugaresi, E. & Montagna, P. (1999): Nocturnal frontal lobe epilepsy. A clinical and polygraphic overview of 100 consecutive cases. *Brain* **122**, 1017–1031.

Saenz, A., Galan, J., Caloustian, C., Lorenzo, F., Marquez, C., Rodriguez, N., Jimenez, M.D., Poza, J.J., Cobo, A.M., Grid, D., Prud'homme, J.F. & Lopez de Munain, A. (1999): Autosomal dominant nocturnal frontal lobe epilepsy in a Spanish family with a Ser252Phe mutation in the CHRNA4 gene. *Arch. Neurol.* **56**, 1004–1009.

Scheffer, I.E., Bhatia, K.P., Lopes-Cendes, I., Fish, D.R., Marsden, C.D., Andermann, F., Andermann, E., Desbiens, R.R., Cendes, F., Manson, J.I. & Berkovic, S.F. (1994): Autosomal dominant frontal epilepsy misdiagnosed as sleep disorder. *Lancet* **343**, 515–517.

Scheffer, I.E., Bhatia, K.P., Lopes-Cendes, I., Fish, D.R., Marsden, C.D., Andermann, E., Andermann, F., Desbiens, R., Keene, D., Cendes, F., Manson, J.I., Constantinou, J.E.C., McIntosh, A. & Berkovic, S.F. (1995): Autosomal dominant nocturnal frontal lobe epilepsy. A distinctive clinical disorder. *Brain* **118**, 61–73.

Semah, F., Picot, M.C., Adam, C., Broglin, D., Arzimanoglou, A., Bazin, B., Cavalcanti, D. & Baulac, M. (1998): Is the underlying cause of epilepsy a major prognostic factor for recurrence? *Neurology* **51**, 1256–1262.

Shewmon, D.A. & Erwin, R.J. (1988): Focal spike-induced cerebral dysfunction is related to the after-coming slow wave. *Ann. Neurol.* **23**, 131–137.

Smith, M.L., Kates, M.H. & Vriezen, E.R. (1992): The development of frontal-lobe functions. In: *Handbook of Neuropsychology*, vol. 7, pp. 309–330, eds. S.J. Segalowitz & I. Rapin. Amsterdam: Elsevier Science Publishers.

Steinlein, O.K., Mulley, J.C., Propping, P., Wallace, R.H., Phillips, H.A. & Sutherland, G.R. (1995): A missense mutation in the neuronal nicotinic acetylcholine receptor 4 subunit is associated with autosomal dominant nocturnal frontal lobe epilepsy. *Nat. Genet.* **11**, 201–203.

Steinlein, O.K., Magnusson, A., Stoodt, J., Bertrand, S., Weiland, S., Berkovic, S.F., Nakken, K.O., Propping, P. & Bertrand, D. (1997): An insertion mutation of the CHRNA4 gene in a family with autosomal dominant nocturnal frontal lobe epilepsy. *Hum. Mol. Genet.* **6**, 943–947.

Steriade, M. & Contreras, D. (1998): Spike-wave complexes and fast components of cortically generated seizures. I. Role of neocortex and thalamus. *J. Neurophysiol.* **80**, 1439–1455.

Thomas, E. & Lytton, W.W. (1998): Computer model of antiepileptic effects mediated by alterations in $GABA_A$-mediated inhibition. *Neuro. Rep.* **9**, 691–696.

Tinuper, P. (2003): Ictal video-EEG features in children with nocturnal frontal lobe seizures. In: *Frontal seizures and epilepsies in children*, eds. A. Beaumanoir, F. Andermann, P. Chauvel, L. Mira & B. Zifkin, pp. 113–119. Mariani Foundation Paediatric Neurology Series, vol. 11. Paris, London: John Libbey Eurotext.

von Krosigk, M., Bal, T. & McCormick, D.A. (1993): Cellular mechanisms of a synchronized oscillation in the thalamus. *Science* **261**, 361–364.

Williamson, P.D. (1992): Frontal lobe seizures - Problems of diagnosis and classification. In: *Advances in Neurology*, vol. 57, pp. 289–309, eds. P. Chauvel, A.V. Delgado-Escueta, E. Halgren & J. Bancaud. New York: Raven Press.

Chapter 7

Can we classify frontal lobe seizures?

Patrick Chauvel

*Clinical Neurophysiology Service and Neurophysiology & Neuropsychology Laboratory, EMIU 9926,
La Timone Hospital, Boulevard Jean-Moulin, 13385 Marseille cedex 5, France
pchauvel@ap-hm.fr*

A general trend influenced by the development of epilepsy surgery has been to separate temporal from extra-temporal seizures as two distinct entities (Williamson *et al.*, 1997). Over the last 10 years, frontal lobe seizures have been intensively studied and significant advances have been made in understanding frontal lobe epilepsy (Chauvel *et al.*, 1992). The human frontal lobe is a very large part of the cerebral cortex, accounting for approximately 40 per cent of its total volume, and the question of subdividing frontal lobe seizures is posed according to different criteria. Based on thalamo-cortical connections, the frontal lobe is classically bound by the central fissure, and may be separated from caudal to rostral into precentral, premotor and prefrontal cortex. Which localization-related frontal epileptic syndromes have really been identified?

The clinical picture of precentral seizures was fully described at the end of the nineteenth century by Hughlings Jackson. The sudden onset of tonic-clonic involvement of distal muscles, the ascending march of the seizure towards proximal muscles, and the different modes of ipsilateral and contralateral spread to the limbs and the face, with post-ictal motor deficits, defined 'convulsions beginning unilaterally' (Loiseau, 1992). They were localized to the motor cortex and differentiated from 'epileptiform seizures', which in this scheme were more bilateral and proximal, and were believed to originate more rostrally in the frontal lobes.

Penfield and his colleagues at the Montreal Neurological Institute later performed stimulation studies of the exposed central region and reported the anatomo-physiological organization underlying the so-called 'Jacksonian' seizures (Penfield & Boldrey, 1937). Because of its heuristic value, the Jacksonian focal seizure obscured the clinical reality of precentral seizures. More tonic, complex, and bilateral but asymmetrical patterns were identified by Ajmone-Marsan & Goldhammer (1973). Trottier (1972) and Chauvel *et al.* (1992) in patients with atrophic lesions of the posterior frontal cortex. Similarly, Bancaud and colleagues studied reflex seizures mimicking startle, or beginning with a startle followed by a tonic attack, in patients with infantile hemiplegia. These seizures were investigated with intracerebral electrodes and attributed to tonic discharges in precentral and premotor cortex (Chauvel *et al.*, 1992; Vignal *et al.*, 1998).

Apart from the seizure patterns in these patients with large non-tumoral lesions, the clinical semiology of precentral seizures is dominated by clonic involvement of distal muscles, which may appear as more or less continuous twitches or jerks. Such seizures have been described under different names according to the syndrome in which they occur: Kojevnikov's syndrome (Bancaud, 1992), Rasmussen's syndrome; epilepsia partialis continua; and cortical (reflex) myoclonus (Hallett et al., 1979). The myoclonic jerks have been shown to originate in the motor cortex (Chauvel et al., 1992) and the classification of the different related syndromes has been clarified (Biraben & Chauvel, 1997).

Premotor seizures have been gradually recognized as a distinct seizure type as a result of studies on 'adversive seizures' (Förster) and of the discovery by Penfield and Welch (1951) of the supplementary motor area (SMA). Förster had earlier proposed that seizures from lateral area 6 resulted in head and eye turning. After Penfield and co-workers proved that stimulating the medial aspect of area 6 elicited the same pattern, with raising of the contralateral arm and vocalization resembling a 'fencing posture', frontal adversion was generally considered to originate from the SMA. Unfortunately, what Penfield and Welch had written in the same paper about a marked difference between seizures elicited by SMA stimulation and spontaneous seizures was therefore ignored. Later, Ajmone-Marsan & Goldhammer (1973), Morris et al. (1988) and Chauvel et al. (1992) emphasized the polymorphic character of SMA seizures and the difficulties in reaching a positive diagnosis. Nevertheless, some common traits can be extracted.

Moving forward from precentral to premotor cortex leads to different motor patterns: attacks are mainly tonic and postural, and as such first involve proximal musculature, bilaterally but asymmetrically. That lateral area 6 and area 8 involvement determines head and eye adversion has been demonstrated by Chauvel et al. (1996). This is also the privileged pathway for generalization.

Distinctions between premotor and prefrontal seizures certainly are difficult to draw, because discharge spread can link both regions, and a coronal compartmentalization remains purely hypothetical. A subtype named 'intermediate' frontal lobe seizures by Bancaud & Talairach (1992) reflects how indistinct the separation can be between anterior and posterior frontal lobe seizures. These are generally characterized by the association of 'automatic' and tonic-postural motor manifestations.

Interestingly, the identification of prefrontal seizures took more than 10 years after a first pioneering paper by Tharp (1972). He reported clinical manifestations in five children, and hypothesized that the seizures were generated in the orbital part of the frontal lobe. The so-called 'orbital frontal seizures' had the following features. They tended to occur as nocturnal episodes, in clusters. Their frequency during symptomatic periods was high. Secondary generalisations never occurred. They were characterised by prominent early signs of autonomic dysfunction: children seemed frightened, would run searchingly about the room and frequently became agitated when restrained. Some fits consisted in repetitive, semipurposeful motor activity and vocalization, either unintelligible screaming or loud expletives of single words or short sentences. A few years later, Ludwig, Van Buren and Ajmone-Marsan (1975) described a similar picture in adult patients investigated with intracerebral electrodes, and followed Tharp in the same hypothesis of 'seizures of probable frontal origin'. They claimed that ictal automatisms occurred simultaneously with recorded orbital discharges in three patients with no concurrent involvement of, or spread to, temporal structures. It took some time until this new interpretation of anatomo-clinical correlations with gestural automatisms generated outside of the temporal lobe was definitively admitted.

However, stimulation of a limited part of anterior cingulated gyrus (area 24) in epileptic patients during SEEG could induce a complex motor behaviour made by arousal and mood changes, gestural stereotypies of hands and fingers, and coordinated complex movements of hands and mouth, generally contralateral to the stimulation (Talairach *et al.*, 1973). This led to the concept of frontal-temporal epilepsies (Talairach *et al.*, 1974) for patients presenting early gestural automatisms simultaneous with discharges in the frontal lobe, even though they could secondarily spread to the temporal lobe. Clinical observations of frontal lobe seizures with video-EEG during scalp recordings attempted to differentiate frontal lobe from temporal lobe seizures on the basis of semiology (Geier *et al.*, 1977). In a famous paper on a 'pure culture' of frontal lobe epilepsies (cured after surgery), Rasmussen (1975) found only automatisms in 30 per cent of the cases, and Quesney *et al.* (1990) specified that they occurred in seizures from the anterolaterodorsal convexity of the frontal lobe and spread to the temporal lobe. One indirect but strong argument in favour of the role of frontal lobe structures in generating automatisms was given by Walsh and Delgado-Escueta (1984) reporting failures of temporal lobe surgery in their type II complex partial seizures (which were characterized by this type of motor manifestations, considered distinct from temporal lobe automatisms – type I). Thereafter, a clear description of 'complex partial seizures of frontal lobe origin' was proposed by Williamson *et al.* (1985) on the basis of depth recordings. They showed a stereotyped pattern, and could be so bizarre that they could appear as hysterical. As from the description from Tharp and later Ludwig, they found that patients presented with frequent seizures, often in clusters, many per day; they were brief, under 1 minute, followed by short post-ictal period with rapid clearing. The most characteristic trait was the occurrence of prominent motor automatisms, usually complex, often beginning suddenly, with the possibility of aggressive sexual automatisms, as part of motor automatisms; vocalization was frequent, with variable complexity from simple hum to shouted obscenities. Warnings were usually nonspecific but sometimes complex with psychic and illusional qualities. Localisation within the frontal lobe remained to be understood.

Chauvel & Bancaud (1994), from their experience of patients implanted with intra-cerebral electrodes, considered as the two best-defined patterns of prefrontal seizures the dorsal prefrontal seizures on one hand, and the orbito-frontal seizures on the other hand.

Some symptoms suggest the origin of seizures in the dorsal region: forced thinking, 'eye-directed' automatism and pseudo-compulsive behaviour, and tonic deviation of the eyes preceding head deviation indicating frontal eye field involvement. Complex visual hallucinations can occur. Ictal discharge can secondarily involve premotor and motor areas and secondary generalization is frequent.

The orbito-frontal seizures (Munari & Bancaud, 1992) corresponded to the pattern described as 'complex partial seizures (CPSs) of frontal origin' (Williamson *et al.*, 1985). They are characterized by sudden onset with loss of contact and more or less elaborate automatisms (Geier *et al.*, 1977): complex gestural sequences with bizarre gesticulations, and eupraxic pseudointentional behaviour. Some seizures start with vocalization, intense fear (or the appearance of fear), and violent movements mimicking fearful behaviour or hallucination. This emotional or pseudoemotional behaviour is associated with autonomic signs: facial flush, mydriasis, respiratory changes. Peri-ictal urination is typical in these seizures. Some patients may report an olfactory hallucination at the onset of seizures. However, olfactory hallucination is not specific for these seizures since they are also observed in seizures primarily involving limbic temporal structures implicated in olfactory function (Acharya *et al.*, 1998).

That the so-called automatisms, in fact very different from temporal lobe automatisms, could not be put in a unique category appeared evident.

The next step in ensuring sublobar localisation of these CPSs of frontal lobe origin was made by reviewing the clinical semiology in patients investigated with SEEG, and seizure-free after surgery. The results in this new 'pure culture' was reported by Chauvel *et al.* (1995). They separated gestural automatisms into stereotypies and forced acting, based on their clinical aspect. Transition signs from premotor to prefrontal areas were the emergence of these motor behaviours preceding or associated with postural and tonic signs, and the presence of emotional or autonomic signs associated with motor signs. Clinical patterns depended on predominant involvement of frontal lateral or medial regions. A clear correlation actually was established between the site of operation and the previous occurrence of these manifestations: all the operations had been performed in the prefrontal region, and preferentially in its medial or medio-basal part.

An interesting distinction between two clinical patterns seems important. Indeed, the description given by previous authors represents in fact only part of the possible observed patterns. Two main categories could be distinguished. The first one has been called 'purposeless', 'dyspraxic' forced acting. Body movements are driven by the proximal musculature, and appear aimless. General aspect is that of a gestural uninhibited behaviour, with marked asocial traits, apparent strong emotional implication and neglect of environmental stimuli. This corresponds well to the description of 'hyper-motor seizures' by Lüders and his co-workers: 'Seizures consisting of complex organized movements which affect mainly the proximal portions of the limbs, leading to a marked increase in motor activity. Consciousness may be preserved' (Holthausen et al., 2000). The second, at the opposite end, is made of 'semi-purposeful', 'eupraxic' forced acting. Movements are distally driven, patient behaviour appears as stimulus-bound, object-oriented, with a compulsive character, associated or not with moderate emotional disturbance. This last pattern is very close to the definition of stereotypy by the experimental psychologists: 'excessive production of one type of motor act, or mental state, which necessarily results in repetition' (Ridley, 1994). Stereotypy may be driven by excessive internal motivational states even if these are not related to the environment in the usual adaptive, 'purposeful' way. Recent results of correlations between anatomical origin and spread of ictal discharges and clinical semiology show that the first pattern is linked with disorganisation of prefrontal medial-ventral cortex (Trébuchon, 2002).

Table 1. Proposed classification for frontal lobe seizures

Central
- Medial (foot area ± SMA)
- Lateral
  - Dorsal central (arm area ± BA 6)
  - Ventral central (face area + perisylvian)

Premotor
- Medial (SMA + pre-SMA)
- Lateral (BA 6 + FEF)

Prefrontal
- Medial
  - Dorsal PreFM (BA 24 + 9 (± SMA)
  - Ventral PreFM (BA 32, 25, 10, 14, 13 +...)
- Lateral
  - Dorsal PreFL (BA 9-46 +/- FEF)
  - Ventral PreFL (BA 11, 47-12, 44/45, IFG +/- frontal operculum)
- Prefrontal-temporal
  - Medial (OF + ACG + Am)
  - Lateral (OF + INS + TP = anterior perisylvian)

Abbreviations: foot-arm-face areas, subdivisions of primary motor area (MI); SMA, Supplementary Motor Area; BA, Brodmann areas; FEF, Frontal Eye Field (BA 8); PreFM, prefrontal medial; PreFL, prefrontal lateral; IFG, inferior frontal gyrus; OF, orbito-frontal; ACG, anterior cingulated gyrus; Am, amygdala; INS, insular cortex; TP, temporal pole.

In conclusion, a strict classification of frontal lobe seizures today cannot be more than a working hypothesis (Table 1). However, general trends may appear along the anteroposterior (from prefrontal to precentral) and mediolateral axes of frontal lobe topography. Distinction between three rostrocaudal compartments (precentral, premotor, prefrontal) according to ictal clinical patterns seems to be valid. Medial *vs* lateral subtypes have been well documented in the precentral (paracentral lobule *vs* hand or face motor area) and in the premotor (SMA *vs* lateral area 6) regions. A further subdivision between dorsal and ventral parts is likely to be supported by careful analysis of prefrontal seizures, and can be extended posteriorly to the separation of seizures originating from the inferior frontal gyrus and perisylvian cortex ventrally, from seizures arising from the dorsolateral cortex of areas 6 and 8 dorsally. This separation can easily be prolonged to the central region, where seizures involving primarily the face and mouth area are well differentiated from those involving the arm and hand area at the onset.

References

Acharya, V., Acharya, J & Lüders, H. (1998): Olfactory epileptic auras. *Neurology* **51**, 56–61.

Ajmone-Marsan, C. & Goldhammer, L. (1973) Clinical patterns and electrographic data in cases of partial seizures of frontal-central-parietal origin. In: *Epilepsy, its phenomena in man*, ed. M.A.B. Brazier, pp. 235–258. New York, Academic Press.

Bancaud, J. (1992): Kojewnikow's syndrome (epilepsia partialis continua) in children. In: *Epileptic syndromes in infancy, childhood and adolescence*, eds. J. Roger, M. Bureau, C. Dravet, F. Dreifuss, A. Perret & P. Wolf, pp. 363–380. London: John Libbey & Company.

Bancaud, J. & Talairach, J. (1992) Clinical semiology of frontal lobe seizures. *Adv. Neurol.* **57**, 3–58.

Biraben, A.& Chauvel, P. (1997): Epilepsia partialis continua. In: *Epilepsy: a comprehensive textbook*, eds. J. Engel Jr. & T. Pedley, pp. 2447–2453. New York: Lippincott-Raven.

Chauvel, P. & Bancaud, J. (1994): The spectrum of frontal lobe seizures: with a note on frontal lobe syndromatology. In: *Epileptic seizures and syndromes*, ed. P. Wolf. London: John Libbey & Company.

Chauvel, P., Delgado-Escueta, A., Halgren, E. & Bancaud, J. (1992a): Frontal lobe seizures and epilepsies. *Adv. Neurol.* **57**, 331–334.

Chauvel, P., Trottier, S., Vignal, J. & Bancaud, J. (1992b): Somatomotor seizures of frontal lobe seizures. *Adv Neurol.* **57**, 185–232.

Chauvel, P., Kliemann, F., Vignal, J., Chodkiewicz, J., Talairach, J. & Bancaud, J. (1995): The clinical signs and symptoms of frontal lobe seizures. Phenomenology and classification. *Adv. Neurol.* **66**, 115–125.

Chauvel, P.Y., Rey, M., Buser, P. & Bancaud, J. (1996): What stimulation of the supplementary motor area in humans tells about its functional organization. *Adv. Neurol.* **70**, 199–209.

Delgado-Escueta, A., Swartz, B., Maldonado, H., Walsh, G., Rand, R. & Halgren, E. (1987): Complex partial seizures of frontal origin. In: *Presurgical evaluation of epileptics*, eds. H.-G. Wieser & C. Elger, pp. 268–299. New York: Springer-Verlag.

Geier, S., Bancaud, J., Talairach, J., Bonis, A., Szikla, G. & Enjelvin, M. (1977): The seizures of frontal lobe epilepsy. A study of clinical manifestations. *Neurology* **27**, 951–958.

Hallett, M., Chadwick, D. & Marsden, C.D. (1979): Cortical reflex myoclonus. *Neurology* **29**, 1107–1125.

Holthausen, H. & Hoppe, M.. (2000) Hypermotor seizures In: *Epileptic Seizures*, eds. H.O. Lüders & S. Noachtar, pp. 439–448. Philadelphia: Churchill Livingstone.

Jasper, H., Riggio, S. & Goldman-Rakic, P. (1995): *Epilepsy and the functional anatomy of the frontal lobe*. New York: Raven Press.

Loiseau, P. (1992): The Jacksonian model of partial motor seizures. *Adv. Neurol.* **57**, 181–184.

Morris, H., Dinner, D., Lüders, H., Wyllie, E. & Krainer, R. (1988): Supplementary motor area seizures: clinical and electroencephalographic findings. *Neurology* **38**, 1075–1082.

Ludwig, B., Ajmone-Marsan, C. & Van Buren, J. (1975): Cerebral seizures of probable orbitofrontal origin. *Epilepsia* **16**, 141–158.

Munari, C. & Bancaud, J. (1992): Electroclinical symptomatology of partial seizures of orbital frontal origin. *Adv. Neurol.* **57**, 257–265.

Penfield, W. & Welch, K. (1951): The supplementary motor area of the cerebral cortex: a clinical and experimental study. *Arch. Neurol. Psychiatry* **66**, 289–317.

Quesney, L.F., Constain, M., Fish D.R. & Rasmussen, T. (1990): The clinical differentiation of seizures arising in the parasagittal and anterolaterodorsal frontal convexities. *Arch. Neurol.* **47**, 677–679.

Rasmussen, T. (1975): Surgery of frontal lobe epilepsy. In: *Neurosurgical management of epilepsies*, eds. D. Purpura, J. Penry J. & R. Walter, pp. 197–205. New York: Raven Press.

Talairach, J., Bancaud, J., Geier, S., Bordas-Ferrer, M., Bonis, A., Szikla, G. & Rusu, M. (1973) The cingulate gyrus and human behaviour. *Electroencephalogr. Clin. Neurophysiol.* **34** (1), 45–52.

Talairach, J., Bancaud, J., Szikla, G., Bonis, A., Geier, S. & Vedrenne, C. (1974) Approche nouvelle de la neurochirurgie de l'épilepsie (méthodologie stéréotaxique et résultats thérapeutiques). *Neurochirurgie* **20** (Suppl. 1), 240 pp.

Talairach, J., Bancaud, J. & Geier, S. et al. (1992): Surgical therapy of frontal epilepsies. *Adv. Neurol.* **57**, 707–732.

Tharp, B.R. (1972): Orbital frontal seizures. An unique electroencephalographic and clinical syndrome. *Epilepsia* **13**, 627–642.

Trébuchon, A. (2002): *Rôle du cortex préfrontal dans l'expression de la peur critique.* Thèse de Médecine, Marseille.

Trottier, S. (1972): *Sémiologie clinique des accès épileptiques à point de départ rolandique.* Thèse de Médecine, Paris.

Vignal, J., Biraben, A., Chauvel, P. & Reutens, D. (1998): Reflex partial seizures of sensorimotor cortex (including cortical reflex myoclonus and startle epilepsy). *Adv. Neurol.* **75**, 207–226.

Walsh, G.O. & Delgado-Escueta, A.V. (1984): Type II complex partial seizures: poor results of anterior temporal lobectomy. *Neurology* **34**, 1–13.

Williamson, P., Engel, J. & Munari, C. (1997): Anatomic classification of localization-related epilepsies. In: *Epilepsy: a comprehensive textbook*, eds. J. Engel Jr. & T. Pedley. Philadelphia: Lippincott-Raven.

Williamson, P.D., Spencer, D.D., Spencer, S.S., Novelly, R.A. & Mattson, R.H. (1985): Complex partial seizures of frontal lobe origin. *Ann Neurol.* **18**, 497–504.

Chapter 8

Dorsolateral frontal lobe seizures: validity and usefulness of compartmentalization

François Dubeau

Department of Neurology and Neurosurgery, Montreal Neurological Institute and Hospital, Room 138, 3801 University St., Montreal, Québec H3T 1R2, Canada
francois.dubeau@muhc.mcgill.ca

Summary

Frontal lobe seizures are divided – compartmentalized – into attacks originating from the primary motor, supplementary motor, dorsolateral frontal, opercular, fronto-polar, orbito-frontal, and cingulate cortices. Seizures originating in the dorsolateral frontal lobe typically consist of partial attacks with tonic or, more rarely, clonic signs, and versive eye and head movements. The latter are consistent with the representation of the frontal eye fields. The symptoms of frontal lobe epilepsy depend mainly on seizure propagation and rarely represent the expression of a strictly confined and easily identifiable epileptogenic area within the frontal lobe. Because of the organization and connections of the dorsolateral frontal lobe, and the anatomical and functional overlap that exists with adjacent primary motor areas and high-order non-primary motor and cognitive fields, we should expect dorsolateral frontal lobe seizures to have highly heterogeneous semiology and patterns.

Although frontal lobe semiology now appears relatively clear, it is difficult or impossible to use the available clinical information in any given patient to localize exactly the source generator to a specific frontal lobe compartment. The problem is even more likely to be unresolved when no lesion is found. In an attempt to further validate the compartmentalization concept, we reviewed the clinical and laboratory data of 46 consecutive patients with clinical features characteristic of frontal lobe epilepsy. We compared the type and frequency of ictal manifestations of dorsolateral frontal lobe seizures with those of seizures originating in other frontal compartments. We found that some clinical features clustered and indicated the anatomical site of the source generator allowing a certain degree of compartmentalization of seizures involving the dorsolateral frontal lobe. Whether a surgical approach should be considered on the basis of clinical and electrographic data only, without a visible structural lesion, remains a matter of considerable debate.

The investigation of patients with epilepsy due to a presumed frontal lobe (FL) epileptic generator remains difficult. The ictal behavioural manifestations of frontal lobe epilepsy (FLE) usually do not provide sufficiently reliable localization of the ictal epileptogenic area (Rasmussen, 1983; Talairach *et al.*, 1992; Quesney *et al.*, 1995). The bizarre appearance of certain clinical ictal patterns during FL seizures may also lead to difficulty in differentiating them from psychiatric, movement or sleep disorders, or from other, often temporal, seizures (Chauvel, 1994). FLE is also often associated with poorly localized scalp EEG interictal and ictal discharges (Quesney *et al.*, 1995; Battista *et al.*, 1998; Gross *et al.*, 2000).

The classification of FL seizures has been derived from intracranial EEG studies (Ajmone-Marsan & Goldhammer, 1973; Bancaud & Talairach, 1992; Quesney *et al.*, 1995; Salanova *et al.*, 1995; Van Ness, 1996), from neurosurgical series (Rasmussen, 1983; Talairach *et al.*, 1992; Olivier, 1995) and more recently, from neuroimaging using high-resolution magnetic resonance (Cascino, 1995; Kuzniecky & Graham, 1995; Fish, 1996). There is a semiological classification of FL seizures (Penfield & Kristiansen, 1951; Penfield & Jasper, 1954; Delgado-Escueta *et al.*, 1987; Waterman *et al.*, 1987; Williamson *et al.*, 1985; Salanova *et al.*, 1995), which divides them into three broad categories often overlapping with each other, reflecting the interconnections that exist between functionally related frontal and extra-frontal, e.g. temporal, areas: (i) focal motor (clonic or tonic) seizures; (ii) asymmetrical tonic, postural seizures (often identified as supplementary motor area seizures); and (iii) frontal lobe complex partial seizures. Appendix I of the 1985 Classification of the Epilepsies and Epileptic Syndromes, revised in 1989, proposes an anatomical classification (compartmentalization) of FL seizures dividing them into seven categories:

(1) *peri-Rolandic*, or primary motor: contralateral partial motor seizures without march or Jacksonian seizures, speech arrest, vocalization, or swallowing, frequent generalization. The ipsilateral leg may be involved in paracentral seizures. Todd's paralysis is frequent;

(2) *supplementary motor*: postural, focal tonic seizures, with vocalization, speech arrest and fencing postures;

(3) *dorsolateral frontal*, or premotor: simple focal tonic or clonic seizures, with versive eye and head movements and speech arrest;

(4) *opercular*: mastication, salivation, swallowing, laryngeal symptoms, speech arrest, epigastric aura, fear, and autonomic phenomena. Partial clonic facial seizures may be ipsilateral, and gustatory hallucinations are common;

(5) *anterior fronto-polar*: forced thinking, initial loss of contact, adversive and subsequent contraversive movements of head and eyes, axial clonic jerks, falls and autonomic signs with frequent generalized tonic-clonic seizures;

(6) *orbito-frontal*: complex partial seizures with initial motor and gestural automatisms, olfactory hallucinations or illusions, and autonomic signs; and

(7) *cingulate* seizures: complex partial with initial complex gestural automatisms, sexual features, vegetative signs, and changes in mood. Seizures originating from the dorsolateral FL (DLFL) are relatively frequent and were described in approximately 12 and 10 per cent of patients, respectively, in the frontal lobe series from Hôpital Sainte-Anne (Paris) and the Montreal Neurological Hospital (Bancaud & Talairach, 1992; Quesney *et al.*, 1992).

Brief review of the structural and functional anatomy of the frontal lobe and the dorsolateral frontal region in particular

The frontal lobe cortex is divided into four regions (Wieser *et al.*, 1992): the primary motor (precentral) cortex (Brodmann's area, 4), the premotor cortex (areas 6, 8, 44 and 45), the prefrontal cortex (areas 9 to 12, 45 to 47) and the limbic and paralimbic cortices (23 to 25, 32 and 33). The frontal lobe has major connections with subcortical, thalamic and mesencephalic structures (Buruss *et al.*, 2000). Each frontal region has a distinct cortical-subcortical organization and also intense cortico-cortical connectivity with other parts of the cerebral cortex, in particular with the limbic system, the amygdala, the temporal neocortex and parietal lobe, *via* preferential pathways such as the corpus callosum, the superior and inferior longitudinal fasciculi, the uncinate fasciculus and the cingulum.

Motor areas of the frontal lobe

The frontal lobe consists of several functionally different motor areas (Tanji, 1994, 1996; Freund, 1996 a, b). In addition to the primary motor area (MI) and premotor cortex (PMC) situated on the lateral convexity, there are four frontal motor areas located on the medial aspect of the hemisphere: the supplementary motor area proper (SMA) and the pre-SMA, and two (anterior and posterior) cingulate motor areas (CMA). The primary motor cortex is involved in concrete, executive and volitional tasks. The premotor cortex and the SMA (pre-SMA and SMA proper) are two non-primary, high-order function, motor fields that have many similarities: they have pronounced effects on postural tasks and regulation. They also influence the temporal control of sequential motor activity and the adjustment between movements of the two sides (Freund, 1996a, 1996b). The SMA is important for self-initiated motor behaviour, and the premotor cortex is involved in motor learning, sensory cueing of movement, and fine temporal adjustment of motor acts. The cingulate cortex is part of the limbic areas and of the limbic system (Broca, 1878; MacLean, 1990). The cingulate gyrus plays a role in emotion and motor functions (anterior cingulate), and in visuo-spatial and memory functions (posterior cingulate). The anterior cingulate cortex is subdivided into 'affective' and 'cognitive' components and appears to play a crucial role in initiation, motivation, and goal-directed behaviours (Devinsky et al., 1995). This area is usually included in the orbitomedial region (see below) and as a whole is also involved in attention, emotional behaviour and visceral control (Fuster, 2003). Finally, the cognitive division of the anterior cingulum includes a cingulate motor area. It has premotor functions and is important for motor response selection and for the expression of specific movement sequences.

Prefrontal cortex

The prefrontal cortex is an association cortex divided into two major regions: orbitomedial and dorsolateral. It is not involved in concrete tasks but supports the temporal organization of sequential actions: it assimilates data from other parts of the brain, integrates this information into an understandable past and present experience, and creates a plan of action (Goldman-Rakic, 1987; Fuster, 1989, 2003; Buruss et al., 2000).

The dorsolateral prefrontal cortex is located in the anterior convexity of the frontal lobe (Fuster, 2003). It is included in the dorsolateral frontal region, which is not a clearly defined anatomical entity (Fig. 1). It is bordered rostrally by the anterior polar region, posteriorly by the peri-Rolandic region (which includes the premotor and motor cortices), inferiorly by frontal and opercular regions (third frontal convolution, or F3) and superiorly and medially by the supplementary motor area. It includes parts of the first and third frontal convolutions (F1 and F3), all of the second frontal convolution (F2), and shares anatomical and functional connectivity with all adjacent structures. For example, the frontal eye field (area 8) is often considered to be part of the premotor cortex but is also transitional between agranular and granular cortex in the posterior portion of the middle frontal gyrus, and could therefore be labelled prefrontal (Wieser et al., 1992; Kotagal & Arunkumar, 1998). Finally, depending on how the DLFL is defined, it contains at least in part Brodmann's areas 6, 8, 9, 10 and 46 and, if F3 is included, Brodmann's areas 44 and 45 (opercular region and inferior frontal gyrus) as well.

Neurons from Brodmann's areas 9 and 10 are the source and termination of the dorsolateral circuit. They project to subcortical structures (caudate, globus pallidus, substantia nigra, thalamic nuclei and subthalamic nucleus), and at each level of the system *via* reciprocal connections, to distant cortical areas such as the temporal, parietal and occipital association cortices, and to the limbic system (Cummings, 1995; Burruss et al., 2000). The dorsolateral circuit is involved in organization and planning, and in attention.

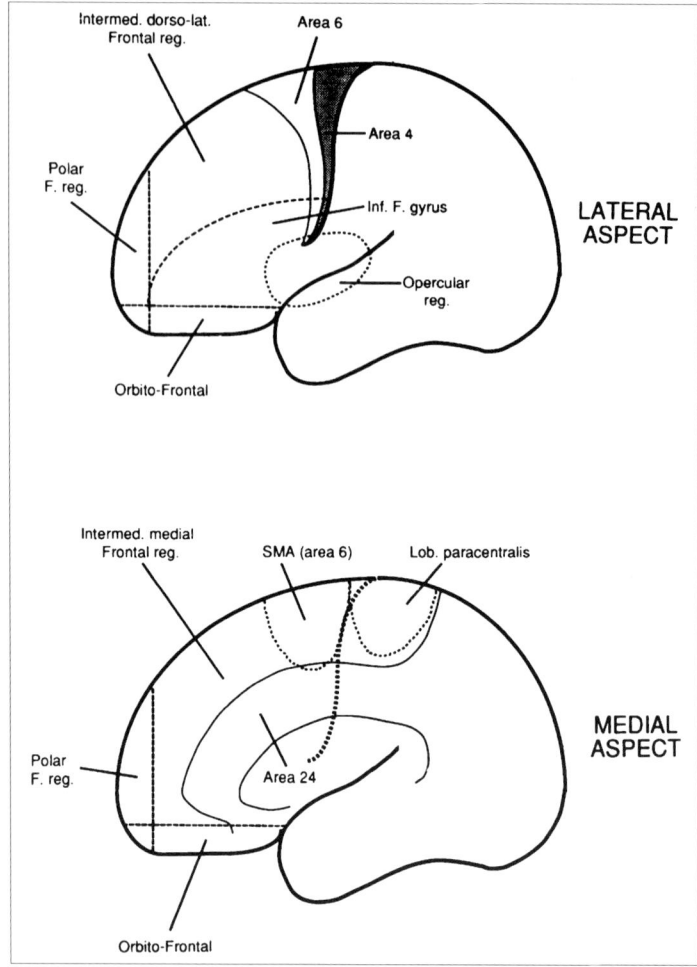

Fig. 1. Anatomical division of the frontal lobe. [From Bancaud & Talairach, 1992, with permission.]

Semiology of dorsolateral seizures: a review of the literature

From a strictly semiological point of view, it is very difficult to study the DLFL alone. The symptoms of FLE depend mainly on seizure propagation and rarely represent the expression of a strictly confined and easily identifiable epileptogenic area within the frontal lobe. Epileptic activity arising from the motor and premotor cortices very likely results in pure motor phenomena. However, prefrontal seizures (dorsolateral, orbito-frontal, fronto-polar and even cingulate), are expected to be more complex or elaborate and to be more likely associated with impairment of consciousness, changes in emotion and behaviour, and with atypical motor behaviour and automatisms. Because of the organization of the DLFL, and the anatomical and functional overlap that exists with adjacent primary motor areas and high-order non-primary motor and cognitive fields, we should expect DLFL seizures to have highly heterogeneous semiology and patterns.

Bancaud & Talairach (1992) reviewed the clinical characteristics of frontal lobe seizures in 210 patients with intractable epilepsy studied at Sainte-Anne's Hospital. They adopted an anatomical classification of epileptic seizures and divided the frontal lobe into eight anatomical regions:

(1) areas 4 and 6;

(2) inferior frontal gyrus;

(3) intermediate medial frontal region;

(4) intermediate DLFL;

(5) anterior cingulate gyrus, or area 24;

(6) fronto-polar region;

(7) orbito-frontal region; and

(8) operculo-insular region (Fig. 1).

They categorized the patients according to the topographic distribution of seizure origin as defined by stereoencephalography (SEEG). They found 25 patients (61 seizures analysed) with seizures originating in the intermediate DLFL. The proportion of patients who underwent surgery, and their outcome, were not reported.

Tonic adversive eye turning followed by contralateral head turning was the most significant and frequent inaugural sign. These authors also described face and arm motor manifestations, visual hallucinations and illusions, forced thinking and complex postural patterns. According to them, forced thinking, and forced acts of frontal lobe origin were easy to differentiate from manifestations of temporal lobe origin; the obsessive thoughts had a more 'ideational' and 'intentional' aspect in the former compared to an 'emotional' or 'affective' content in the latter. They commented that visual phenomena, when not overshadowed by motor signs, are observed early during an attack, are different from those of occipital origin, and never consist of simple hallucinations. They reported frequent early tonic-clonic generalization, and autonomic features in the late stages of the seizure.

Wieser et al. (1992, 1995) reviewed the semiology of seizures originating in the prefrontal area, i.e. from the DLFL, the fronto-polar, orbito-frontal and cingulate regions, and summarized previous observations (Penfield & Kristiansen, 1951; Ajmone-Marsan & Ralston, 1957; Bancaud et al., 1965; Ajmone-Marsan & Goldhammer, 1973; Walsh & Delgado-Escueta, 1984). They found that initial signs of complex partial seizures of DLFL origin commonly consist of impaired consciousness with, at onset, widened palpebral fissures, brief tonic elevation of the head, contraversive head and eye movements, mild facial clonic contractions and non-fluent aphasia. Subsequent seizure semiology depended on propagation of the discharge to adjacent structures, in particular to the primary motor area (simple partial focal seizures), SMA (asymmetric or symmetric posturing), cingulate gyrus (with autonomic signs) and amygdala (with oro-alimentary signs). Wieser also reported that DLFL seizures may occur without motor signs and consist of isolated brief episodes of loss of awareness.

Quesney et al. (1990, 1992) reported a group of 40 patients with seizures arising from the DLFL. The patients had been surgically treated and were seizure-free for more than 2 years after selective removal of the superior parasagittal frontal convexity (10 patients), anterofrontal (21) or fronto-opercular regions (9). Seizures originating in the superior aspect of the frontal lobe convexity had a high incidence of somatosensory warnings (60 per cent), partial motor clonic or tonic manifestations (100 per cent), conscious head- or eye-turning, usually contralateral (32.5 per cent), and sometimes a typical SMA seizure pattern (20 per cent), but no automatisms. Seizures arising in the fronto-opercular area (part of the intermediate portion of the lateral frontal convexity including mostly the second frontal convolution, Brodmann's area 8, and parts of areas 6 and 9) began with various types of aura, sometimes temporal-like (epigastric sensation), associated with or followed by often conscious and always contralateral head- or eye-turning (44 per cent), and by motor manifestations (partial motor attacks or automatisms) in less than half. Seizures originating in the anterofrontal region had even less specific features, somewhat resembling temporal lobe attacks with an occasional characteristic warning sensation (epigastric sensation, fear), arrest of activity (24 per cent), and automatisms (33 per cent). Head or eye turning, usually unconscious and contralateral, was described in 24 per cent of the patients in this subgroup, and focal motor attacks or posturing were infrequent (< 30 per cent of the patients) compared to the other two groups.

Validation of the concept of compartmentalization of frontal lobe seizures

The definition of frontal lobe semiology is now relatively clear. It is difficult however to use the available clinical information in any given patient in order to define in which frontal lobe the source generator is located. It is even more difficult and sometimes impossible, particularly in non-lesional cases, to determine the exact location of this source within one frontal lobe. In an attempt to further validate the compartmentalization concept, we reviewed the clinical and laboratory data of 46 consecutive patients with clinical features characteristic of FLE. We itemized their ictal symptoms and signs according to the anatomical classification proposed by the ILAE Classification of Epilepsies and Epileptic Syndromes (1985, 1989). We compared the type and frequency of ictal manifestations of DLFL seizures with those of seizures originating in other FL compartments.

Analysis of frontal lobe seizures

Patients

The patients (23 men, 23 women) were investigated between 1995 and 2000 at the Montreal Neurological Hospital because of intractable seizures. Their age at first seizure and at evaluation was 12.4 ± 10.2 (range, 11 months to 35 years) and 26.5 ± 11.9 years (mean ± SD), respectively. Past medical history was remarkable for: premature birth, three patients; low birth weight, one; febrile convulsions, two; probable chronic encephalitis, one; tuberculous meningitis, one; and head trauma, seven. Three patients had had brain surgery for intractable seizures prior to this evaluation; one had a left SMA resection, and the remaining two a left and right anterior temporal resection, respectively. Positive family history of seizures was found in 15 patients. They all had extensive scalp EEG evaluation and prolonged telemetry monitoring, and all except four had at least one seizure recorded (377 seizures were recorded with an average of 11 per patient). In addition to high-resolution MRI studies, 16 patients had interictal ^{18}fluorodeoxyglucose (FDG) positron emission tomography (PET) studies, negative in 14. Eleven had interictal and ictal ^{99m}Tc-hexamethyl-propyleneamine oxime (HMPAO) SPECT imaging, four showing ictal regional frontal increased blood flow. Finally, 15 had intracranial depth electrode recordings (208 seizures recorded with an average of 16 per patient). Twenty-six patients (56 per cent) had no lesion, seven (15 per cent) had uni- or bilateral frontal atrophy, five (11 per cent) post-traumatic epilepsy with frontal encephalomalacia, atrophy and gliosis, five (11 per cent) focal cortical dysplasia, two unilateral focal periventricular nodular heterotopia, and one (2 per cent) a frontal arteriovenous malformation. Finally, 14 were treated surgically; all had a visible lesion on MRI, and 10 had a presurgical invasive intracranial evaluation.

Methods

The patients were divided into different topographical frontal groups (Tables 1 and 2 a-f) according to the anatomical criteria proposed by the Classification of Epilepsies and Epileptic Syndromes (1985, 1989). The decision to assign a patient to a specific group was based first on the constellation of ictal clinical features described by the patient, second on the observations by the medical and nursing staff and relatives, and third on review of the available video recordings. The decision was then guided by the electroencephalographic (including SEEG) results, the imaging findings and

Table 1. Anatomical subdivisions and demographic data in 46 patients with FLE

Frontal cortical regions		Rolandic	Premotor		Prefrontal	
Anatomical divisions	Not classifiable	C	SMA	DL	Cing.	OF
Number of patients	12	10	5	8	6	5
Family history of seizures	4	4	2	1	1	3
Mean age at seizure onset in years	9.3	12.8	17.8	10.2	16.7	8.5
(range)	(18mo-20)	(1-27)	(4-33)	(1-30)	(5-40)	(18mo-16)
Lesion	4	5	0	5	4	2
SEEG	4	2	1	4	1	1
Surgery	5	3	0	3	2	1
*Outcome I-II	1	1	–	2	1	1
III-IV	4	2		1	1	0

C = central region; Cing. = cingulate region; DL = dorsolateral region; OF = orbito-frontal region; SEEG = stereoencephalography; SMA = supplementary motor area. * = Engel's classification.

when available by the surgical outcome. We defined a group of patients that included unclassifiable cases including those with heterogeneous or poorly characterized events, and those with multiple seizure patterns. We did not include a fronto-polar category because we found it difficult to distinguish fronto-polar seizure semiology from that of DL, orbito-frontal or cingulate attacks. Also, we found no patients with seizures suggesting opercular origin; they may have been included in the central and DL groups. Patients were thus divided into six categories:

(1) unclassifiable frontal lobe seizures, 12 patients;

(2) central (or Rolandic) seizures, 10;

(3) SMA seizures, five;

(4) DLFL seizures, eight;

(5) cingulate seizures, six; and

(6) orbito-frontal seizures, five. Table 1 summarizes the main demographic data, and Table 2 contains a detailed description of the ictal semiology in each patient and of the different FL epilepsy groups.

Results

Ictal semiology and frequency of symptoms and signs are summarized in Table 3. Most patients (63 per cent) experienced a warning at the onset of all or some of their seizures. The highest incidence of aura was found in the central group (80 per cent) compared to 33 to 50 per cent in the others. Auras usually provided little or no reliable localizing or lateralizing information (Table 4). Somatosensory auras were the exception however, and were described by 10 patients, mostly of the central group (six patients). They had localizing features suggesting implication of the central region in nine cases, and in others suggesting involvement of the post central cortex: two patients (#15 and 16) described a clearly lateralized sensory march, four (#7, 12, 21 and 23) had a localized sensory feeling in a portion of one limb, two a sensation in the tongue (#13, 17); one had ocular and periorbital pain (#35), and one had bilateral ascending paraesthesiae (#14). Fear was the second most frequent aura and was uniformly distributed in patients with seizures from different frontal compartments. Viscerosensory and visceromotor auras (e.g. an epigastric sensation and palpitations) were described almost exclusively in patients with seizures considered to originate in mesial frontal and orbito-frontal cortices. Two patients, both in the central seizure group, described a gustatory

Table 2 a. Seizure semiology: patients not classifiable, n = 12

Patients	MRI lesion	Aura	Ictal	Post-ictal
1. S.G., f	R F, AVM and scar tissue	Déjà vu; epigastric	Not responsive, 'absence' → sec. gen.	Confusion, if sec. gen.
2. N.S., m	None	None	Initially responsive, heavy breathing, frowning, → discrete bipedal and manual aut. and elevation of arms, H + E → R, → sec. gen.	Confusion, if sec. gen.
3. D.G., m	None	Body sensation	Moans, myoclonic jerks H and L arm, → agitation	No confusion
4. M.P., m	Bil F, atrophy and gliosis	None	Staring spells with or without salivation, at times H → L or R, → sec. gen. (occ.)	± confusion
5. M.D., m	None	Fear	3 patterns: 1) confusional state; 2) unresponsiveness and arrest of activity, → pedaling mvts and elevation both arms, E → L; 3) as 2) except E → R, → H + E → L, → sec. gen.	Confusion
6. J.V., f	None	None	Brief staring, → tonic H + E → R, diffuse tonic posturing, → sec. gen.	Confusion
7. L.R., f	L F3, FCD; remote L SMA resection	Numb feeling R face	Heavy breathing → apnoea, → R arm tonic elevation and extension, unresponsive, → L arm ADD and flexion	Numb feeling, R arm
8. J.D., f	None; remote L T resection	Fear (occ.)	4 patterns: 1) fear, 'mamama', unresponsive, anxiety, oral aut.; 2) moans, vocalization, heavy breathing and thrashing; 3) L hemibody tonic posturing → clonic, → sec. gen.; 4) gen. at onset	Confusion with 1), 2) and 4)
9. A.M.J., f	None	None	2 patterns: 1) stares, 'dadada', → elevation L or R arm; 2) brief staring spell, → tonic H + E → R, moaning, heavy breathing, → R arm flexed, diffuse clonic activity	1) No confusion; 2) confusion
10. C.B., f	None	Dizziness	2 patterns: 1) tonic H + E → R, not conscious, apnoea, cyanosis, → diffusely tonic, may fall; 2) tonic H + E → L, ? conscious, → L tonic hemibody and rotation of trunk → L, 1) and 2) → sec. gen. (occ.)	1) Confusion, dysphasic; 2) no confusion
11. A.L., m	R OF, FP, atrophy and gliosis	None	Arousal, 'bahbahbah', → tremor-like L > R body, eyes blinking, tonic posturing L → R, → sec. gen.	Confusion
12. N.N., f	None	Numb feeling, L elbow; flashbacks; palpitations	2 patterns: 1) somatosensory aura, → vocalization 'fuck, OK', → H → R or L, → tonic posturing L > R, → bimanual and bipedal aut. 2) experiential aura and palpitations, fear, unresponsive; → sec. gen. (occ.)	± confusion

Legend for table 2 a, b, c, d, e, f: abd. = abdominal; ABD = abduction; ADD = adduction; AF = anterior frontal; ant. = anterior; aut. = automatism; AVM = arteriovenous malformation; bil = bilateral; C = central; cing. = cingulate; E = eye; F = frontal; F1 = first frontal convolution; F3 = third frontal convolution; FCD = focal cortical dysplasia; FP = frontopolar; H = head; hem. = hemispheric; L = left; LOC = loss of consciousness; mvts = movements; occ. = occasional ; OF = orbitofrontal; operc. = frontal operculum; PNH = periventricular nodular heterotopia; porenceph. = porencephalic; R = right; sec. gen. = secondary generalized; SMA = supplementary motor area; T = temporal; wm = white matter.

Table 2 b. Seizure semiology: patients with seizures of central origin, n = 10

Patients	MRI lesion	Aura	Ictal	Post-ictal
13. S.R., m	R operc., C, FCD	Electric shock, Tongue	Tonic extension of L arm and leg, → bil eye blinking L > R, clonus R leg	Todd, L arm; no confusion
14. M.B., m	R F, porenceph. cyst	Ascending bil paraesthesia; metallic taste	L eye clonus, → L arm and leg clonus, → H → L	Todd, L hemibody; no confusion
15. K.P., f	None	Pulsation, R hand; 'feeling' R arm → body → leg	2 patterns: 1) aura → speech problems; 2) aura → R arm and leg tonic posturing, → H → R and sec. gen.	1) No confusion 2) Todd, R arm
16. A.M.C., f	None	Numb feeling, R hand → arm → body and leg	R hemiparesis, → clonus R face and arm, no LOC	Todd, R arm; dysarthric and dysphasic
17. M.P., m	L PNH, body and F horn	Bad taste; fear; thick tongue; Cephalic	2 patterns: 1) no aura, R face clonus; 2) aura, → dysarthria, ? dysphasia, → R face clonus, → sec. gen. (rare)	No confusion
18. H.S., m	L FT, encephalomalacia	Cephalic; Dizziness	Speech arrest, and arrest of activity, → R arm clonus and tonic elevation, → H + E →R, sec. gen.	Todd, R hemibody
19. M.K.P., f	None	None	3 patterns: 1) L leg clonus often reflex → foot, → L arm, and L face, no LOC; 2) L arm clonus; 3) L face clonus	No confusion
20. S.H., f	R C, atrophy	Fear; epigastric	Tonic L leg → arm, may fall but no LOC; reflex seizures (occ.)	No confusion
21. J.L., f	None	Paraesthesia, R thigh and buttock	Arousal, clonic mvts of pelvis and R thigh and kicking, → tonic extension R arm, clonus R arm, →H + E → and sec. gen. (occ.)	No confusion
22. L.B., m	None	None	Bil periorbital twitches, pulling L side of the mouth, H → L, → clonic and tonic L hemibody, sometimes pedaling	No confusion; Todd L (occ.)

Table 2 c. Seizure semiology: patients with SMA seizures, n = 5

Patients	MRI lesion	Aura	Ictal	Post-ictal
23. D.T., f	None	'Bad feeling', L leg	L leg mvts, unresponsive, → H → L, fencing, → eyelid fluttering, diffuse clonus, → sec. gen.	Confusion
24. C.P., f	None	Palpitations; fear; panic; epigastric	Pulling L face, → fencing, → sec. gen.	Confusion
25. M.G., m	Bil FC, atrophy and gliosis	None	H + E → L and LOC, → symmetrical or asymmetrical tonic posturing, screaming	No confusion
26. E.B., m	None	None	2 patterns: 1) arousal, moaning, → pedaling; 2) arousal, symmetrical tonic posturing, moaning, 'athetoid-like' mvts of both hands and fingers	No confusion
27. E.S., f	none	'Diffuse body feeling' (occ.)	2 patterns: 1) aura → falls, no LOC; 2) no aura, arousal, → tonic symmetrical or asymmetrical posturing, → H → R or L, fencing, screaming	Confusion

Table 2 d. Seizure semiology: patients with dorsolateral frontal seizures, n = 8

Patients	MRI lesion	Aura	Ictal	Post-ictal
28. D.N., m	L hem., atrophy	None	Arousal, staring, → H → L (often early, and sometimes R), → tonic posturing L hemibody, → pedaling, fumbling with fingers, → sec. gen. (rare)	No confusion; no recollection
29. J.M., m	L F, atrophy	Epigastric (occ.)	Screaming, H → L, tonic posturing L hemibody, H + E → R, bil tonic posturing R > L, → sec. gen.	Confusion, if sec. gen.
30. S.G., f	R F1-F2, FCD	Epigastric; dizziness	2 patterns: 1) screaming, E → L, body → L, face flushing, tonic posturing L arm and leg; 2) screaming, E and body → L, fencing or asymmetrical tonic posturing, sometimes pedaling, → sec. gen. (rare)	± confusion
31. A.R., m	Bil F, atrophy	None	2 patterns: 1) H → R, sometimes with E → R, elevation R arm, trunk → R, → dystonic L arm and leg, rocking, moaning; 2) H → R rocking motion of the trunk, elevation of both arms, moaning, → sec. gen. (occ.)	1) ± confusion 2) no confusion
32. S.S., m	L FT, atrophy and gliosis	None	H → R, extension and ABD R arm, screaming, → rotation → R, → sec. gen.	Dysphasia; confusion if sec. gen.
33. G.N., f	None	Sensation of falling; lightheaded	2 patterns: 1) arousal, H + E → R, → clonus R face, → tonic posturing R hemibody, no LOC; 2) same → asymmetrical tonic posture R > L, ? LOC, → sec. gen. (occ.)	Confusion, if repetitive or sec. gen.
34. D.L., m	R F, atrophy; L OF, gliosis	None	Arrest of activity, mute, palor eyes ↑, → E + H → R, clonus R face → R hemibody, may fall, → sec. gen.	Confusion
35. L.P., f	None	Pain, L periorb. and eye	H → R, ABD and extension R arm, → bil tonic extension L > R, → sec. gen. (occ.)	Confusion

Table 2 e. Seizure semiology: patients with cingulate seizures, n = 6

Patients	MRI lesion	Aura	Ictal	Post-ictal
36. V.O., m	None	Palpitations; fear	Screaming, agitation, H → R, asymmetric tonic posturing L arm and leg, → sec. gen. (rare)	Confusion
37. E.M., f	L AF, FCD	Palpitations; thoracic pressure; urge to void; impression of dying	2 patterns: 1) aura → urinary incontinence; 2) arousal, pedaling and pelvic thrusting, urinary incontinence, swearing	No confusion
38. J.M.H., m	None	None	Intense agitation, screaming and thrashing, complex gestural aut., → sec. gen.	Confusion
39. T.O., m	L ant. cing., FCD	Fear	Screaming, agitation, turning from side to side, kicking, pedaling, complex gestural aut.	No confusion
40. S.P., f	L AF, wm signal	None	High-pitched cry, bil leg mvts, palor, hands over face, → tonic posturing both legs, → sec. gen. (occ.)	± confusion; no recollection
41. C.B., f	None	Fear; abd. and throat sensation	Agitation, thrashing, screaming, → H → R and sec. gen. (occ.)	Confusion, if sec. gen.

Table 2 f. Seizure semiology: patients with orbitofrontal seizures, n = 5

Patients	MRI lesion	Aura	Ictal	Post-ictal
42. K.D., f	None	None	Heavy breathing, → laughing and vocalizations, screaming, agitation, → bipedal and bimanual aut., pelvic thrusting	No confusion; no recollection
43. J.B., m	None; remote RT resection	None	Screams, H side to side, claps hands, → agitation, walking on his knees, loud vocalizations, pelvic thrusting	No confusion; no recollection
44. C.L., m	None	Epigastric (occ.)	2 patterns: 1) agitation, ambulatory aut., headstand, jumping, running, ± conscious; 2) H → R, rotation → R > L, then → 1)	No confusion
45. S.L., m	L PNH, F horn	Choking sensation	LOC, 'gnagnagna', pointing with R index, → fear, bimanual and ambulatory aut., → sec. gen.	Dysphasic, slow, ambulatory aut.
46. J.B., f	Bil OF, gliosis	Epigastric (occ.)	Arrest of activity and 'strange laugh', unresponsive, urinary incontinence (occ.), → sec. gen. (rare)	No confusion; no recollection

aura. Dizziness, a non-specific body sensation, and a cephalic aura were described in patients with seizures originating in posterior frontal regions (motor and premotor cortices, including SMA). Experiential auras (*déjà vu* and flashbacks), usually considered to indicate temporal or limbic origin, were rare and described in only two patients. Finally, no patient reported forced thinking, olfactory, auditory or visual hallucinations, or illusions.

Table 3. Ictal semiology in 46 patients with FLE (per cent)

Aura	63
Secondary generalization	63
Head- or eye-turning	56
Nocturnal	50
No postictal confusion	50
Vocalization	41
Autonomic features	41
Partial motor tonic	39
Automatisms	35
Symmetric or asymmetric tonic posturing	33
Partial motor clonic	26
Hypermotor	22
Arrest of activity only	17

Autonomic manifestations were relatively frequent and were described in 41 per cent of patients (Table 5). They varied widely, usually consisting of an aura (epigastric sensation, palpitations, urge to void, thoracic sensation and choking), and were devoid of localizing value. As expected, however, they were found mainly in patients with seizures considered to originate in anteromesial frontal (cingulate) and orbito-frontal cortices.

Motor manifestations are the most salient clinical manifestations of FL seizures. There are many clinical patterns, reflecting the extension and complexity of the different motor areas implicated in the production of simple executive tasks or of complex high-order motor functions. The seizures may consist of relatively simple, usually unilateral, patterns such as myoclonus or clonus if they originate in M1, or of more complex motor activities such as unilateral or bilateral postures, with fencing and other postural tonic seizures involving the upper and lower extremities if the premotor cortex and SMA are involved. They may also mimic sophisticated movement sequences if they originate in or involve the prefrontal cortices (e.g. DL, orbito-frontal and anterior cingulate areas).

Table 4. Auras in FLE, by anatomical regions

Types of aura*	Anatomical regions						
	Nc	C	SMA	DL	Cing.	OF	Total
Somatosensory	2	6	1	1	–	1	11
Fear	2	2	1	–	4	-	9
Epigastric	1	1	1	2	2	2	9
Autonomic	1	-	1	–	2	1	5
Dizziness	1	1	–	1	–	–	3
Body sensation	1	–	1	1	–	–	3
Cephalic	–	2	–	–	–	–	2
Experiential	2	–	–	–	–	–	2
Taste	–	2	–	–	–	–	2
None	5	2	2	4	2	2	17
(per cent)	(42)	(20)	(40)	(50)	(33)	(40)	(37)

* numbers refer to number of patients. A patient may have more than one type of aura. Nc = not classified; C = central (or Rolandic); SMA = supplementary motor area; DL = dorsolateral; Cing. = cingulate; OF = orbito-frontal.

Table 5. Viscerosensory and visceromotor manifestations in FLE, by anatomical regions

Autonomic nervous system manifestations*	Anatomical regions						
	Nc	C	SMA	DL	Cing.	OF	Total
Epigastric	1	1	1	1	1	2	7
Palpitations	1	–	1	–	2	–	4
Skin colour changes	1	–	–	2	1	–	4
Respiratory changes	2	–	–	–	–	1	3
Urge to void, incontinence	–	–	–	–	1	1	2
Thoracic sensation	–	–	–	–	1	–	1
Choking	–	–	–	–	–	1	1
Salivation	1	–	–	–	–	–	1
None	6	9	1	6	2	1	28
(Per cent)	(50)	(90)	(80)	(75)	(33)	(20)	(59)

* numbers refer to number of patients. A patient may have more than one type of autonomic nervous system manifestations. Nc = not classified; C = central (or Rolandic); SMA = supplementary motor area; DL = dorsolateral; Cing. = cingulate; OF = orbito-frontal.

This is obviously a simplified view of a much more complex problem. Nevertheless, our findings (Fig. 2 a) seem to support such a caudo-rostral hierarchy of epileptic motor symptomatology. For instance, rhythmic clonic seizures involving the face or the extremities, usually unilaterally, and unilateral tonic attacks were considered to represent seizures of central and DL origin (or motor and premotor origin excluding SMA). In contrast, symmetrical and asymmetrical bilateral tonic postures, complex gestural acts, agitation and archaic movements were far more frequently found in seizures thought to originate in mesial frontal or prefrontal regions. If these signs are clustered with other clinical manifestations, it may be possible to further specify the type and origin of an epileptic attack. For example, the association of a somatosensory warning with a postictal Todd's phenomenon and the absence of post-ictal confusion was found mostly in the central group. However, motor symptoms accompanied by vocalizations or autonomic changes indicated a prefrontal origin (Tables 4 and 5, Fig. 2 b).

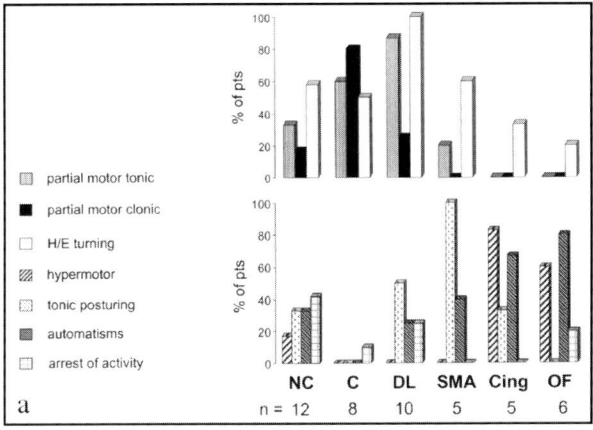

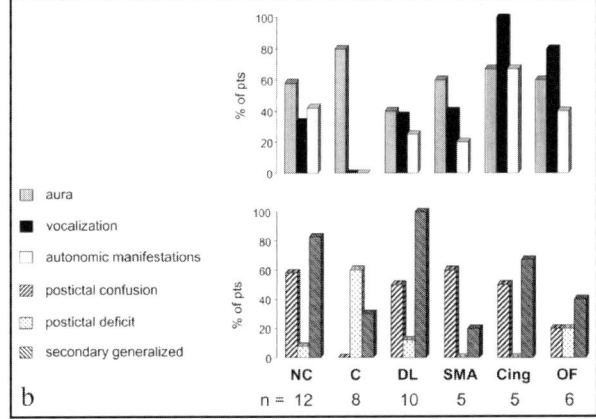

Fig. 2 a, b. Ictal semiology of frontal lobe seizures.

Table 6. Interictal EEG findings in FLE, by anatomical regions

Interictal EEG*	Anatomical regions					
	Nc (n = 12)	C (n = 10)	SMA (n = 5)	DL (n = 8)	Cing. (n = 6)	OF (n = 5)
Unilateral frontal	42 %	50	20	12	17	20
Bilateral frontal synchronous	17	0	0	25	17	20
Bilateral frontal independent	25	0	20	25	17	0
Extra-frontal	42	0	20	25	17	24
None	17	50	60	37	50	40

* Numbers refer to percentage of patients. A patient may have more than one type of EEG abnormality. Nc = not classified; C = central (or Rolandic); SMA = supplementary motor area; DL = dorsolateral; Cing. = cingulate; OF = orbito-frontal.

We found a high incidence (56 per cent) of versive head- or eye-turning (Table 3). This represents the second most frequent ictal clinical manifestation, after aura, and is the most frequent motor sign in patients with FLE. Again, we can see a postero-anterior gradient with head- or eye-turning predominating in the DLFL, SMA and central seizure groups compared to the anterior frontal regions (Fig. 2 a). The incidence of head-turning ranged from 20 to 100 per cent, clearly predominating in the DLFL. We included here early and late, conscious and unconscious, as well clonic or tonic versive movements whether associated or not with other motor features. Five of the DLFL patients had an early, conscious or unconscious, head or eye deviation presumably contralateral to the focus, but 11 had late versive eye or head movements often preceding secondary generalization and clearly indicating ictal discharge propagation.

Because of the nature of this study, we could not analyse adequately arrest of activity, speech disorders and disturbances of consciousness. Direct examination of the patient is mandatory to evaluate the type and degree of altered consciousness (Gloor, 1986), and the information available including review of videotapes was insufficient to allow accurate interpretation. Nevertheless, some patients (17 per cent) had as the main clinical feature of their seizures an arrest of activity, an 'absence' or a 'state of confusion' followed or not by other manifestations. Five – one (#45) in the orbito-frontal group, one (#35) with DLFL seizures, and three (#1, 4 and 5) in the unclassified group – had absence-like events or arrest of activity, sometimes repetitive or prolonged, as their main seizure pattern.

Comment

In summary, some clinical features clustered and indicated the anatomical site of the seizure generator allowing a certain degree of compartmentalization of seizures involving the DLFL. Typically, seizures originating in the DLFL consist of simple partial attacks with tonic or clonic signs, and eye- and head-turning. Such versive eye and head movements seem to represent the most consistent motor manifestations of DLFL seizures. Penfield & Kristiansen (1951), Fegersten & Roger (1961), Rasmussen (1963, 1983), Ajmone-Marsan & Goldhammer (1973), and Geier et al. (1977) had already noted that adversive head and eye movements were among the most common manifestations of FL seizures. Bancaud & Talairach concluded that tonic adversive eye-turning followed by contralateral head-turning were the most significant and frequent inaugural signs (1992). Quesney documented (1992) early head-turning not associated with other motor features, usually contralateral (80 per cent of frontal lobe ictal head-turning) to the epileptic generator occurring in approximately 33 per cent of the patients studied. He also suggested that conscious head turning preferentially occurred in seizures arising in the superior and posterior portions of the DLFL whereas unconscious head-turning occurred with seizure onset involving its anterior and inferior aspects.

Considerable controversy exists regarding the utility and value of head and eye movements as reliable lateralizing and localizing signs. Electrical stimulation of the intermediate frontal cortex in humans (approximately Brodmann's areas 6 and 8) produced eye- and head-turning usually contralateral to the side of stimulation (Rasmussen & Penfield, 1947; Penfield & Jasper, 1954). When the stimulus was applied more posteriorly and adjacent to the central sulcus, responses were variable consisting of contralateral as well as ipsilateral eye movements occasionally associated with head-turning (Rasmussen & Penfield, 1947). In addition, head-turning had been described with temporal, parietal, occipital and even generalized seizures (Cotte-Rittaud & Courjon, 1962; King & Ajmone-Marsan, 1977; Robillard et al., 1983; Ochs et al., 1984; Thurston et al., 1985; Quesney, 1986; Wyllie et al., 1986a, b; Gastaut et al., 1986; Rosenbaum et al., 1986; Masson & St-Hilaire, 1986; McLachlan, 1987; Jakayar et al., 1992; Chee et al., 1993; Kernan et al., 1993; Fakhoury & Abou-Khalil, 1995; Abou-Khalil & Fakhoury, 1996; Marks & Laxer, 1998). Several reports indicate that ictal head and eye movements provide no reliable lateralization and localization of seizure onset (King & Ajmone-Marsan, 1977; Robillard et al., 1983; Ochs et al., 1984; Quesney, 1986) while others on the contrary suggested that eye- and head-turning may be reliable localizing and lateralizing ictal signs (Wyllie et al., 1986a, b; McLachlan, 1987; Jakayar et al., 1992; Chee et al., 1993; Kernan et al., 1993; Fakhoury & Abou-Khalil, 1995; Abou-Khalil & Fakhoury, 1996; Marks & Laxer, 1998). As pointed out by Marks & Laxer, the variability in the reliability of this sign could be explained by the subjective nature of observing and classifying head and eye movements (versive *vs* non-versive, conscious or unconscious), consideration of head and eye movement during different phases of the seizure (initial or late, preceded or not by staring, automatisms, etc.), and variability of seizure spread patterns (associated or not with other motor features, with or without secondary generalization). Different cortical (frontal, occipital and parietal) and subcortical (basal ganglia and brainstem) mechanisms may also be involved; this would account for the variability of clinical manifestations. Conscious forced head-turning, usually at onset of a seizure, is generally contralateral to the epileptic focus and hence it seems legitimate to look for a lesion in the contralateral intermediate frontal region. This certainly reflects the specific organization of the lateral frontal convexity in relation to the frontal eye field, or Brodmann's area 8 (Foerster & Penfield, 1930; Penfield & Kristiansen, 1951). Head-turning associated with loss of awareness, non-versive head movements, and late version are probably not reliable indicators of the epileptic focus.

According to Quesney and his colleagues (1990, 1992), patients with seizures originating in the superior aspect of the DLFL (F1) had symptoms in keeping with the proximity of primary motor and premotor cortices, and the SMA, and with spread to these structures. It was difficult to distinguish origin from spread of discharge. However, patients with seizures originating from more inferior and anterior portions of the frontal convexity had clinical features that may reflect spread of the epileptic discharge to the temporal lobe. Auras were common and occurred in 62 per cent of Quesney's patients, and in 63 per cent of this series with a high incidence of somatosensory auras, particularly when seizures originate in the central region or in the superior convexity of the DLFL and propagate rapidly to the adjacent supplementary motor area. Mesial or neocortical temporal lobe auras were also frequent: fear, epigastric sensations, auditory and visual hallucinations and dizziness were described by the patients, and may be explained by the links to temporal lobe structures *via* the uncinate fasciculus and the cingulum (Quesney *et al.*, 1992).

Other relatively frequent clinical features of DLFL seizures included arrest of activity which could be an isolated manifestation, forced thinking (not found in our series), and automatic behaviour occurring only in seizures originating from the lateral convexity and not in those from the more superior parasagittal region. Subsequent ictal semiology depends on the propagation of the ictal discharge and can resemble focal motor attacks, SMA or temporal lobe seizures and, as with attacks originating in other FL regions, these seizures often become secondarily generalized.

Conclusions

The interpretation of FL epileptic semiology is difficult, often subjective, depends on the observer's knowledge, experience and skill, and is time-consuming. Only 24-hour monitoring of the seizures can allow a complete, uniform and reliable collection of data indicating the symptoms and signs of the pre-ictal, ictal and post-ictal epileptic phases. This information may then be used for the analysis and classification of FL seizures. Simultaneous scalp EEG recording helps define an appropriate hypothesis of the source, origin and propagation of the ictal discharges. Frontal lobe epilepsy, however, is often associated with poorly localized, absent or scanty, scalp EEG interictal epileptiform activity of poor localizing value, often widespread or multifocal, and with frequent bilateral synchrony or generalization (Table 6, Quesney *et al.*, 1995; Battista *et al.*, 1998; Gross *et al.*, 2000).

Whether a surgical approach should be considered based on clinical and electrographic data only, in the absence of an identifiable structural lesion, is hotly debated. In many centres, surgery is not currently considered in such patients. Alternatively, a major and as complete as possible frontal resection may be considered when the side of origin is clearly lateralized. Such an approach is repugnant to conservative surgeons though it was often effective in the hands of Rasmussen during an era when high-quality imaging was not available. In such cases one is concerned about creating a behavioural deficit amounting to a frontal lobe syndrome. In many patients with FLE such a deficit is already present and the risks have to be weighed against the often considerable burden of intractable FLE itself. Certainly in patients with extensive post-traumatic frontal damage following a depressed fracture, extensive resection of fronto-polar and lateral frontal damaged tissue yields excellent results (Cukiert, *et al.*, 1996; Kazemi *et al.*, 1997).

In clinical practice, attempts at compartmentalization of FL seizures represent a difficult or artificial exercise and help only to some extent in defining the exact epileptogenic source. With the exception of seizures originating in the motor strip, and perhaps of those from the SMA, the delineation of the clinical syndrome and its correlation with a well identifiable electrical source is often impossible unless a structural lesion can be found. Invasive intracranial recording may help define the epileptogenic zone, but again the difficulty here is to elaborate a good working hypothesis, which is often only determined by the clinical information available. Surgical outcome is far better in patients with lesional *vs* non-lesional FLE. The use of high resolution MR techniques clearly affects the decision-making process in surgical candidates, the type of diagnostic evaluation (including the indications and types of intracranial EEG monitoring), and the therapeutic approach and outcome.

Acknowledgments: The author thanks Dr. Frederick Andermann for thoughtful comments.

References

Abou-Khalil, B. & Fakhoury, T. (1996): Significance of head turn sequences in temporal lobe onset seizures. *Epilepsy Res.* **23**, 245–250.

Ajmone-Marsan, C. & Goldhammer, L. (1973): Clinical ictal patterns and electrographic data in partial seizures of frontal-central-parietal origin. In: *Epilepsy: its phenomena in man*, ed. Brazier, pp. 235–258. New York/London: Academic Press.

Ajmone-Marsan, C. & Ralston, B.L. (1957): *The epileptic seizure: its functional morphology and diagnostic significance.* Springfield, IL: Charles C. Thomas.

Bancaud, J. & Talairach, J. (1992): Clinical semiology of frontal lobe seizures. In: *Advances in Neurology*, vol. 57, eds. P. Chauvel, A.V. Delgado-Escueta, E. Halgren & J. Bancaud, pp. 233–244. New York: Raven Press.

Bancaud, J., Talairach, J., Bonis, A., Schaub, C., Szikla, G., Morel, P. & Bordas-Ferrer, M. (1965): *La stéréo-encéphalographie dans l'épilepsie.* Paris: Masson.

Battista, R.E.D., Spencer, D.D. & Spencer, S.S. (1998): EEG findings in frontal lobe epilepsies. *Neurology* **50**, 1765–1771.

Broca, P. (1878): Anatomie comparée des circonvolutions cérébrales: le grand lobe limbique et la scissure limbique dans la série des mammifères. *Rev. Anthrop.* **1**, 385–498.

Burruss, J.W., Hurley, R.A., Taber, K.H., Rauch, K.A., Norton, R.E. & Hayman, L.A. (2000): Functional neuroanatomy of the frontal lobe circuits. *Radiology* **214**, 227–230.

Cascino, G.D. (1995): Magnetic resonance imaging in frontal lobe epilepsy. In: *Advances in Neurology*, vol. 66, eds. H.H. Jasper, S. Riggio & P.S. Goldman-Rakic, pp. 199–211. New York: Raven Press.

Chauvel, P. & Bancaud, J. (1994): The spectrum of frontal lobe seizures: with a note on frontal lobe syndromatology. In: *Epileptic seizures and syndromes*, ed. P. Wolf, pp. 331–334. London: John Libbey.

Chee, M.W.L., Kotagal, P., Van Ness, P.C., Gragg, L., Murphy, D. & Lüders, H.O. (1993): Lateralizing signs in intractable partial epilepsy: blinded multiple-observer analysis. *Neurology* **43**, 2519–2525.

Commission on Classification and Terminology of the International League Against Epilepsy (1985): Proposal for classification of epilepsies and epileptic syndromes. *Epilepsia* **26**, 268–278.

Commission on Classification and Terminology of the International League Against Epilepsy (1989): Proposal for revised classification of epilepsies and epileptic syndromes. *Epilepsia* **30**, 389–399.

Cotte-Rittaud, M.R. & Courjon, J. (1962): Semiological value of adversive epilepsy. *Epilepsia* **3**, 151–166.

Cummings, J.L. (1995): Anatomic and behavioural aspects of frontal-subcortical circuits. *Ann. N.Y. Acad. Sci.* **769**, 1–13.

Cukiert, A., Olivier, A. & Andermann, F. (1996): Post-traumatic frontal lobe epilepsy with structural changes: excellent results after cortical resections. *Can. J. Neurol. Sci.* **23**, 114–117.

Delgado-Escueta, A., Swartz, B.E., Maldonado, H.M., Walsh, G.O., Rand, R.W. & Halgren, E. (1987): Complex partial seizures of frontal lobe origin. In: *Presurgical evaluation of epileptics: basics, techniques, implications*, eds. H.G. Wieser & C.E. Elger, pp. 268–299. New York: Springer-Verlag.

Devinsky, O., Morrell, M.J. & Vogt, B.A. (1995): Contributions of anterior cingulate cortex to behaviour. *Brain* **118**, 279–306.

Fakhoury, T. & Abou-Khalil, B. (1995): Association of ipsilateral head turning and dystonia in temporal lobe seizures. *Epilepsia* **36**, 1065–1070.

Fegersten, L. & Roger, A. (1961): Frontal epileptogenic foci and their clinical correlations. *Electroencephalogr. Clin. Neurophysiol.* **13**, 905–913.

Fish, D.R. (1996): Magnetic resonance imaging and supplementary motor area epilepsy. In: *Advances in Neurology*, vol. 70, ed. H.O. Lüders, pp. 341–351. Philadelphia: Lippincott-Raven Publishers.

Foerster, O. & Penfield, W. (1931): The structural basis of traumatic epilepsy and results of radical operation. *Brain* **53**, 99–119.

Freund, H.J. (1996a): Functional organization of the human supplementary motor area and dorsolateral premotor cortex. In: *Advances in Neurology*, vol. 70, ed. H.O. Lüders, pp. 263–269. Philadelphia: Lippincott-Raven Publishers.

Freund, H.J. (1996b): Historical overview. In: *Advances in Neurology*, vol. 70, ed. H.O. Lüders, pp. 17–27. Philadelphia: Lippincott-Raven Publishers.

Fuster, J.M. (1989): *The prefrontal cortex: anatomy, physiology, and neuropsychology of the frontal lobe*. 2nd ed. New York: Raven Press.

Fuster, J.M. (2003): Functional anatomy of the prefrontal cortex. In: *Frontal seizures and epilepsies in children*, eds. A. Beaumanoir, F. Andermann, P. Chauvel, L. Mira & B. Zifkin, pp. 1-10. Mariani Foundation Paediatric Neurology Series, vol. 11. Paris, London: John Libbey Eurotext.

Gastaut, H., Aguglia, U. & Tinuper, P. (1986): Benign versive or circling epilepsy with bilateral 3-cps spike-and-wave discharges in late childhood. *Ann. Neurol.* **19**, 301–303.

Geier, J., Bancaud, J., Talairach, J., Bonis, A., Szikla, G. & Enjelvin, M. (1977): The seizures of frontal lobe epilepsy. *Neurology* **27**, 951–958.

Gloor, P. (1986): Consciousness as a neurological concept in epileptology: a critical review. *Epilepsia* **27** (Suppl. 2), S14–S26.

Goldman-Rakic, P.S. (1987): Circuitry of primate prefrontal cortex and regulation of behaviour by representational memory, mechanisms of emotion and attention. In: *Handbook of physiology. Section I, The Nervous System*, vol. 5, *Higher functions of the brain*, ed. F. Plum, pp. 373–417. Bethesda: American Physiological Society.

Gross, D., Dubeau, F., Quesney, L.F. & Gotman, J. (2000): Closely spaced electrodes in frontal lobe epilepsy. *J. Clin. Neurophysiol.* **17**, 414–418.

Jakayar, P., Duchowny, M., Resnick, T. & Alvarez, L. (1992): Ictal head deviation: lateralizing significance of the pattern of head movement. *Neurology* **42**, 1989–1992.

Kazemi, N.J., So, E.L., Mosewich, R.K., O'Brien, T.J., Cascino, G.D., Trenerry, M.R. & Sharbrough, F.W. (1997): Resection of frontal encephalomalacias for intractable epilepsy: outcome and prognostic factors. *Epilepsia* **38**, 670–677.

Kernan, J.C., Devinsky, O., Luciano, D.J., Vasquez, B. & Perrine, K. (1993): Lateralizing significance of head and eye deviation in secondary generalized tonic-clonic seizures. *Neurology* **43**, 1308–1310.

Kotagal, P. & Arunkumar, G.S. (1998): Lateral frontal lobe seizures. *Epilepsia* **39** (Suppl. 4), S62–S68.

Kuzniecky, R.I. & Jackson, G.D. (1995): Frontal lobe epilepsy. In: *Magnetic resonance in epilepsy*, eds. R.I. Kuzniecky & G.D. Jackson, pp. 183–202. New York: Raven Press.

MacLean, P.D. (1990): *The triune brain in evolution: role in paleocerebral functions*. New York: Plenum Press.

Marks, W.J. & Laxer, K.D. (1998): Semiology of temporal lobe seizures: value in lateralizing the seizure focus. *Epilepsia* **39**, 721–726.

Masson, H. & Saint-Hilaire, J.M. (1986): Contraversive seizures in occipital epilepsy. *Neurology* **36**, 1543–1544 (letter).

McLachlan, R.S. (1987): The significance of head and eye turning in seizures. *Neurology* **37**, 1617–1619.

Ochs, R., Gloor, P., Quesney, L.F., Ives, J. & Olivier, A. (1984): Does head-turning during a seizure have lateralizing or localizing significance? *Neurology* **34**, 884–890.

Olivier, A. (1995): Surgery of frontal lobe epilepsy. In: *Advances in Neurology*, vol. 66, eds. H.H. Jasper, S. Riggio & P.S. Goldman-Rakic, pp. 321–352. New York: Raven Press.

Olivier, A. (1996): Surgical strategies for patients with supplementary motor area epilepsy: the Montreal experience. In: *Advances in Neurology*, vol. 66, eds. H.H. Jasper, S. Riggio & P. Goldman-Rakic, pp. 429–444. New York: Raven Press.

Penfield, W. & Jasper, H.H. (1954). *Epilepsy and the functional anatomy of the human brain*. Boston: Little, Brown.

Penfield, W. & Kristiansen, K. (1951): Seizure patterns. In: *Epileptic seizure patterns*, pp. 16–46. Springfield, IL: Charles C Thomas.

Quesney, L.F., Cendes, F., Olivier A., Dubeau, F. & Andermann, F. (1995): Intracranial electroencephalographic investigation in frontal lobe epilepsy. In: *Advances in Neurology*, vol. 66, eds. H.H. Jasper, S. Riggio & P.S. Goldman-Rakic, pp. 243–260. New York: Raven Press.

Quesney, L.F., Constain, M., Fish, D.R. & Rasmussen, T. (1990): The clinical differentiation of seizures arising in the parasagittal and anterodorsal frontal convexities. *Arch. Neurol.* **47**, 677–679.

Quesney, L.F., Constain, M. & Rasmussen, T. (1992): Seizures from dorsolateral frontal lobe. In: *Advances in Neurology*, vol. 57, eds. P. Chauvel, A.V. Delgado-Escueta, E. Halgren & J. Bancaud, pp. 233–244. New York: Raven Press.

Rasmussen, T. (1983): Characteristics of a pure culture of frontal lobe epilepsy. *Epilepsia* **24**, 482–493.

Rasmussen, T. (1963): Surgical therapy of frontal lobe epilepsy. *Epilepsia* **4**, 181–198.

Rasmussen, T. & Penfield, W. (1947): Movements of the head and eyes from stimulation of human frontal cortex. *Res. Publ. Assoc. Res. Nerv. Ment. Dis.* **27**, 346–361.

Robillard, A., Saint-Hilaire, J.M., Mercier, M. & Bouvier, G. (1983): The lateralizing and localizing value of adversion in epileptic seizures. *Neurology* **33**, 1241–1242.

Rosenbaum, D.H., Siegel, M. & Rowan, A.J. (1986): Contraversive seizures in occipital lobe epilepsy: case report and review of the literature. *Neurology* **36**, 281–284.

Salanova, V., Morris, H.H., Van Ness, P., Kotagal, P., Wyllie, E. & Lüders, H. (1995): Frontal lobe seizures: electroclinical syndromes. *Epilepsia* **36**, 16–24.

Talairach, J., Bancaud, J., Bonis, A., Szikla, G., Trottier, S., Vignal, J.P., Chauvel, P., Munari, C. & Chodkiewicz, J.P. (1992): Surgical therapy for frontal epilepsies. In: *Advances in Neurology*, vol. 57, eds. P. Chauvel, A.V. Delgado-Escueta, E. Halgren, J. Bancaud, pp. 707–732. New York: Raven Press.

Tanji, J. (1994): The supplementary motor area in the cerebral cortex. *Neurosci. Res.* **19**, 251–268.

Tanji, J. (1996): Contrast of neuronal activity between the supplementary motor area and other cortical motor area. In: *Advances in Neurology*, vol. 70, ed. H.O. Lüders, pp. 95–103. Philadelphia: Lippincott-Raven Publishers.

Thurston, S.E., Leigh, R.J. & Osorio, I. (1985): Epileptic gaze deviation and nystagmus. *Neurology* **35**, 1518–1521.

Van Ness, P.C. (1996): Invasive electroencephalography in the evaluation of supplementary motor area seizures. In: *Advances in Neurology*, vol. 70, ed. H.O. Lüders, pp. 319–340. Philadelphia: Lippincott-Raven Publishers.

Walsh, G.O. & Delgado-Escueta, A.V. (1984): Type II complex partial seizures: poor results of anterior temporal lobectomy. *Neurology* **34**, 1–13.

Waterman, K., Purves, S.J., Kosaka, B., Strauss, E. & Wada, J.A. (1987): An epileptic syndrome caused by mesial frontal lobe foci. *Neurology* **37**, 577–582.

Wieser, H.G., Swartz, B.E., Delgado-Escueta, A.V., Bancaud, J., Walsh, G.O., Maldonado, H. & Saint-Hilaire, J.M. (1992): Differentiating frontal lobe seizures from temporal lobe seizures. In: *Advances in Neurology*, vol. 57, eds. P. Chauvel, A.V. Delgado-Escueta, E. Halgren & J. Bancaud, pp. 267–285. New York: Raven Press.

Wieser, H.G. & Hajek, M. (1995): Frontal lobe epilepsy: compartmentalization, presurgical evaluation, and operative results. In: *Advances in Neurology*, vol. 66, eds. H.H. Jasper, S. Riggio & P.S. Goldman-Rakic, pp. 297–319. New York: Raven Press.

Williamson, P.D., Spencer, D.D., Spencer, S.S., Novelly, R.A. & Mattson, R.H. (1985): Complex partial seizures of frontal lobe origin. *Ann. Neurol.* **18**, 497–504.

Wyllie, E., Lüders, H., Morris, H.H., Lesser, R.P. & Dinner, D.S. (1986): The lateralizing significance of versive head and eye movements during epileptic seizures. *Neurology* **36**, 606–611.

Wyllie, E., Lüders, H., Morris, H.H., Lesser, R.P., Dinner, D.S. & Goldstick, L. (1986): Ipsilateral forced head and eye turning at the end of the generalized tonic-clonic phase of versive seizures. *Neurology* **36**, 1212–1217.

Chapter 9

Cingulate and mesial frontal seizures

Adriana Magaudda and Carol di Perri

Centro Interdipartimentale per la Diagnosi e Cura dell'Epilessia,
First Neurology Clinic, University Polyclinic, via Consolare, 98013 Gazzi-Messina, Italy
adriana.magaudda@libero.it

Summary

The term mesial frontal seizures has frequently been used as a synonym for orbito-frontal seizures. We propose limiting the definition of mesial frontal seizures to those originating in the mesial frontal cortex, posterior to the orbito-frontal region. These seizures can then be subdivided into medial intermediate frontal lobe seizures, including frontal absences and complex motor seizures, and supplementary motor seizures (SMSs). SMSs are characterized by predominantly nocturnal seizures with abrupt tonic posturing of one or more limbs, retained consciousness and absence of post-ictal confusion. SMSs may also present as complex partial seizures without tonic posture with typical frontal automatisms. Interictal and ictal EEG may be normal or non-specific and the absence of EEG abnormalities may lead to a misdiagnosis of pseudoseizures. Asymmetric tonic posturing and intact awareness may lead to confusion with paroxysmal kinesigenic choreoathetosis/dyskinesias (PKC/PKD) and paroxysmal dystonic choreoathetosis/non-kinesigenic dyskinesias (PDC/PNKD). The tonic posture, which may involve all four limbs, and clonic movements which may be observed in the final phase of SMSs, can also lead to misdiagnosis of generalized tonic-clonic seizures.

Cingulate seizures are characterized by intense fear, precocious and dramatic automatisms, bizarre gesturing and vigorous, possibly obscene or aggressive, verbalization. Dystonic posturing and versive movements may occur. Consciousness is maintained. Genital manipulation and urinary incontinence may also be seen.

Seizures originating in the cingulate gyrus are rare. The dramatic clinical manifestations, without loss or impairment of consciousness, may lead to confusion of cingulate seizures with pseudoseizures and panic attacks.

The classification of epilepsy and epileptic syndromes (Commission on classification, 1989) subdivides frontal lobe seizures as follows: supplementary motor seizures, cingulate seizures, fronto-polar seizures, orbito-frontal seizures, dorsolateral seizures, opercular seizures, motor cortex seizures.

This subclassification is based on the anatomical localization of the onset of the ictal discharge. However, this is of little help to the clinician because the symptomatology of a seizure depends on the spread of the ictal discharge and on the connections between the cerebral regions involved. This is particularly true of the frontal lobe where the discharge spreads extremely rapidly and because some frontal regions, such as the orbito-frontal region, are clinically silent. Thus, no clinical symptoms occur until the discharge extends to other areas.

In addition there is confusion over the terminology regarding the definition of orbito-frontal and mesial frontal seizures. Waterman *et al.* (1987) described seizures characterized by bilateral coordinated movements of the limbs, axial movements, vocalization and oral non-masticatory activity as 'an epileptic syndrome caused by mesial frontal lobe seizure foci'. They attributed these seizures to activity in the frontal lobes, within the sagittal-fissure or orbital area, and also implicated the mesial frontal cortex in the origin of these attacks. Following this report, the terms orbito-frontal seizures and mesial frontal seizures have been used synonymously, supported by the observation that seizures starting in the orbito-frontal cortex only become evident when the ictal discharge spreads to the mesial frontal areas. Munari & Bancaud (1992) recorded ictal discharges beginning in the orbito-frontal regions which remained clinically silent for 6–60 seconds.

It would seem opportune to limit the use of the term orbito-frontal seizures to the ones described by Waterman *et al.* (1987) primarily characterized by bimanual, bipedal complex automatisms. The term mesial frontal seizures should be reserved for those originating in the mesial frontal cortex, posterior to the orbito-frontal region.

Mesial frontal seizures

Mesial frontal seizures can be subdivided as follows:
- medial intermediate frontal lobe seizures,
- supplementary motor seizures (SMSs).

Medial intermediate frontal lobe seizures

These are further subdivided into frontal absences and complex motor seizures (Bancaud & Talairach, 1992).

Frontal absences are characterized by impairment of consciousness, speech arrest, movement arrest, simple gestural automatisms, deviation of the head and eyes, and immediate recovery of consciousness.

Complex motor seizures are characterized by altered consciousness, deviation of the head and eyes, abduction and raising of the upper limbs, head and trunk manifestations, autonomic signs, simple gestural automatisms and tonic-clonic generalization (Chauvel *et al.*, 1995).

Supplementary motor seizures

SMSs usually begin without warning. However, a localized or generalized feeling of tightness or paraesthesias may signal their onset. This is followed by abrupt tonic posturing. Morris *et al.* (1988) studied 11 patients with seizures arising in the supplementary motor area (SMA) and reported that the tonic posturing could involve one or more limbs; rhythmic or clonic movements of the extremities could occur at the end of the tonic posturing and writhing or twisting body movements could occur during the tonic phase.

Five of the eight patients with SMSs reported by Jobst *et al.* (2000) had predominantly tonic seizures. Four had asymmetric tonic posturing while one had symmetric tonic seizures. However, asymmetric tonic posturing can also be observed in frontal lobe seizures beginning outside the SMA. In these cases seizure onset was never explosive and lateralization was inconsistent. Vocalization, considered a typical sign of SMSs, is not always present. Speech may or may not be maintained during seizures. Consciousness is maintained in most patients with SMSs. This may be difficult to appreciate in patients with speech arrest. Contraversive movements may occur later on in the seizure and were observed in only two of the eleven patients reported by Morris *et al.* (1988).

SMSs may also present as complex partial seizures. Two of the eight patients with SMS reported by Jobst *et al.* (2000) had seizures characterized by typical frontal automatisms without tonic posturing. SMSs occur frequently and are predominantly nocturnal. The interictal scalp EEG may show sharp waves at (or next to) the midline or may be normal (Morris *et al.*, 1988). Figs. 1 and 2 show the interictal EEG of two patients with SMSs. During the seizure the scalp EEG may show a focal discharge at the midline, or generalized delta or theta activity (Morris *et al.*, 1988). However, the ictal EEG may be uninformative (Williamson, 1995). Fig. 3 shows the ictal pattern of a SMS.

Distinguishing supplementary motor seizures from pseudoseizures

The following characteristics of SMSs make it difficult to distinguish them from pseudoseizures:
- no loss of consciousness during motor ictal activity involving all four limbs;
- atypical nature of motor activity during the seizure;
- frequent absence of interictal and/or ictal EEG abnormalities;
- frequently poor response to antiepileptic medication.

The differential diagnosis of SMSs and pseudoseizures was studied by Kanner *et al.* (1990). They analysed videotapes of 63 SMSs in 12 patients and 111 pseudoseizures in 44 patients and attempted to assess the value of clinical phenomena in distinguishing between SMSs and pseudoseizures. They found that SMSs are brief, stereotypic, tend to occur in sleep, and are often marked by tonic contraction of the upper extremities in abduction. Conversely, pseudoseizures are longer, not stereotyped and occur in wakefulness. This distinction is based solely on ictal symptoms. Global evaluation of the patient is of vital importance for correct diagnosis. Psychiatric evaluation is necessary to establish the presence of those psychiatric disorders which may provoke pseudoseizures.

Distinguishing supplementary motor seizures from paroxysmal kinesigenic choreathetosis/dyskinesias (PKC/PKD)

PKC/PKD consists of brief and frequent dyskinetic attacks (Bhatia, 1999). The distinction between SMSs and PKC/PKD is based on the triggering of dyskinetic attacks by sudden movement in PKC/PKD. However, SMSs may also be provoked by startle (Serles *et al.*, 1999) although the stimulus is usually auditory. Spontaneous seizures can occur together with startle seizures. In paroxysmal dystonic choreoathetosis/*non-kinesigenic* dyskinesias (PDC/PNKD), attacks are induced by factors including coffee, tea, alcohol and fatigue, but not by startle (Bhatia, 1999). The main difference between these events and SMSs is their duration; PDC may last several minutes but SMSs are briefer (Morris *et al.*, 1988).

SMSs may also be confused with generalized tonic-clonic seizures because the tonic posture of SMSs may involve all four limbs and be followed by clonic movements in the final phase of the attack. Differential diagnosis is more difficult if the SMS is followed, as often occurs, by secondary generalization. The main criteria for differential diagnosis are retained consciousness during SMSs and the absence of confusion or post-ictal coma in SMSs that have not generalized.

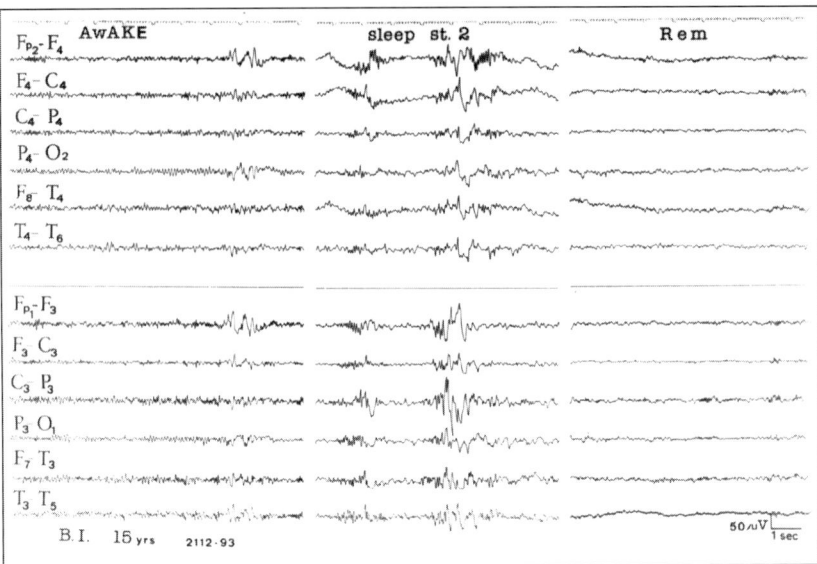

Fig. 1. Interictal EEG in a patient with SMSs and normal MRI: sharp waves are localized to both frontal regions. These are activated during stage 2 sleep but disappear during REM sleep.

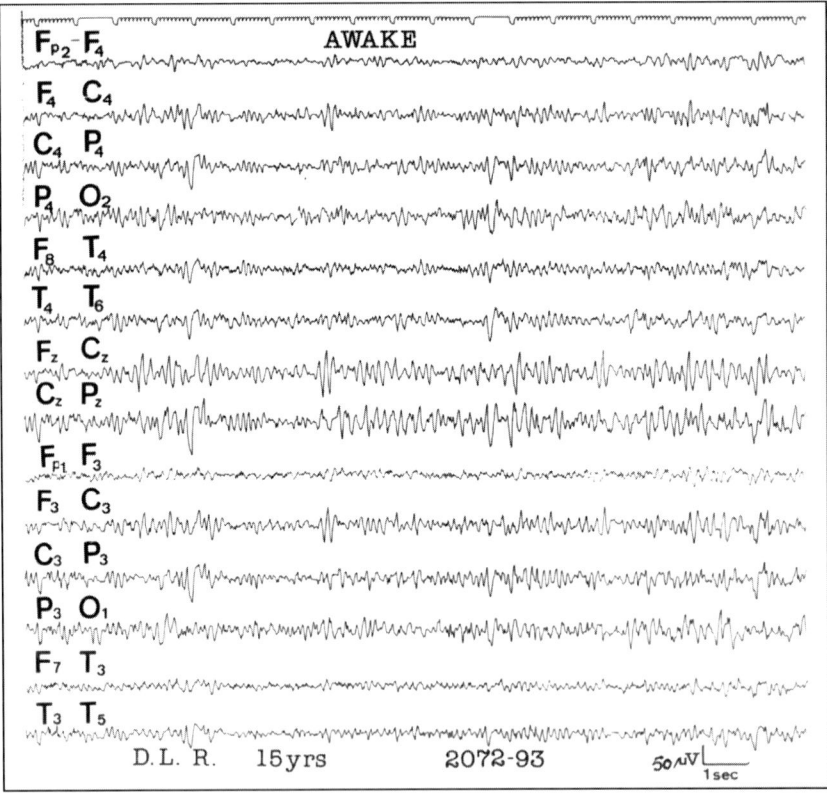

Fig. 2. Interictal EEG in a patient with SMSs and abnormality in the right insula on MRI: sharp waves localized to the vertex regions.

Chapter 9 Cingulate and mesial frontal seizures

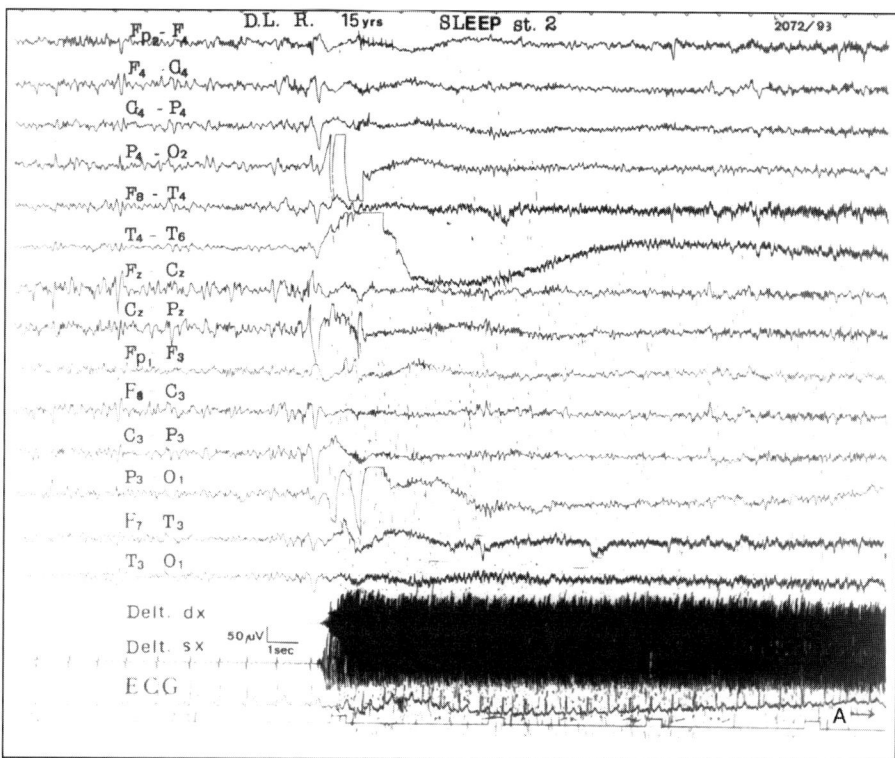

Fig. 3 (A-E). Recording of a SMS in the same patient as in Fig. 2: the patient is sleeping. There is sudden abduction of the upper limbs, then stretching of the neck, slow relaxation of the upper limbs, and head-turning, first to the right and then to the left. The patient then removes the bedclothes and tries to get out of bed. Finally he lies down again.

A. Before seizure onset the EEG shows an increased frequency of spikes in the vertex region. The seizure begins with a high-voltage diffuse sharp wave followed by flattening and subsequently by low voltage rapid rhythm which progressively increases in amplitude and decreases in frequency. The EMG of the right and left deltoids shows tonic activity. The ECG shows an increase in the heart-rate.

B. Tonic EMG activity progressively disappears. The EEG rapid rhythms progressively slow down.

C. Ictal EEG activity is slower. EMG activity corresponds to the movements of the patient as he tries to get out of bed.

D. The EEG shows many movement artifacts. E. At the end of the seizure, the EEG shows a marked increase of the spikes in the vertex regions, which spread to both hemispheres.

(Follows on pages 88–89.)

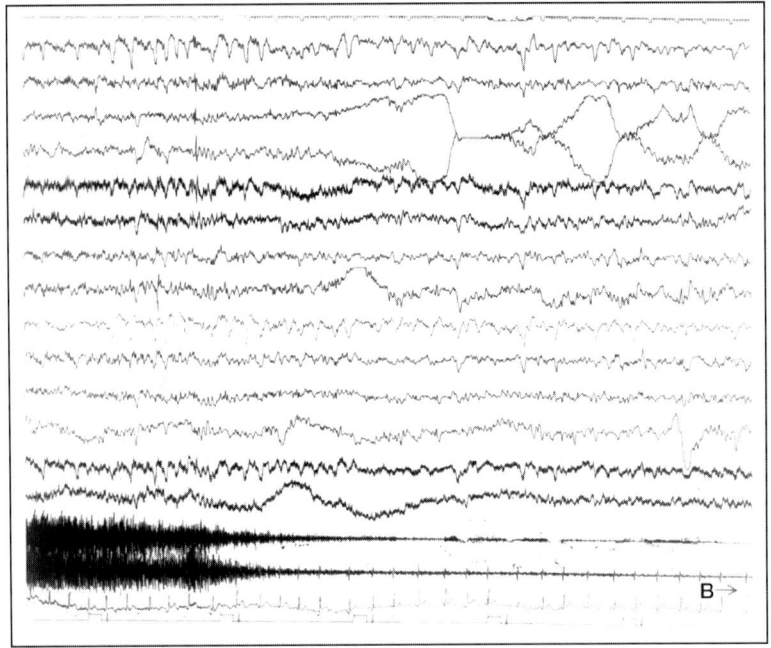

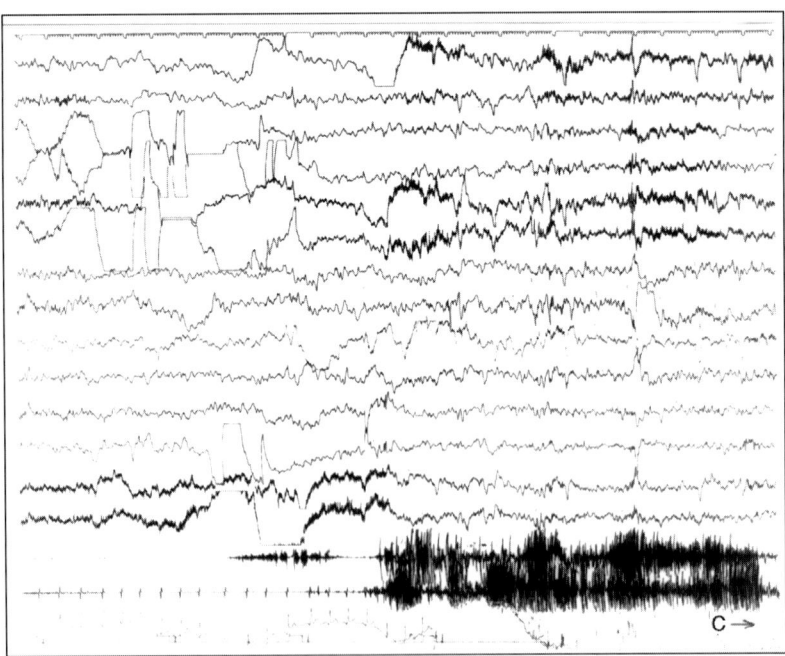

Figure 3 – follows

Chapter 9 Cingulate and mesial frontal seizures

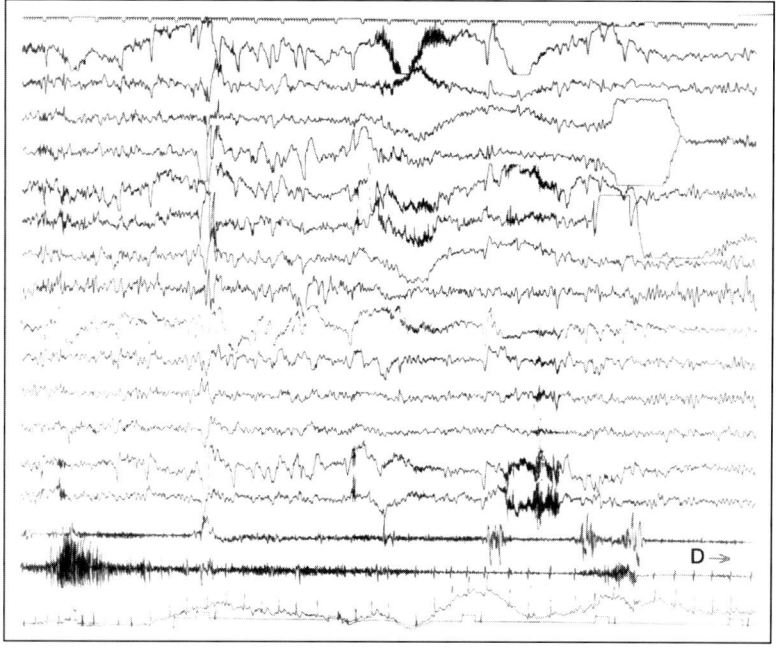

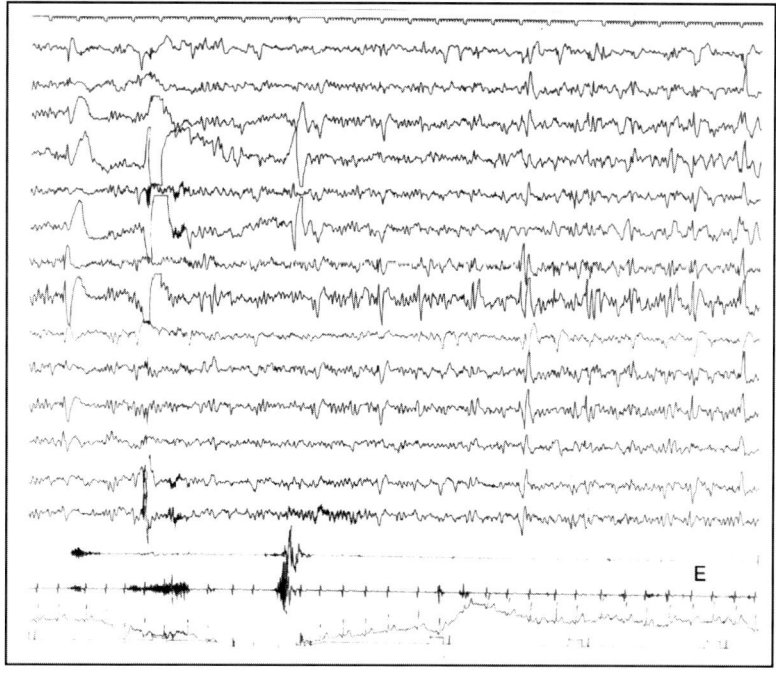

Figure 3 – follows

Cingulate seizures

Cingulate seizures are characterized by intense fear, early and dramatic automatisms, autonomic phenomena, complex repetitive motor automatisms, bizarre gesturing, and vigorous verbalization, which may be obscene or aggressive. Dystonic posturing and versive movements may also occur. Consciousness is maintained and the patient is aware of this activity. Sexual manifestations may also be seen.

Seizures confined to the cingulate gyrus are rare. The discharge often spreads, producing bizarre motor phenomena (Veilleux *et al.*, 1992). Seizures originating in the cingulate gyrus are also seldom observed. Salanova *et al.* (1995) reported eight patients with complex partial seizures starting in the frontal lobes; in none of these patients did the ictal discharge begin in the cingulate gyrus. In a study analysing the characteristics of seizures recorded by intracranial video-EEG monitoring in 26 patients with intractable frontal lobe epilepsy, not one seizure started in the cingulate gyrus (Jobst *et al.*, 2000).

Mihara *et al.* (1997) reported eight patients with complex partial seizures of frontal lobe origin. Of these, only one had seizures originating in the cingulate gyrus. This patient had focal cortical dysplasia in the anterior cingulate cortex. The seizures consisted of an indefinable intense fear, automatic behaviour reactive to the surroundings, and urinary incontinence. The patient remained conscious. Stoffels *et al.* (1980) analysed the genital and sexual manifestations in 42 seizures recorded in 15 patients. The origin of the ictal discharge was localized in four patients to the anterior cingulate gyrus. In those seizures there were no evident early sexual manifestations, but at the end of the ictal discharge masturbation was noted. Fondling the genitals was noted immediately after the post-ictal phase.

Although it is rare for ictal discharges to begin in the cingulate gyrus, it is not uncommon for a discharge originating outside the frontal lobe to spread there. During the late stages of inferomesial temporal lobe seizures, ictal discharges may spread to the anterior or posterior cingulate region (Wieser, 1992).

Distinguishing cingulate seizures from non-epileptic disorders

Cingulate seizures may be difficult to distinguish from pseudoseizures and panic attacks, given the characteristic sensation of extreme fear, the elaborate and bizarre motor phenomena, obscene verbalization and urinary incontinence without loss or impairment of consciousness. We stress that global evaluation of the patient is a fundamental tool of differential diagnosis. It is necessary to evaluate whether a conversion disorder exists, which could give rise to pseudoseizures, or if an anxiety disorder is present, which may be related to panic attacks. The problem of differential diagnosis between panic attacks and epileptic seizures has been widely studied. Panic attacks are discrete periods of intense fear or discomfort, in which four or more of the following symptoms develop abruptly and reach a peak within 10 minutes (DSM-IV):

    (1) palpitations, pounding heart, or accelerated heart rate;
    (2) sweating;
    (3) trembling or shaking;
    (4) sensation of shortness of breath or smothering;
    (5) feeling of choking;
    (6) chest pain or discomfort;
    (7) nausea or abdominal distress;

(8) feeling dizzy, unsteady, light-headed, or faint;

(9) derealization or depersonalization;

(10) fear of losing control or going crazy;

(11) fear of dying;

(12) paraesthesias;

(13) chills or hot flushes.

The sudden onset of these symptoms, and the presence of autonomic manifestations and symptoms of derealization and depersonalization, which may be confused with impaired consciousness, may lead to suspicion of an epileptic seizure.

The symptom of fear is not only found in cingulate seizures but is also present in approximately one-third of patients with temporal lobe seizures (Young *et al.*, 1995). Panic attacks have also been reported as manifestations of parietal lobe seizures (Alemayehu *et al.*, 1995). Five patients with brief simple partial seizures mimicking panic disorders were reported by Young *et al.* (1995). Each patient had a mesial temporal structural lesion, in the right temporal lobe in two patients and in the left temporal lobe in the remaining three. Frequent attacks of sudden and unprovoked fear often associated with autonomic symptoms, a sensation of unreality, and chest discomfort were the main manifestations of their seizures. The features that differentiated these seizures from panic attacks were:

- the sensation of fear lasted only a few seconds;
- the seizures were stereotyped while in panic attacks symptoms may vary in the same patient;
- some seizures progressed to typical complex partial seizures;
- aphasia and dysmnesia occurred during seizures in some patients.

When panic attacks and epileptic seizures are present in the same patient, differential diagnosis is more difficult (Weilburg *et al.*, 1987; McNamara, 1993). In these cases EEG monitoring is often necessary to make the diagnosis. The principal features of epileptic seizures which enable differential diagnosis from panic attacks are as follows:

- epileptic seizures are generally briefer;
- they are not usually provoked by emotional factors;
- they are stereotyped in the same patient;
- they respond to antiepileptic drugs and not to serotonin re-uptake inhibitors useful in panic disorder;
- they may include automatisms or a generalized tonic-clonic phase which do not occur in panic attacks;
- interictal and ictal EEGs are usually abnormal in epileptic seizures.

References

Alemayehu, S., Bergey, G.K., Barry, E., Krumholz, A., Wolf, A., Fleming, C.P. & Frear E.J. Jr. (1995): Panic attacks as ictal manifestations of parietal lobe seizures. *Epilepsia* **36**, 824–830.

Bancaud, J. & Talairach, J. (1992): Clinical semeiology of frontal lobe seizures. In: *Advances in Neurology*, eds. P. Chauvel, A.V. Delgado-Escueta. E. Halgren & J. Bancaud, vol. 57, pp. 3–58. New York: Raven Press.

Bhatia, K.P. (1999): The paroxysmal dyskinesias. *J. Neurol.* **246**, 149–155.

Chauvel, P., Kliemann, F., Vignal, J.P., Chodkiewicz, J.P., Talairach, J. & Bancaud, J. (1995): The clinical signs and symptoms of frontal lobe seizures: phenomenology and classification. In: *Advances in Neurology*, eds. H.H. Jasper, S. Riggio & P.S. Goldman-Rakic, vol. 66, pp. 115–126. New York: Raven Press.

Commission on classification and terminology of the International League Against Epilepsy (1989): Proposal for revised classification of epilepsies and epileptic syndromes. *Epilepsia* **30**, 389–399.

Diagnostic and Statistical Manual of Mental Disorders, Fourth Edition – Washington, DC, American Psychiatric Association, 1994.

Jobst, B.C., Siegel, A.M., Thadani, V.M., Roberts, D.W., Rhodes, H.C. & Williamson, P.D. (2000): Intractable seizures of frontal lobe origin: clinical characteristics, localizing signs, and results. *Epilepsia* **41**, 1139–1152.

Kanner, A.M., Morris, H.H., Luders, H., Dinner, D.S., Wyllie, E., Medendorp, S.V. & Rowan, A.J. (1990): Supplementary motor seizures mimicking pseudoseizures: some clinical differences. *Neurology* **40**, 1404–1407.

McNamara, M.E. (1993): Absence seizures associated with panic attacks initially misdiagnosed as temporal lobe epilepsy: the importance of prolonged EEG monitoring in diagnosis. *J. Psychiatr. Neurosci.* **18**, 46–48.

Mihara, T., Tottori, T., Kazumi, M., Otsubo, T., Inoue, Y., Yagi, K. & Seino, M. (1997): Analysis of seizure manifestations of 'pure' frontal lobe origin. *Epilepsia* **38**, 42–47.

Morris, H.H., Dinner, D.S., Luders, H., Wyllie, E. & Kramer, R. (1988): Supplementary motor seizures: clinical and electroencephalographic findings. *Neurology* **38**, 1075–1082.

Munari, C. & Bancaud, J. (1992): Electroclinical symptomatology of partial seizures of orbital frontal origin. In: *Advances in Neurology*, eds. P. Chauvel, A.V. Delgado-Escueta, E. Halgren & J. Bancaud, vol. 57, pp. 257–265. New York: Raven Press.

Salanova, V., Morris, H.H., Van Ness, P., Kotagal, P., Wyllie, E. & Luders, H. (1995): Frontal lobe seizures: electroclinical syndromes. *Epilepsia* **36**, 16–24.

Serles W., Leutmezer, F., Pataraia, E., Olbrich, A., Groppel, G., Czech, T. & Baumgartner, C. (1999): A case of startle epilepsy and SSMA seizures documented with subdural recordings. *Epilepsia* **40**, 1031–1035.

Stoffels, C., Munari, C., Bonis, A., Bancaud, J. & Talairach, J. (1980): Manifestations génitales et sexuelles lors des crises épileptiques partielles chez l'homme. *Rev. EEG Neurophysiol.* **10**, 386–392.

Veilleux, F., Saint-Hilaire, J.M., Giard, N., Turmel, A., Bernier, G.P., Rouleau, I., Mercier, M. & Bouvier, G. (1992): Seizures of the medial frontal lobe. In: *Advances in Neurology*, eds. P. Chauvel, A.V. Delgado-Escueta, E. Halgren & J. Bancaud, vol. 57, pp. 245–255. New York: Raven Press.

Waterman, K., Purves, S.J., Kosaka, B., Strauss, E. & Wada, J.A. (1987): An epileptic syndrome caused by mesial frontal lobe seizure foci. *Neurology* **37**, 577–582.

Weilburg, J.B., Bear, D.M. & Sachs, G. (1987): Three patients with concomitant panic attacks and seizure disorder: possible clues to the neurology of anxiety. *Am. J. Psychiatry* **144**, 1053–1056.

Wieser, H.G. & Hajek, M. (1995): Frontal lobe epilepsy: compartmentalization, presurgical evaluation, and operative results. In: *Advances in Neurology*, eds. H.H. Jasper, S. Riggio & P.S. Goldman-Rakic, vol. 66, pp. 297–319. New York: Raven Press.

Williamson, P.D. (1995): Frontal lobe epilepsy: some clinical characteristics. In: *Advances in Neurology*, eds. H.H. Jasper, S. Riggio & P.S. Goldman-Rakic, vol. 66, pp. 127–152. New York: Raven Press.

Young, B.G., Chandarana, P.C., Blume, W.T., McLachlan, R.S., Muñoz, D.G. & Girvin, J.P. (1995): Mesial temporal lobe seizures presenting as anxiety disorders. *J. Neuropsychiatry Clin. Neurosci.* **7**, 352–357.

Chapter 10

Reflex frontal lobe epilepsies

Jean-Pierre Vignal and Louis Maillard

*Neurology Service, University Hospital Centre of Nancy, Central Hospital,
29, avenue du Maréchal-de-Lattre-de-Tassigny, c.o. 34, 54035 Nancy Cedex, France*
jp.vignal@chu-nancy.fr

Summary

Seizures in frontal lobe reflex epilepsies are the result of focal hyperexcitability in limited cortical areas including chiefly the primary motor cortex and, in some cases, the primary sensory cortex and the premotor cortex. We describe here several epileptic syndromes characterized by reflex seizures of the frontal lobe: startle epilepsy and epilepsies with seizures provoked by movement or a cutaneous stimulation, with or without trigger zone; and discuss the role of the frontal lobe in seizures induced by reading. Cortical reflex myoclonus is also a sensorimotor cortex seizure and can occur in partial and generalized epilepsies.

The frontal lobe can be divided into the prefrontal cortex, and the motor and premotor cortices. Reflex seizures of the prefrontal cortex have not been described, but premotor cortex and especially the motor cortex play a major part in the organization of several partial reflex seizure types in children and adults. However, to understand this role we must recall that the primary sensory cortex is closely associated with the primary motor cortex and that the majority of these reflex seizures are explained by the involvement of both sensory and motor cortices with possible involvement of the premotor cortex. The sensorimotor cortex is the centre of an anatomical network associating the lemniscal pathways and the pyramidal tract. This network constitutes a transcortical reflex loop (Gioanni *et al.*, 1983, Chauvel *et al.*, 1978; Palmer & Ashby, 1992). Localized hyperexcitability of these areas enables sensory impulses to synchronize a sufficient neuronal volume to start a seizure. We will see that the effective stimulus is not necessarily somaesthetic and can be auditory or visual, as described in startle seizures. It is certain that partial reflex seizures of the sensorimotor cortex reflect both the proximity of the periphery and a low threshold for cortical excitability.

Reflex seizures of the sensorimotor cortex include startle seizures, seizures provoked by cutaneous stimulation, seizures triggered by movement, cortical reflex myoclonus, and one type of reading seizures.

Cortical reflex myoclonus occurs in several localization-related and generalized epileptic syndromes. It can be understood as the motor response of a low-threshold transcortical reflex in connection with a hyperexcitable motor and/or sensory cortex (Chauvel *et al.*, 1992; Lamarche & Vignal, 2000).

Cortical reflex myoclonus also occurs in Kojewnikow's syndrome, which is an epilepsy of the Rolandic cortex.

Apart from the particular case of cortical reflex myoclonus, other frontal lobe reflex seizures are integrated in syndromes that are more complex. However, the limits between some of these are not always clear. Thus, some authors (Gastaut & Tassinari, 1966) classified seizures triggered by movement as a particular case of startle epilepsy. The epilepsies with seizures triggered by cutaneous stimulation and those with seizures induced by movement are closely related, since any movement involves a coactivation of proprioceptive and exteroceptive afferents. Therefore, it is debatable whether one should separate them as two syndromes. We prefer to describe them separately using a detailed phenomenological approach at least for purposes of discussion.

Startle epilepsy

Startle seizures are somatomotor seizures triggered by a sudden and unexpected sensory stimulation, usually auditory. The classic form of startle epilepsy is described in subjects with infantile hemiplegia (Alajouanine & Gastaut, 1955, 1958; Chauvel et al., 1992).

Description of the startle seizures

Startle seizures are brief and sudden tonic seizures, not longer than 30 seconds. Motor manifestations usually combine flexion of the head and trunk with elevation and abduction of the arms, corresponding to a tonic contraction of the proximal muscles. Concomitant hyperextension of the legs often occurs. Thus, this motor activation involves axial and proximal muscles, often bilaterally but typically with predominance on the paretic side. Sometimes the tonic signs are localized to the paretic arm. These sudden events can cause the patient to fall and injury is common. Initial clonic manifestations are rare, noted in only one patient of the 20 reported by Chauvel et al. (1992). In more than half of the cases, deviation of the head and eyes occurs, usually ipsilateral to the paretic side, and rarely contralateral. In half of the cases, consciousness is not altered during the seizure, but speech arrest always occurs. Facial spasm is often noted. Autonomic manifestations such as flushing and bilateral mydriasis are frequent. Postictal mood changes, such as euphoria, or sadness and even crying are rarer. Secondary generalization is rare.

The ictal scalp EEG shows flattening or bilateral low-voltage fast discharges that can sometimes predominate over the right or left fronto-parietal area. In most cases, the ictal discharge is preceded by a high-amplitude evoked spike at the vertex (Gastaut, 1953). Ictal EEG changes may be difficult to discern because of abundant EMG artefact.

Description of the syndrome

Startle seizures are often observed in children with infantile hemiplegia. Early occurrence of a cerebral lesion, before 2 years of age, is much more important than the aetiology in determining the risk of subsequent startle epilepsy (Chauvel et al., 1992). A prenatal origin is sometimes suspected when hemiplegia develops in the first few months and no perinatal event is reported. The aetiology can be ischaemic, inflammatory or infectious.

Neurological examination almost always shows spastic hemiparesis with hemiatrophy. In more than half of the cases, the motor deficit is associated with hemisensory disturbance and mental retardation.

Imaging often shows extensive cortical and subcortical hemispheric lesions. Hemicranial and unilateral cerebral atrophy are common and more rarely a porencephalic cyst is found. The atrophic and often extensive lesions usually involve the Rolandic cortex and, to a variable degree, the premotor and parietal cortices. The lateral cortex appears to be preferentially involved more than the medial and supero-external cortices.

In all cases, spontaneous seizures also occur. Epilepsy begins in childhood, between 8 months and 16 years, and usually around 9 years. Spontaneous seizures generally precede startle seizures. The seizure pattern can change in childhood, but only rarely after age 12 years.

The spontaneous seizures resemble the startle seizures. They are usually tonic motor seizures, more rarely clonic. However, two differences are sometimes reported: the motor signs are more often preceded by somatosensory signs, and the tonic signs are often less explosive and more localized at their onset. Spontaneous seizures are associated with EEG features very similar to those of startle seizures with fast discharge or bilateral flattening sometimes predominating in the frontoparietal area. Other types of seizures can coexist such as cortical reflex myoclonus (Kojewnikow's syndrome), and seizures beginning with complex visual hallucinations (Vignal, 1984).

In the population studied by Chauvel *et al.* (1992), most of the patients had several seizures each day and eight patients out of 20 had status epilepticus at least once.

Apart from the syndrome of startle epilepsy, startle seizures have been reported in several syndromes: Lennox-Gastaut syndrome (Aguglia *et al.*, 1984), Down syndrome (Guerrini *et al.*, 1990), Sturge-Weber syndrome (Nakamura *et al.*, 1975), and also with dysplastic lesions in patients without gross neurological deficit (Manford *et al.*, 1996).

Characteristics of the stimulus

The effective seizure stimuli can be auditory, somatosensory or more rarely visual (Chauvel *et al.*, 1992; Manford *et al.*, 1996). The auditory stimulus must be intense and distinct from surrounding noise. In startle epilepsy, auditory stimuli are effective triggers in all patients but somatosensory stimuli are effective in only half of them (Chauvel *et al.*, 1992). Somatosensory stimuli consist of sudden cutaneous percussion on the paretic side or sudden contact of the paretic foot with an obstacle. Visual stimuli are seldom effective and usually consist of a sudden intrusion of an object into the patient's visual field. When only one type of stimulus is effective, this stimulus is always auditory. Some other patients may be about equally sensitive to all such stimuli. Startle seizure triggers and physiologic startle stimuli share some common features. Regardless of modality, the stimulus must be unexpected, surprising for the subject. Repetition of the stimulus leads to 'habituation', i.e. a reduction in the intensity of the seizures, until the stimulus becomes ineffective. However, in startle seizures, the effective stimulus threshold can be lower and does not necessarily elicit a feeling of surprise, which is in any case less intense than in physiological startle.

Some patients report that an unexpected emotion can trigger a seizure. In this case, surprise is always a decisive factor.

Mechanisms

Although the clinical presentation and the localized cortical origin of startle seizures have been well established from SEEG and corticectomy data by Chauvel *et al.* (1992), the underlying physiological mechanisms remain controversial. The role of a startle as a trigger of the seizures has been debated.

An epilepsy of the motor and premotor cortices

Alajouanine & Gastaut (1955, 1958) postulated that the seizures originate in the Rolandic area based on semiological study of the startle seizure and its association with infantile hemiplegia, and ruled out a temporal or a supplementary motor area (SMA) origin.

Later, Bancaud et al. (1967, 1975) analysed two cases using implanted electrode recordings (SEEG). They confirmed the role of the motor cortex in the organization of startle seizures, but they documented an essential role for the SMA. Further SEEG studies (Chauvel et al., 1992) showed that startle seizures are organized in the motor and premotor cortices. The seizures begin with a high voltage potential located in the motor cortex and/or in the SMA followed by a very high frequency discharge (Figs. 1 and 2). This potential is concomitant with the vertex spike described on the surface EEG. These seizures originated in an injured and reorganized cortex. As noted, the atrophic lesions usually involve the lateral cortex. The seizures involve first the mesial cortex (motor and premotor) and supero-lateral cortex. Activation limited to the lateral cortex is rare. The atrophic lesions, especially if they are extensive, are associated with a spatial and somatotopic reorganization of the motor cortex as shown by electrical stimulation. Electrical stimulation also shows abnormal function of the premotor cortex, especially the SMA (Vignal, 1984). These motor and premotor functional lesions and evidence of reorganization support the hypothesis that the motor signs are directly related to activation of the motor and premotor cortices by the ictal discharge. However, it should be noted that initial extension of the ictal discharge in the premotor and parietal cortices is variable from one subject to another, with the exception of the SMA, which is almost always involved. EEG rapid rhythms usually propagate toward the mesial frontal cortex, especially to the cingulate gyrus, and toward the contralateral posterior frontal cortex. To summarize, SEEG studies show that the usual bilateral tonic motor signs of startle seizures are explained by initial involvement of the motor cortex and even of the SMA, and by secondary involvement of the SMA and then of the motor and premotor cortices of the contralateral frontal lobe. Spontaneous seizures have the same anatomical organization as startle seizures (Fig. 3).

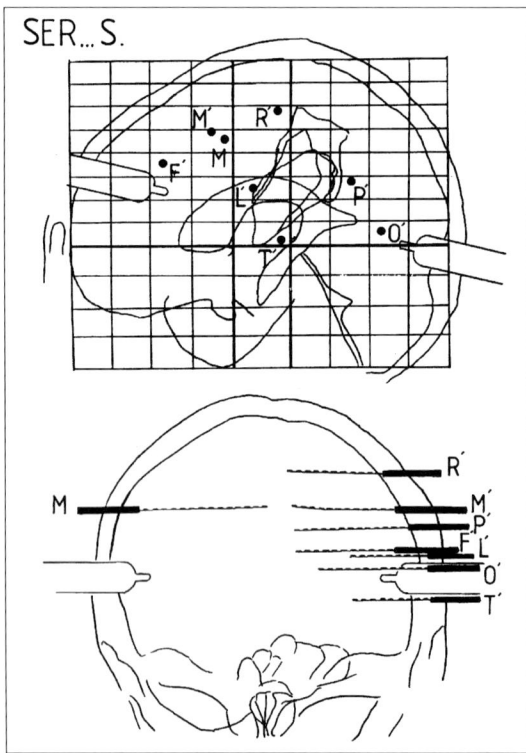

Fig. 1. Diagram of intracerebral electrode implantation (patient in Figs. 2 and 3). Seven electrodes are implanted in the left hemisphere and one electrode in the right hemisphere. R' and L' explore the left motor cortex. M' is situated in the left supplementary motor area (SMA) (medial leads) and second frontal gyrus (lateral leads). M explores the right SMA (medial leads) and second frontal gyrus.

Chapter 10 Reflex frontal lobe epilepsies

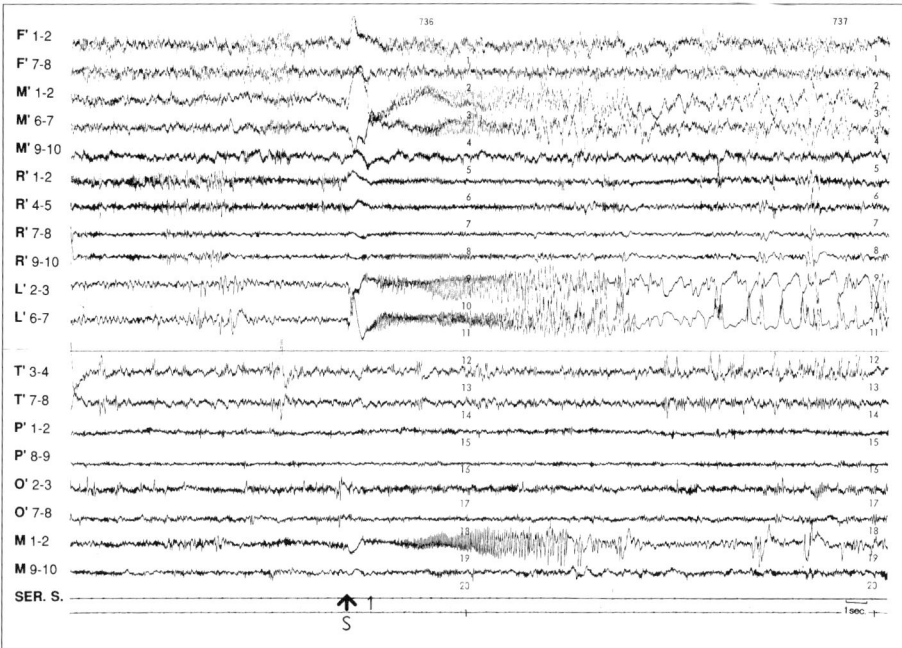

Fig. 2. Startle seizure triggered by an unexpected sound (S). The tonic signs started on the right side but spread to the contralateral upper and lower limb. Recording from intracerebral electrodes shows a paroxysmal potential in the motor cortex (L'), immediately followed by a fast discharge in left motor and premotor cortices (L', M', R'). The fast discharge spread to the right SMA (M1-2).

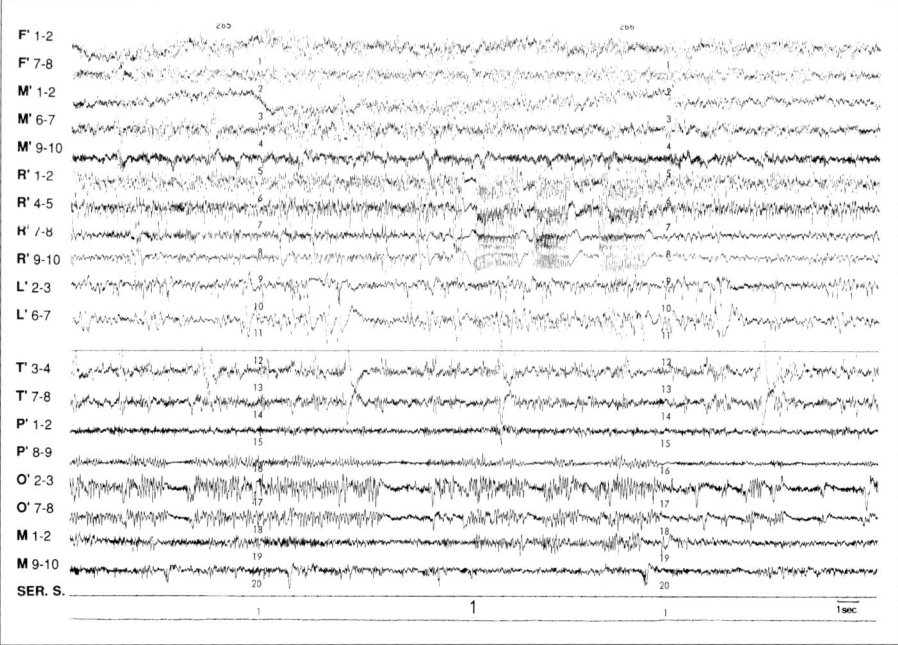

Fig. 3. SEEG recording of a spontaneous clonic seizure limited to the right upper limb in the same patient as in Fig. 2. The seizure is characterized by a clonic discharge in the left motor cortex (R').

97

Description and mechanism of startle

The physiological startle reaction is bilateral and symmetrical, and predominates in flexor muscles (Shimamura, 1973; Wilkins et al., 1986). Physiological startle results from activation of a subcortical loop with a generator located in the reticularis pontis caudalis. This loop is controlled by some cortical areas, in particular by the auditory cortex and by the primary sensory cortex (Ascher, 1965; Liégeois-Chauvel et al., 1989). The startle reaction observed with startle seizures has two characteristics which differentiate it from physiological startle:

- a low threshold for release,
- an asymmetric muscular activation localized to the paretic side or even confined to the deltoid and the biceps.

Two mechanisms have been proposed to explain this startle reaction. The first is an increase in reticulospinal activity among patients who often have marked spasticity (Shimamura, 1973). This is observed among patients with spastic hemiplegia and was described as 'syncinésie-sursaut' by Alajouanine & Scherrer (1952). However, this mechanism is rejected by Chauvel et al. (1992) because the startle reaction is asymmetrical or even localized and there is no evidence suggesting a primary tegmental disturbance. Chauvel et al. suggest a local deterioration of control exerted by the primary sensory cortices over the subcortical generators of the startle. They emphasize the role of atrophic and/or functional lesions of these cortices.

Triggering of the seizures

Chauvel et al. (1992) studied the relations between the muscular activation of the startle reaction, the auditory evoked cortical potential and the fast discharge recorded from intracerebral electrodes in five patients with motor seizures triggered by an unexpected sound. To explain their diverging results, they hypothesized three mechanisms of seizure triggering: one patient reported by Chauvel et al. (1992) showed a paroxysmal evoked potential in the motor cortex, preceding the motor activation. This suggested functional projections of auditory afferents to the motor cortex and possibly an anatomical and functional reorganization of these projections due to perinatal lesions. However, in this particular case, the startle seizure had unusual initial clonic signs. Second, these neurophysiological findings could be explained by auditory afferents projecting to the SMA, which is also known as an area of multimodality convergence (Wiesandanger et al., 1973; Tanji & Kurata, 1983). Recordings of a paroxysmal evoked potential in the auditory cortex preceding the potential in the motor cortex suggested activation of the motor cortex by a cortico-cortical loop from the auditory cortex. The third assumption would be independent of the stimulus modality and would rely on an intermediate pathological startle to a surprising and sudden stimulus. Activation of the muscle and joint receptors by the startle would activate the lemniscal pathway, which would project to the hyperexcitable motor cortex, either directly or indirectly, through the S1 cortex. This is supported by physiological evidence of short latency proprioceptive responses recorded in monkey motor cortex (Rosen & Asanuma, 1972) and anatomical evidence of connections between S1 and the motor cortex (Jones & Powell, 1968).

To summarize, despite their homogeneous clinical and EEG presentation, several mechanisms can explain the triggering of startle seizures in different cases. However, the third mechanism, involving an intermediate pathological startle, would be most often responsible and would explain why, in some patients, stimuli of different modalities are equally effective. Alajouanine & Gastaut (1955, 1958) had already postulated that seizures induced by auditory and somaesthetic stimulation followed an identical mechanism.

Treatment

There is no single antiepileptic drug of choice. Various authors reported that clobazam was remarkably effective (Tinuper et al., 1986; Gimenez-Roldan & Martin, 1979) as was lamotrigine (Faught, 1999).

Surgery can be effective in medically intractable cases. Cortical resection and callosotomy have each been performed for intractable startle seizures. Fronto-parietal resection has a high rate of success in hemiplegic patients (Chauvel et al., 1987; Oguni et al., 1998). It requires presurgical intracerebral recordings to determine the limits of the resection, but the Rolandic cortex and the SMA must always be removed. This does not increase the neurological deficit. Postoperatively there is usually reduction of spasticity, thus improving functional capacities of the patients. Failures are either due to an insufficiently wide resection, or to a contralateral epileptogenic focus.

If motor deficit is mild or absent, callosotomy can be considered. In this case, a lateralized and fronto-parietal epileptogenic focus and unilateral atrophic lesion predict a good postsurgical outcome (Purves et al., 1988).

Epilepsy with seizures provoked by movement

Seizures induced by voluntary or passive movements have been reported for a long time but are rare. Thus, Gowers (1901), Spiller (1917), Wilson (1930) and Cooper (1933) described seizures provoked by a voluntary and usually abrupt movement. Seizures provoked by movement may be confused with paroxysmal kinesigenic dyskinesias (PKDs). PKDs are attacks of dystonic movement or of movements mixing dystonic, choreic and ballic signs, lasting from a few seconds to 2 minutes in most cases and rarely up to several hours in a few. The attacks are induced by an abrupt movement after a period of rest. The interictal EEG is normal. Standard antiepileptic drugs such as phenytoin and carbamazepine are effective, often in low doses (Kertesz, 1967; Demirkiran & Jankovic, 1995; Revol et al., 1989). The possible epileptic nature of these attacks is still discussed (Loiseau & Duche, 1989), but such events were reported as reflex seizures in the past (Burger et al., 1972; Fukayama et al., 1967). PKDs are now usually considered as non-epileptic dyskinesias of subcortical origin because of the type of motor activity, the normal EEG, the preservation of consciousness and the lack of postictal deficit (Demirkiran & Jankovic, 1995). None of these characteristics is specific of the diagnosis on its own; each one can be observed individually in epilepsy (Beaumanoir et al., 1996; Vignal et al., 1998). However, taken together, these characteristics, and especially the normal ictal and postictal EEG, are against a diagnosis of partial seizures and make it necessary to hypothesize a different mechanism (Revol et al., 1989).

Gastaut & Tassinari (1966) classified epileptic seizures induced by movement as a subtype of startle epilepsy. They considered that startle was the result of proprioceptive afferent stimulus elicited by sudden activation of the muscles. They also pointed out that pure proprioceptive stimulation could sometimes induce startle seizures.

Description of the movement

The effective trigger movements are very variable from one subject to another: catching one's foot on an obstacle, starting to walk, putting on a shirt, extending a leg, handling a pen, or striking a tendon can elicit a seizure (Gowers, 1885; Lishman et al., 1962; Falconer et al., 1963; Whitty et al., 1964; Gabor, 1973; Kochen,1989; Pirelli et al., 1997; Vignal et al., 1998). Thus the trigger movement can be voluntary or passive, single or repetitive, simple or complex, and can involve one or several joints.

However, in spite of this great variability three points must be emphasized:
- the articular and muscular group activated to provoke the seizures is always the same for a given patient;
- the movement does not have to be sudden or surprising to provoke a seizure;
- the seizures induced by a single and often sudden movement must be distinguished from the seizures induced by repetitive movements.

Cutaneous stimulation near the activated muscle and joint may be necessary, in association with the proprioceptive stimulus, to elicit a seizure (Vignal et al., 1992). Gabor (1974) reported seizures induced by the thought of initiating movement.

Description of the seizures

Seizures induced by movement begin with somatosensory or somatomotor signs. Sensory symptoms initially involve the skin close to the musculo-articular group that provokes the seizures, and often progress in a Jacksonian march. They are followed by tonic motor signs that begin in the same territory and vary in extent among patients. Speech arrest is frequent, but consciousness is preserved. The reflex seizures can begin with motor signs, usually tonic, involving the limb whose movement provoked the seizure. The progression of motor signs is also variable. Secondary generalization is uncommon (Lishman et al., 1962; Falconer et al., 1963; Whitty et al., 1964; Santiago et al., 1989; Pirelli et al., 1997; Vignal et al., 1998). Seizures beginning with myoclonus (Kochen, 1989), and atonic seizures (Oller-Daurella & Oller Ferrer-Vidal, 1989) have also been reported. All patients can have spontaneous seizures clinically similar to their reflex seizures.

Mechanism

Understanding the mechanism triggering these seizures depends on the hypothesized localization of the epileptogenic cortex. This can be determined from electroclinical studies, and occasionally, from the localization of a lesion. The existence of a hyperexcitable sensorimotor cortex is inferred from the ictal behaviour and from the localization of ictal EEG discharge and interictal paroxysmal activity (Santiago et al., 1989; Vignal et al., 1998). The role of the SMA (Gabor, 1974; Pirelli et al., 1997) is inferred only from the ictal semiology. The observation reported by Falconer et al. (1963) does not permit precise localization of the hyperexcitable cortex.

Two mechanisms can therefore be discussed based on these approaches. First, the seizures could be triggered by the projection of proprioceptive afferents to the sensorimotor cortex. Several studies support this mechanism: Vignal et al. (1998) reported a surface EEG observation of short-lasting rapid discharge over the central area, triggered by movement of the arm. Chauvel et al. (1978) demonstrated the role of proprioceptive afferents in motor seizures triggered by active or passive movement of the limb when the relevant cortical representation is lesioned and made hyperexcitable (see also Lamarche et al., 1978; Gioanni et al., 1981; Gioanni et al., 1983). Thus the seizures can be caused by projection of proprioceptive afferents, either to the primary sensory cortex responsible for somatosensory-onset seizures, or directly to the motor cortex responsible for tonic-onset motor seizures.

Second, seizures could result from activation of a motor program stored in the SMA, and would be initiated and organized from the SMA (Gabor, 1974; Pierelli et al., 1997). In his case report, Gabor dismisses the role of proprioceptive afferent activation because in that patient, seizures could be provoked by pure mental imaging of an arm movement after anaesthesia of the brachial plexus.

Eating seizures

Seizures induced by eating for which the effective stimulus is chewing or movement of the jaws, can be related to seizures provoked by movement. Seizures induced by eating are heterogeneous and include seizures of temporal and extratemporal origin, and seizures triggered by several different stimuli (Rémillard et al., 1998). However in some cases, the effective stimulus seems to be movement of the jaws. The seizures then combine sensorimotor signs of the orofacial and pharyngeal regions with salivation, and deviation of the head, consistent with origin in the opercular Rolandic cortex. Therefore a role for the proprioceptive afferent projections to the opercular cortex has been proposed (Loiseau et al., 1986; Rémillard et al., 1998; Biraben et al., 1999).

Epilepsy with seizures triggered by cutaneous stimulation

Epilepsies with seizures provoked by cutaneous stimulation are closely related to the epilepsies of movement. Coactivation by a movement and a cutaneous stimulus can also occur.

Description of the stimulus

The effective cutaneous stimulus can be a touch, a jolt, a massage, a caress, etc. Some patients are sensitive to a single stimulation and others require repetition of the stimulus. The cutaneous trigger zone is always the same for a given patient but is variable from one patient to another. The stimulus may first provoke paraesthesias, at the site of stimulation. These can also occur spontaneously. These sensory hallucinations are seizures associated with brief but repetitive fast activity recorded in the primary sensory cortex (Vignal et al., 1998). Unlike in startle epilepsy, the stimulus does not have to be surprising to be effective, although Forster et al. (1949) reported seizures induced by a sudden blow without trigger zone or initial dysaesthesia. Goldie & Green (1959) reported a patient with a parietal angioma and seizures induced by rubbing the right side of the face or by the thought of rubbing it. These seizures began with paraesthesias of the left face and left arm.

Description of the seizures

These reflex seizures begin with dysaesthesia or motor signs. Sensory symptoms, such as a feeling of pins and needles, begin in the stimulated area. These may remain localized or extend in a Jacksonian march. Then tonic motor signs begin near the dysaesthetic area. These may remain localized or spread to an arm and leg, even involving all four limbs, the face and the axial muscles. The attacks often end with clonic jerks. Seizures may also begin with localized tonic signs (Vignal et al., 1998). There is no alteration of consciousness and secondary generalization is rare. Speech arrest is frequent.

Two clinical patterns should be distinguished from these observations:
- reflex seizures with initial somatosensory symptoms, provoked by progressive or repeated stimulation of a trigger zone. The patient can often induce these attacks;
- reflex seizures with initial tonic motor signs, triggered by a single and often surprising cutaneous stimulation such as a jolt.

Spontaneous seizures are always possible and clinically similar to the reflex seizures.

Seizures provoked by brushing the teeth

Holmes *et al.* (1982), and O' Brien *et al.* (1996) described seizures triggered by brushing the teeth. Initial symptoms are facial dysaesthesia followed by facial motor signs, salivation and head deviation. We include these among the reflex seizures triggered by repeated sensory stimulation (brushing) applied to a trigger zone (the gums).

Mechanisms

The nature of the stimulus, the existence of a trigger zone, and the initial somatosensory symptoms suggest a localized hyperexcitability of the primary sensory cortex. This is supported by intracerebral studies that localize the origin of the seizures in the postcentral gyrus (Penfield & Erickson, 1941; Forster *et al.*, 1949; Vignal *et al.*, 1998). However, origin in the motor cortex cannot be excluded when the seizures begin with somatomotor signs. Most probably, seizures are provoked by sensory afferents, projecting directly to primary sensory cortex or to motor cortex. This is supported by the demonstration of giant evoked potentials or giant potentials with a short discharge of fast activity in the postcentral gyrus triggered by tapping the trigger zone (Forster *et al.*, 1949; Vignal *et al.*, 1998).

Reading epilepsy

The purpose of this paragraph is not to describe the reading epilepsies (Wolf, 1992; Koutroumanidis *et al.*, 1998), but to discuss the evidence for frontal lobe involvement in the organization of reading-induced seizures. In 1956, Bickford *et al.* first reported seizures induced by reading in eight patients. They distinguished two groups of reading epilepsies: primary reading epilepsy, with seizures consisting of jaw myoclonus only during reading, possibly followed by secondary generalization; and secondary reading epilepsy with seizures which may occur in other circumstances. The electroclinical characteristics are heterogeneous and many mechanisms have been proposed for these seizures. These can be classified in three groups:

- two proprioceptive mechanisms: the seizures would be induced by proprioceptive afferent projections to the motor cortex. This proprioceptive bombardment of the motor cortex would result from movement of the jaws (Bickford *et al.*, 1956) or from ocular movements or saccades (Stevens *et al.*, 1957);
- a visual mechanism: Bingel (1957) suggested that visual interruptions caused by ocular saccades were equivalent to an intermittent light stimulation;
- cognitive mechanisms: either reading seizures are included in a more global disorder of language in which seizures can also be precipitated by writing and speaking (Geschwind & Sherwin, 1967), or reading seizures remain the only manifestation of a limited disorder involving grapheme to phoneme transformation (Stella *et al.*, 1983; Zagury *et al.*, 1989), or related to complexity of the text.

Thus, Bickford *et al.* (1956) postulated a frontal lobe hyperexcitability in primary reading epilepsy. This proprioceptive hypothesis was reviewed and modified by Radhakrishnan *et al.* (1995) to explain the EEG discordance and the heterogeneous characteristics of effective stimuli. These authors made a parallel between myoclonus of the jaw, and cortical and reticular reflex myoclonus. They postulated variable combinations of localized motor cortex hyperexcitability and cortico-reticular hyperexcitability. Koutroumanidis *et al.* (1998) classified reading seizures in two groups: partial reading epilepsies, and myoclonic reading epilepsies. In partial reading epilepsies, seizures would originate from the left posterior or temporo-occipital regions. They discussed a cortical and subcortical neural network for reading and postulated that reading seizures are the result of a global or partial hyperexcitability of this network. They suggested that the myoclonic reading seizures would result from a localized, bilateral and synchronous activation of the opercular motor cortex. Based on this, certain reading epilepsies must be considered as frontal lobe epilepsies. Ritaccio *et al.* (1992) reported a case of reading epilepsy that is incontestably an epilepsy of the frontal lobe. However, this observation is atypical because it was a symptomatic epilepsy with a localized frontal vascular malformation. The EEG showed left frontal spikes during reading. These authors hypothesized a cortical reflex myoclonus with a left premotor origin. They suggested that this reflex myoclonus was not triggered by proprioceptive projections to the motor cortex or SMA, but by a more complex mechanism related to grapheme to phoneme transformation.

References

Aguglia, U., Tinuper, P. & Gastaut, H. (1984): Startle-induced epileptic seizures. *Epilepsia* **25**, 712–720.

Alajouanine, T. & Gastaut, H. (1955): La syncinésie-sursaut et l'épilepsie-sursaut à déclenchement sensoriel ou sensitif inopiné. *Rev. Neurol.* **93**, 29–41.

Alajouanine, T. & Gastaut, H. (1958): La syncinésie-sursaut et l'épilepsie-sursaut à déclenchement sensoriel ou sensitif inopiné : considérations sur les épilepsies dites 'réflexes'. In: *Bases physiologiques et aspects cliniques de l'épilepsie*, pp. 199–231. Paris: Masson.

Alajouanine, T. & Scherrer, J. (1952): Sur une syncinésie-sursaut déclenchée par le bruit. *C. R. Acad. Sci.* **234**, 2008–2010.

Ascher P. (1965): *La réaction de sursaut du chat anesthésié au chloralose*. Paris: Thèse Doctorat Science.

Bancaud, J., Talairach, J. & Bonis, A. (1967): Physiopathologie des épilepsies-sursaut (à propos d'une épilepsie de l'AMS). *Rev. Neurol.* **3**, 441–453.

Bancaud, J., Talairach, J., Lamarche, M., Bonis, A. & Trottier, S. (1975): Hypothèses neurophysiopathologiques sur l'épilepsie-sursaut chez l'homme. *Rev. Neurol.* **8**, 559–571.

Beaumanoir, A., Mira, L. & van Lierde, A. (1996): Epilepsy or paroxysmal kinesigenic choreoathetosis. *Brain Dev.* **18**, 139–141.

Bickford, R.G., Whelan, J.L., Klass, D.W. & Corbin, K.B. (1956): Reading epilepsy: clinical and electroencephalographic studies of a new syndrome. *Trans Am. Neurol. Assoc.* **81**, 100–102.

Bingel, A. (1957): Reading epilepsy. *Neurology* **7**, 752–756.

Biraben, A., Scarabin, J.M., de Toffol, B., Vignal, J.P. & Chauvel, P. (1999): Opercular reflex seizures: a case report with stereo-electroencephalographic demonstration. *Epilepsia* **40**, 655–663.

Burger, L.J., Lopez, R.I. & Elliot, F.A. (1972): Tonic seizures induced by movement. *Neurology* **22**, 656–659.

Chauvel, P., Louvel, J. & Lamarche, M. (1978): Transcortical reflexes and focal motor epilepsy. *EEG Clin. Neurophysiol.* **45**, 309–318.

Chauvel, P., Vignal, J.P., Liegeois-Chauvel, C., Chodkiewicz, J.P., Talairach, J. & Bancaud, J. (1987). Startle epilepsy with infantile brain damage: the clinical and neurophysiological rationale for surgery. In: *Presurgical evaluation of epileptics*, eds. H.G. Wieser & C.E. Elger, pp. 306–307. Berlin, Heidelberg: Springer-Verlag.

Chauvel, P., Trottier, S., Vignal, J.P. & Bancaud, J. (1992): Somatomotor seizures of frontal lobe origin. In: *Frontal lobe seizures and epilepsies*, eds. P. Chauvel, A.V. Delgado-Escueta, E. Halgren, J. Bancaud, pp. 185–232. *Advances in Neurology*, vol. 57. New York: Raven Press.

Demirkiran, M. & Jankovic, J. (1995): Paroxysmal dyskinesias: clinical features and classification. *Ann. Neurol.* **38**, 571–579.

Falconer, M.A., Driver, M.V. & Serafetinides, E.A. (1963): Seizures induced by movement. Report of case relieved by operation. *J. Neurol. Neurosurg. Psychiatry* **26**, 300–307.

Faught E. (1999): Lamotrigine for startle-induced seizures. *Seizure* **8**, 361–363.

Forster, F.M., Penfield, W., Jasper, H. & Madow, L. (1949): Focal epilepsy, sensory precipitation and evoked cortical potentials. *EEG Clin. Neurophysiol.* **1**, 349–356.

Fukuyama, S. & Okada, R. (1967): Hereditary kinesigenic reflex epilepsy. Report of five families of peculiar seizures induced by sudden movements. *Adv. Neurol. Sci.* **11**, 168–197.

Gabor, A.J. (1974): Focal seizures induced by movement without sensory feedback mechanisms. *EEG Clin. Neurophysiol.* **36**, 403–408.

Gastaut, Y. (1953): Les pointes négatives évoquées sur le vertex, leur signification psychophysiologique et pathologique. *Rev. Neurol.* **89**, 382–399.

Gastaut, H. & Tassinari, C.A. (1966): Triggering mechanisms in epilepsy. The electroclinical point of view. *Epilepsia* **7**, 85–138.

Geschwind, N. & Sherwin, I. (1967): Language-induced epilepsy. *Arch. Neurol.* **16**, 25–31.

Gimenez-Roldan, S. & Martin, M. (1979): Effectiveness of clonazepam in startle-induced seizures. *Epilepsia* **20**, 555–561.

Gioanni, Y., Lamarche, M., Chauvel, P. & Encabo, H. (1981): Réflexes transcorticaux d'origine proprioceptive et épilepsie motrice. *Rev. EEG Neurophysiol.* **11**, 317–323.

Gioanni, Y., Everett, J. & Lamarche, M. (1983): The transcortical reflex triggered by cutaneous or muscle stimulation in the cat with a penicillin epileptic focus: relative importance of regions 3a and 4. *Expl. Brain Res.* **51**, 57–64.

Goldie, L. & Green, J.A. (1959): A study of the psychological factors in a case of sensory reflex epilepsy. *Brain* **82**, 505–524.

Gowers, W.R. (1901): *Epilepsy and other chronic convulsive diseases: their causes, symptoms and treatment*. London: J&A Churchill.

Guerrini, R., Genton, P., Bureau, M., Dravet, C. & Roger, J. (1990): Reflex seizures are frequent in patients with Down syndrome and epilepsy. *Epilepsia* **31**, 406–417.

Holmes, G.L., Blair, S., Eisenberg, E., Scheebaum, R., Margraf, J. & Zimmerman, A.W. (1982): Tooth-brushing-induced epilepsy. *Epilepsia* **23**, 657–661.

Jones, E.G. & Powell, T.P.S. (1968): The ipsilateral cortical connexions of the somatic sensory areas in the cat. *Brain Res.* **9**, 71–94.

Kertesz, A. (1970): Paroxysmal kinesigenic choreoathetosis: an entity within the paroxysmal choreoathetosis syndrome: description of 10 cases, including 1 autopsied. *Neurology* **17**, 680–690.

Kochen, S. (1989): Reflex epilepsy induced by movement. A case report. In: *Reflex seizures and reflex epilepsies*, eds. A. Beaumanoir, H. Gastaut & R. Naquet, pp. 115–117. Genève: Éditions Médecine et Hygiène.

Koutroumanidis, M., Koepp, M.J., Richardson, M.P., Camfield, C., Agathonikou, A., Ried, S., Papadimitriou, A., Plant, G.T., Duncan, J.S. & Panayiotopoulos, C.P. (1998): The variants of reading epilepsy. A clinical and video-EEG study of 17 patients with reading induced seizures. *Brain* **121**, 1409–1427.

Lamarche, M. & Chauvel, P. (1978): Movement epilepsy in the monkey with an experimental motor focus. *EEG Clin. Neurophysiol (Suppl.)* **34**, 323–328.

Lamarche, M. & Vignal, J.P. (2000): Boucle transcorticale réflexe et ses implications en épileptologie. *Epileptic Disord* **2** (special issue 1), 25–44.

Liégeois-Chauvel, C., Morin, C., Musolino, A., Bancaud, J. & Chauvel, P. (1989): Evidence for a contribution of auditory cortex to audiospinal facilitation in man. *Brain* **112**, 375–301.

Lishman, W.A., Symonds, C.P., Whitty, C.W.H. & Willison, R.G. (1962): Seizures induced by movement. *Brain* **85**, 93–108.

Loiseau, P. & Duche, B. (1989): Seizures induced by movement. In: *Reflex seizures and reflex epilepsies*, eds. A. Beaumanoir, H. Gastaut & R. Naquet, pp. 109–114. Genève: Éditions Médecine et Hygiène.

Loiseau, P., Guyot, M., Loiseau, H., Rougier, A. & Desbordes, P. (1986): Eating seizures. *Epilepsia* **27**, 161–163.

Manford, M.R.A., Fish, D.R. & Shorvon, S.D. (1996): Startle-provoked epileptic seizures: features in 19 patients. *J. Neurol. Neurosurg. Psychiatry* **61**, 151–156.

Nakamura, M., Kanai, H. & Miyamoto, Y. (1975): A case of Sturge-Weber syndrome with startle epilepsy. *Brain Nerve* **27**, 325–329.

O'Brien, T.J., Hogan, R.E., Sedal, L., Murrie, V. & Cook, M.J. (1996): Toothbrushing epilepsy: a report of a case with structural and functional imaging and electrophysiology demonstrating a right frontal focus. *Epilepsia* **37**, 694–697.

Oguni, H., Hayashi, K., Usui, N., Osawa, M. & Shimizu, H. (1998): Startle epilepsy with infantile hemiplegia: reports of two cases improved by surgery. *Epilepsia* **39**, 93–98.

Oller-Daurella, L. & Oller Ferrer-Vidal, F. (1989): Seizures induced by voluntary movements In: *Reflex seizures and reflex epilepsies*, eds. A. Beaumanoir, H. Gastaut & R. Naquet, pp. 139–146. Genève: Éditions Médecine et Hygiène.

Palmer, E. & Ashby, P. (1992): Evidence that a long latency stretch reflex in humans is transcortical. *J. Physiol.* **449**, 429–440.

Penfield, W. & Erickson, T.C. (1941): *Epilepsy and cerebral localization*, pp. 27–28. Springfield, IL: Charles C. Thomas.

Pierelli, F., Di Gennaro, G., Gherardi, M., Spanedda, F. & Marciani, M.G. (1997): Movement-induced seizures: a case report. *Epilepsia* **38**, 941–944.

Purves, S.J., Wada, J.A., Woodhurst, W.B., Moyes, P.D., Strauss, E., Kosaka, B. & Li, D. (1988): Results of anterior corpus callosum section in 24 patients with medically intractable seizures. *Neurology* **38**, 1194–1201.

Radhakrishnan, K., Silbert, P.L. & Klass, D.W. (1995): Reading epilepsy. An appraisal of 20 patients diagnosed at the Mayo Clinic, Rochester, Minnesota, between 1949 and 1989, and delineation of the epileptic syndrome. *Brain* **118**, 75–89.

Rémillard, G.M., Zifkin, B.G. & Andermann, F. (1998): Seizures induced by eating. In: *Reflex epilepsies and reflex seizures*, eds. B.G. Zifkin, F. Andermann, A. Beaumanoir & A.J. Rowan, pp. 227–240, *Advances in Neurology*, vol. 75. Philadelphia: Lippincott-Raven.

Revol, M., Moreau, T., Isnard, H., Gilly, R. & Langue, J. (1989): Report of five cases and review of the literature. In: *Reflex seizures and reflex epilepsies*, eds. A. Beaumanoir, H. Gastaut & R. Naquet, pp. 131–138. Genève: Éditions Médecine et Hygiène.

Ritaccio, A.L., Hickling, E.J. & Ramani, V. (1992): The role of dominant premotor cortex and grapheme to phoneme transformation in reading epilepsy: a neuroanatomic, neurophysiologic, and neuropsychological study. *Arch. Neurol.* **49**, 933–939.

Rosen, I. & Asanuma, H. (1972): Peripheral afferent inputs to the forelimb area of the monkey motor cortex: input-output relations. *Exp. Brain Res.* **14**, 257–273.

Santiago, M., Sampaio, M.J.F. & Keating, J. (1989): Movement-induced epilepsy: a study of 2 cases. In: *Reflex seizures and reflex epilepsies*, eds. A. Beaumanoir, H. Gastaut & R. Naquet, pp. 147–148. Genève: Éditions Médecine et Hygiène.

Shimamura, M. (1973): Neural mechanisms of startle reflex in cerebral palsy, with special reference to its relationship with spino-bulbo-spinal reflexes. In: *New developments in electromyography and clinical neurophysiology: human reflexes, pathophysiology of motor systems, methodology of human reflexes*, ed. J.E. Desmedt, pp. 761–766. Basel: Kruger.

Spiller, W.G. (1927): Subcortical epilepsy. *Brain* **50**, 171–187.

Stella, L., Fels, A., Pillo, G., Fragassi, N., Buscaino, G.A. & Striano, S. (1983): Primary reading epilepsy. Clinical and EEG study of a case and characteristics of the effective stimulus. *Acta Neurol. Napoli* **5**, 426–431.

Stevens, H. (1957): Reading epilepsy. *N. Engl. J. Med.* **257**, 165–170.

Tanji, J. & Kurata, K. (1983): Functional organization of supplementary motor area. In: *Motor control mechanisms in health and disease*, ed. J.E. Desmedt, pp. 393–420. New York: Raven Press.

Tinuper, P., Aguglia, U. & Gastaut, H. (1986): Use of clobazam in certain forms of status epilepticus in startle epileptic seizures. *Epilepsia* **27**, Suppl. 1, 18–26.

Vignal, J.P. (1984): *Epilepsie-sursaut. Sémiologie critique et aspect physiopathologique*. Paris: Thèse Doctorat Médecine.

Vignal, J.P., Biraben, A., Chauvel, P. & Reutens, D.C. (1998): Reflex partial seizures of sensorimotor cortex (including cortical reflex myoclonus and startle epilepsy). In: *Reflex epilepsies and reflex seizures*, eds. B.G. Zifkin, F. Andermann, A. Beaumanoir & A.J. Rowan, pp. 207–226. *Advances in Neurology*., vol. 75. Philadelphia: Lippincott-Raven.

Wiesendanger, M., Seguin, J.J. & Kunzle, H. (1973): The supplementary motor area: a control system for a posture? In: *Control of posture and locomotion*, pp. 331–346. New York: Plenum.

Whitty, C.W.M., Lishman, W.A. & Fitzgibbon, J.P. (1964): Seizures induced by movement: a form of reflex epilepsy. *Lancet* **1**, 1043–1045.

Wilkins, D.E., Hallet, M. & Wess, M.M. (1986): Audiogenic startle reflex of man and its relationship to startle syndromes. A review. *Brain* **109**, 561–573.

Wilson, S.A.K. (1930): Nervous semiology with special reference to epilepsy. *Br. Med. J.* **2**, 53–90.

Wolf, P. (1992): L'épilepsie à la lecture. In: *Les syndromes épileptiques de l'enfant et de l'adolescent*, eds. J. Roger, M. Bureau, C. Dravet, F.E. Dreifuss, A. Perret & P. Wolf, pp. 281–298. London: John Libbey & Company.

Zagury, S., Daniele, O. & Salas-Puig, J. (1989): Primary reading epilepsy. In: *Reflex seizures and reflex epilepsies*, eds. A. Beaumanoir, H. Gastaut & R. Naquet, pp. 275–282. Genève: Éditions Médecine et Hygiène.

Chapter 11

Frontal lobe epilepsy in infancy

Olivier Dulac, Jean-Paul Rathgeb and Perrine Plouin

Paediatric Clinic, Neuropediatrics Service, Saint-Vincent-de-Paul Hospital, 74-82, avenue Denfert-Rochereau, 75674 Paris, France

Summary

Frontal lobe seizures in infancy are clinically similar to those occurring later in life, though less elaborate. Some infants also have infantile spasms, or a combination of focal discharge and a cluster of spasms within the same seizure. Various causes, particularly malformations, are implicated in these more complex forms. Cases without evidence of a brain lesion occur; it is among these patients that the unusual condition of migrating partial seizures is encountered. In contrast, no case of infantile frontal lobe epilepsy is on record with a benign outcome. The role of maturation is critical to explain poor outcome in patients with lesions affecting the frontal lobe and involving other areas of the brain.

Partial epilepsy has long been known, but has been recognized in infancy for no more than 20 years (Duchowny *et al.*, 1987; Luna *et al.*, 1987), and the relations between semiology and the location of the epileptic discharge remain poorly investigated. Very few infants with focal epilepsy investigated with video-EEG in the first months of the disease undergo cortical resection. Therefore, there are few opportunities to correlate the semiology to the topography of the ictal discharge. Epilepsy in infants has various causes, distinct from epilepsy in adults. This chapter will address the issues of semiology and aetiology in infants, based on published and personal, unpublished data.

Seizure semiology

This study was based on frame by frame study of split screen video-EEG recordings. Several seizures could be recorded in each individual.

Patients with purely frontal lobe discharge

Two seizure patterns could be identified in infants with purely frontal discharge. The first began with arrest of activity and continued with hypertonia and pedalling movements of all four limbs. This was followed either by slow rhythmic clonic movements of the head and eyelids with lateral deviation of the head and eyes, or by slow rhythmic clonic movements of the whole body, thus quite distinct from the clonic phase of a tonic-clonic seizure. There was no evidence of loss of consciousness and no post-ictal phase. The seizures lasted from half a minute to two minutes. In the second type, there was initially only arrest of activity, with no movement of the limbs, followed by jerks of the eyelids or automatisms of the hands. Again, there was no evidence of loss of consciousness and the seizures were very brief with no post-ictal phase.

Seizures in which there is a combination of a frontal lobe discharge with spasms in clusters

The combination of a focal discharge with a cluster of spasms is now well recognized. This may occur in infants with West syndrome and frontal lobe involvement. In these cases, the focal discharge may precede the onset of the spasms, coincide with the first spasm, or follow the cluster. Although the clinical seizure pattern combined with the focal discharge in these cases has the same characteristics as described earlier for patients with isolated frontal lobe discharges, arrest of activity is the major component of the seizure, and focal EEG discharge is the only feature confirming frontal lobe involvement.

Seizures in infants with other types of focal seizure and frontal lobe discharges

In infants with other types of focal seizures, seizures related to frontal lobe discharge are mainly characterized by unilateral hypertonia of upper and lower limbs (Coppola *et al.*, 1996). These frontal lobe seizures are also usually brief but the precise mode of onset is difficult to identify because very frequent seizures involving other areas of the brain are combined with the frontal lobe discharges. Similarly, the post-ictal phase is difficult to evaluate. These infants are markedly hypotonic and make poor eye contact.

Types of epilepsy affecting the frontal lobe in infancy

Focal epilepsy of the frontal lobe

Five infants in our series had frontal lobe seizures only. As in older children, seizures are frequent, occurring several times a day. However, the relation with sleep is not clear.

Cortical malformation is the major cause of frontal lobe epilepsy in infants. Some patients with cortical malformation and very early seizure onset begin with frontal lobe seizures, but then go on to have spasms in clusters, and later focal frontal lobe seizures. In our experience, patients treated with vigabatrin from the first seizures occurring very early in life do not develop infantile spasms at the usual age for this syndrome, although they may continue to have focal seizures. In other instances, onset is later with a combination of spasms and frontal lobe seizures. In patients with other kinds of lesion, tumours or pre- or post-natal, mainly destructive lesions, and for those with ring chromosome 20, onset of epilepsy is usually later, after the age of 3 years.

Neuroimaging shows no brain lesion in some cases and the cause remains unknown. We could find no personal or reported case with family history suggestive of familial nocturnal frontal lobe epilepsy starting in infancy, and no case of benign partial epilepsy in infancy affecting the frontal lobe.

Frontal lobe epilepsy combined with West syndrome

Onset in these patients is usually with spasms in clusters, but focal seizures may precede the occurrence of spasms in clusters. Monitoring shows that the seizure consists of a combination of a focal discharge with the series of spasms (Bour *et al.*, 1986). In addition, 24-hour recordings can show that these patients have focal discharges in addition to clusters of spasms (Plouin *et al.*, 1993).

Lesions in these patients are either destructive, due to a prenatal more often than perinatal cause, or dysplastic, such as cortical dysplasia or porencephaly with microgyria. The age at seizure onset for patients with West syndrome combined with a focal brain lesion has been shown to be later for those with frontal lesions than for those with occipital lesions (Koo & Hwang, 1996). In some patients, frontal lobe involvement in seizures occurs several months after seizure onset in other parts of the brain, particularly in occipital areas. This is especially so in tuberous sclerosis, as tubers in the posterior areas may become epileptogenic earlier than those in the frontal lobe. The combination of frontal and posterior tubers increases the risk of the epilepsy becoming intractable (Jambaqué *et al.*, 1991). However, such age-dependency does not seem to apply to patients with focal cortical dysplasia (Lortie *et al.*, 2002).

Patients with porencephaly usually develop infantile spasms as the first seizure type. Outcome depends on the extent of the lesion, with more favourable outcome for a lesion involving only the occipital or Rolandic areas, whereas frontal involvement is more likely to produce persisting infantile spasms (Cusmai *et al.*, 1988).

Migrating partial seizures in infancy

This is a rare and still poorly understood condition (Coppola *et al.*, 1996). It begins in the first 6 months of life, with a peak around 4 months, and is rarely present at birth. Focal seizures first occur every week or so in infants with no evidence of previous psychomotor retardation, although it is difficult to be sure of normal development in such young infants. The first seizures involve occipital or temporal areas, not the frontal lobes. After a few weeks, four on average, seizure frequency increases. Seizures occur daily and then nearly continuously. Seizures affect various parts of the brain, one seizure starting before the previous one is over. Thus, there is a very complex semiology that results from the combination of several focal seizures involving distinct parts of the brain at the same moment. Only one patient in our series of 24 cases had clusters of spasms, and there was no major inter-ictal paroxysmal EEG activity in this case. At this stage, the frontal lobes are involved in most cases.

Seizures then occur in clusters lasting from several days to a few weeks during which seizures seem particularly frequent, with severe psychomotor deterioration. Then, seizure frequency decreases for a few days and the child recovers slightly, regaining eye contact and possibly some head control, but the next cluster soon appears with loss of all skills. As time goes on, the seizures tend to become generalized.

The aetiology of this condition is unknown. All neuroradiological, biochemical and chromosomal investigations have been negative, and in two autopsied cases no lesion could be identified except for neuronal depopulation in Ammon's horn that most likely was unrelated to the cause of the epilepsy but followed repeated episodes of ischaemia due to status epilepticus.

Discussion

The frontal lobe may be involved in several different infantile epilepsies, and there can be no such concept as 'frontal lobe epilepsy' at this early age. Frontal lobe involvement includes various conditions. Some are clearly focal and others are both focal and generalized, particularly in West syndrome. In this case, the epilepsy seems to predominate in the frontal lobes although there is diffuse involvement of the brain.

The semiology of frontal lobe seizures becomes progressively more complex. The appearance of new ictal features has been reported with partial seizures, whatever the topography of the discharge (Luna *et al.*, 1987; Nordli *et al.*, 2001). This applies particularly to the frontal lobe and seems to be related to brain development. Although there is a change in the clinical patterns through infancy and childhood, and although semiology is richer in childhood than it is in infancy, the characteristics of frontal lobe seizures are recognizable and quite specific from a very early age. Thus, arrest of activity is often encountered in older patients, including adults. The same applies to lateral deviation of the eyes and head, and to asymmetric tonic motor activity. Thus, the frontal lobes seem to acquire progressively the characteristics that will be those of seizures occurring in adulthood.

Age of onset of infantile spasms seems to be later when the epileptic zone is in the frontal lobes than when it is in the occipital area. The frontal cortex matures later than posterior areas of the brain, and this process begins in the second half of the first year of life, persisting throughout the first decade (Chugani *et al.*, 1986; Chiron *et al.*, 1992). This could explain the longer duration and frequent intractability of epilepsy in patients with frontal lobe porencephaly (Cusmai *et al.*, 1988). In our experience this does not seem to apply to frontal lobe seizures due to dysplasia. The reason is not clear, but involvement of the mesial aspect of the frontal lobe could be one explanation (Lortie *et al.*, 2002). It could also be due to the large size of epileptogenic dysplastic lesions in our series.

Recognition of migrating partial epilepsy is challenging (Coppola *et al.*, 1996). One may be led initially to diagnose a focal epilepsy because in the early stage seizures may be of a single type, before they become migrating several weeks or months later (Gérard *et al.*, 1999). However, in these early cases with frequent and apparently focal seizures, the discharges affect the temporal lobe, not the frontal lobe. Therefore, it is very unlikely that a patient with frontal lobe epilepsy would go on to develop migrating partial epilepsy in infancy.

We could find no benign partial epilepsy affecting the frontal lobe in infancy, although infantile benign partial epilepsy has been shown to affect the Rolandic strip and the temporal lobe (Vigevano *et al.*, 1992; Watanabe *et al.*, 1990).

References

Bour, F., Chiron, C., Dulac, O. & Plouin, P. (1986): Caractéristiques électrocliniques des crises dans le syndrome d'Aicardi. *Rev. Electroencephalogr. Neurophysiol. Clin.* **16**, 341–353.

Chiron, C., Raynaud, C., Mazière, B., Zilbovicius, M., Laflamme, L., Masure, M.C., Dulac, O., Bourguignon, M. & Syrota, A. (1992): Changes in regional cerebral blood flow during brain maturation in children and adolescents. *J. Nucl. Med* **33**, 696–703.

Chugani, H. & Phelps, M.H. (1986): Maturational changes in cerebral function in infants determined by [18]FDG positron emission tomography. *Science* **231**, 840–843.

Coppola, G., Plouin, P., Robain, O., Chiron, C. & Dulac, O. (1995): Migrating partial seizures in infancy: a malignant disorder with developmental arrest. *Epilepsia* **36**, 1017–1024.

Cusmai, R., Dulac, O. & Diebler, C. (1988): Lésions focales dans les spasmes infantiles. *Rev. Electroencephalogr. Neurophysiol. Clin.* **18**, 235–241.

Duchowny, M. (1987): Complex partial seizures of infancy. *Arch. Neurol.* **44**, 911–914.

Dulac, O., Lemaitre, A. & Aubourg, P. (1983): *Épilepsie dans les syndromes neurocutanés. Journées Parisiennes de Pédiatrie*, pp. 77–84. Paris: Masson.

Gérard, F., Kaminska, A., Echenne, B. & Dulac, O. (1999): Focal seizures *vs* focal epilepsy in infancy: a challenging distinction. *Epileptic Disord.* **1**, 135–139.

Jambaqué, I., Cusmai, R., Curatolo, P., Cortesi, F., Pierrot, C. & Dulac, O. (1991): Neuropsychological aspects of tuberous sclerosis: relation to epilepsy and MRI findings. *Dev. Med. Child Neurol.* **33**, 698–705.

Koo, B. & Hwang, P. (1996): Localization of focal cortical lesions influences age of onset of infantile spasms. *Epilepsia* **37**, 1068–1071.

Lortie, A., Plouin, P., Chiron, C., Delalande, O. & Dulac, O. (2002): Focal cortical dysplasia in infancy. *Epilepsy Res.* **51**, 133–145.

Luna, D., Dulac, O. & Plouin, P. (1989): Ictal characteristics of cryptogenic partial epilepsies in infancy. *Epilepsia* **30**, 827–832.

Nordli, D.R., Kuroda, M.M. & Hirsch, L.J. (2001): The ontogeny of partial seizures in infants and young children. Presented at the Amalfi meeting on inborn errors of metabolism and epilepsy in infancy.

Plouin, P., Jalin, C., Dulac, O. & Chiron, C. (1993): Twenty-four-hour ambulatory EEG monitoring in infantile spasms. *Epilepsia* **34**, 686–691.

Vigevano, F., Fusco, L., Di Capua, M., Ricci, S., Sebastianelli, R. & Lucchini, P. (1992): Benign infantile familial convulsions. *Eur. J. Pediatr.* **151**, 608–612.

Watanabe, K., Yamamoto, N., Negoro, T., Takahashi, I., Aso, K. & Maehara, M. (1990): Benign infantile epilepsy with complex partial seizures. *J. Clin. Neurophysiol.* **7**, 406–416.

Chapter 12

Ictal video-EEG features in children with nocturnal frontal lobe seizures

Paolo Tinuper

Department of Neurological Sciences, University of Bologna, via Ugo Foscolo 7, 40123 Bologna, Italy
tinuper@neuro.unibo.it

Summary

Nocturnal frontal lobe epilepsy (NFLE) is a syndrome that includes paroxysmal episodes of different semiology, intensity and duration, representing different aspects of the same epileptic condition. Video-polysomnographic recordings in young patients disclosed four main patterns. *Paroxysmal arousals* are brief simple motor phenomena, similar to sudden arousal, recurring several times per night. *Hypermotor seizures* (previously known as short-lasting nocturnal paroxysmal dystonia) are more complex motor episodes; the violent and often bizarre behaviour, with vocalization, screaming, fearful expression, and repetitive movements of the trunk and limbs resemble orbitofrontal seizures, whereas *asymmetric, bilateral tonic seizures* suggest mesial frontal seizures. In some patients, the seizures can mimic sleepwalking episodes. Because the EEG during these episodes shows continuous epileptiform activity, we named these *epileptic nocturnal wanderings*.

Nocturnal seizures arise from non-REM sleep, are very frequent, and sometimes become quasi-periodic during some portions of sleep. Ictal and interictal EEG, as often happens in frontal epilepsies, can be inconclusive. Video-polygraphic recording of nocturnal episodes is extremely useful in differentiating NFLE seizures from paroxysmal non-epileptic phenomena arising from sleep.

History

In 1981, Lugaresi and Cirignotta first described unusual paroxysmal motor attacks during sleep in otherwise healthy subjects. They labelled this condition nocturnal hypnogenic, and later, nocturnal paroxysmal dystonia (Lugaresi *et al.*, 1986). This has been the subject of many papers by the Bologna school (Tinuper *et al.*, 1990, 1997, 1999, 2002; Montagna *et al.*, 1990; Montagna, 1992; Sforza *et al.*, 1993; Plazzi *et al.*, 1995; Provini *et al.*, 1999, 2000a, b,) and by others (Godbout *et al.*, 1985; Lee *et al.*, 1985; Peled & Lavie, 1986; Berger *et al.*, 1987; Meierkord *et al.*, 1993; Vigevano & Fusco, 1993; Sheffer *et al.*, 1994, 1995; Oldani *et al.*, 1996, 1998; Thomas *et al.*, 1998; Sheffer, 2000). Recently, autosomal dominant inheritance was shown although sporadic cases are common.

Provini *et al.* (1999) reviewed the semiology of the seizures of nocturnal frontal lobe epilepsy (NFLE) in 100 patients. In this series, 70 per cent were males. Age at onset ranged from 1 to 64 years (mean 14 ± 10). A personal history of parasomnias was found in 34 per cent, and at least 40 per cent of cases had at least one first-degree relative with parasomnic episodes. A family history of epilepsy was found in one-quarter of the patients, one-third of them having nocturnal frontal lobe seizures. Seizures were very frequent and almost all of them occurred during non-REM sleep. The seizure pattern was remarkably stereotyped in each patient. Neurological and neuropsychological examinations were normal in 86 per cent of patients. Interictal EEGs were normal in 55 per cent of cases and there were no clear-cut epileptiform discharges in more than half the patients. Carbamazepine proved to be the treatment of choice although it was ineffective in one-third of the patients.

Based on videopolysomnographic recordings of the seizures it is possible to distinguish four main ictal patterns: asymmetric, bilateral tonic seizures, hypermotor seizures, very brief motor seizures (paroxysmal arousals), and prolonged seizures (epileptic wanderings) (Table 1).

Table 1. Seizures in nocturnal frontal lobe epilepsy

Very brief motor seizures
Bilateral and axial involvement resembling a sudden arousal
Opening of the eyes
Sitting up in bed
Sometimes frightened expression
Hypermotor seizures
Body movements that can start in the limbs, head or trunk
Complex, often violent behaviour
Often with a dystonic-dyskinetic component
Sometimes with cycling or rocking or repetitive body movements, prevalent in the trunk or legs
The patient may vocalize, scream or swear
Fear is a frequent expression
Asymmetric, bilateral tonic seizures
Sustained uncustomary forced position
Prolonged seizures
Same beginning as above
Semi-purposeful ambulatory behaviour
Mimicking sleepwalking

Asymmetric, bilateral tonic seizures

In younger children, as described by Vigevano *et al.* (1993), an asymmetric tonic component may be prominent at the beginning of the attacks (Fig. 1) followed, as in adults, by repetitive movements of the limbs and trunk. In some cases, the onset of the seizures may be dramatic, with seizures becoming increasingly frequent and mimicking an acute encephalopathy. In rare cases, seizures can also appear during wakefulness. When seizures occur exclusively during sleep, and particularly if they are elaborate, it may be difficult to distinguish them from parasomnias or physiological movements of sleep. The interictal EEG is often normal; ictal EEG is more often abnormal than in adults, showing clear-cut epileptiform discharges consisting of diffuse or lateralized recruiting fast activity (Fig. 2). In children as in adults, carbamazepine is the most effective drug, but drug-resistant cases also occur, with progressive psychological and behavioural impairment and language disturbances.

Hypermotor seizures (FHS)

These attacks are characterized by a sudden arousal from non-REM sleep followed by complex body movements that can start in the limbs, head, or trunk, often with a dystonic-dyskinetic component. Other motor activity may consist of kicking or bicycling movements of all limbs, or rocking

Chapter 12 Ictal video-EEG features in children with nocturnal frontal lobe seizures

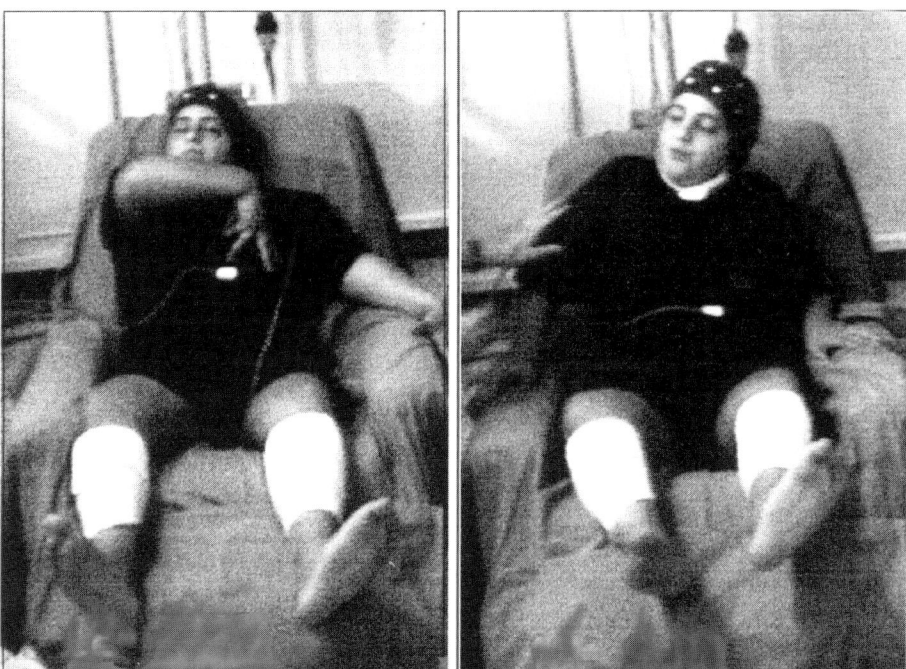

Fig. 1. Asymmetric postural seizure in a 8-year-old child. The tonic contraction is more evident on the right side, with the right arm flexed and adducted. Note the facial grimace and the splaying of the feet.

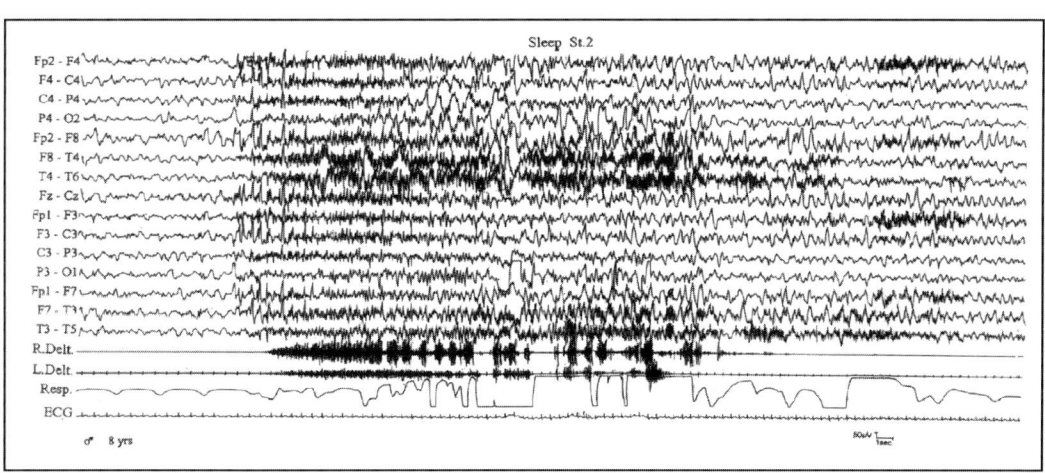

Fig. 2. Ictal EEG during an asymmetric postural seizure in a 8-year-old child. The ictal discharge starts from stage 2 sleep and is characterized by paroxysmal recruiting sharp wave activity predominant over both frontal regions. Polygraphic channels show an asymmetric tonic contraction of the deltoid muscle, more intense on the right. Tachycardia and breathing irregularities are also present.

of the trunk, sometimes with semipurposeful repetitive movements mimicking sexual activity (Fig. 3). The patient may vocalize, scream, or swear. Sometimes the motor activity may be very violent with injury or a fall from bed. Sudden autonomic activation with tachycardia and hypertension accompanies the episodes. Seizures last several seconds and there is no post-ictal confusion.

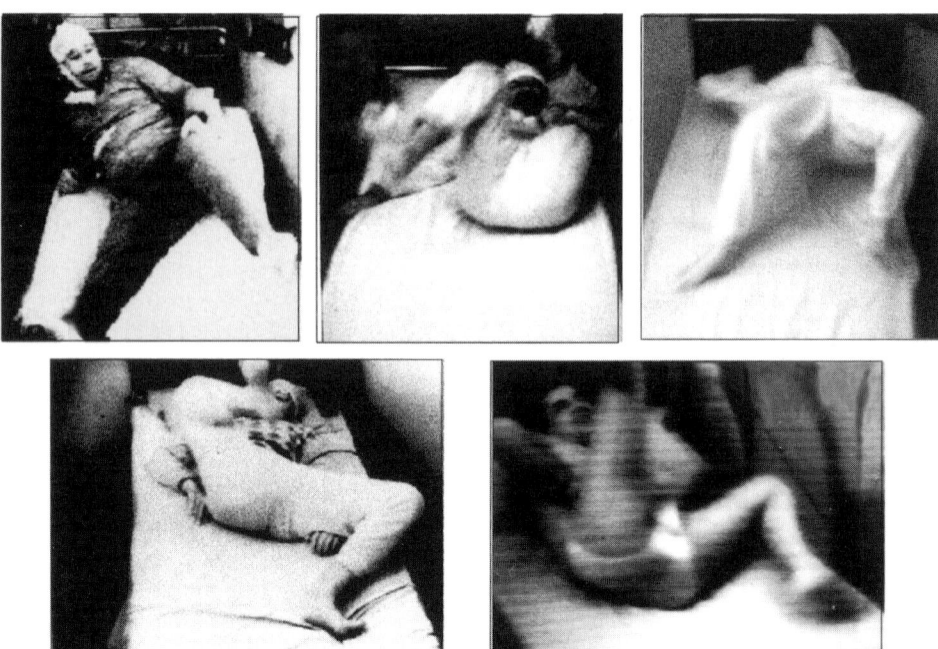

Fig. 3. Five photographs of nocturnal frontal seizures in five different patients. Note the similar movement of the legs that are splayed and flexed in a repetitive cycling movement. There are repetitive movements of the trunk. The patients appear frightened and scream.

If questioned, the patient may or may not recall a motor attack. The seizure pattern is very similar among patients, and in each patient the episodes remain stereotyped without changing during the night or from one night to another. Seizures may recur several times each night; some patients had seizures of different intensity in the same night, representing fragments of the entire attack, recurring in a quasi-periodic sequence for much of sleep (Tinuper *et al.*, 1990; Sforza *et al.*, 1993).

As frequently observed with frontal foci, interictal EEG abnormalities may be scanty, and ictal tracings may be misleading because clear-cut spike and wave activity over the frontal regions is rare and the EEG is often masked by muscle artefact during the event. Polygraphically, the onset of the attack coincides with an abrupt transition from non-REM sleep to wakefulness, often preceded by a K complex. Tachycardia and breathing irregularities are also recorded.

Very brief motor seizures (epileptic arousals – EA)

These attacks, arising from stage 2 sleep, were first described in 1990 (Montagna *et al.*, 1990) and are characterized by a sudden bilateral and axial involvement resembling a sudden arousal. The patient opens his eyes and often sits up in bed with a frightened expression. Some slight dystonic posture or finger movements may occur (Fig. 4), as may a brief vocalization. The attacks are stereotyped in the same patient and, as in the patients with hypermotor seizures, may recur every night and sometimes several times nightly. Seizures are very short, up to 3-5 seconds, and in almost 25 per cent of patients recur periodically every 20-30 seconds for prolonged segments of non-REM sleep. The episode is preceded in the EEG by a K complex; the tracing is partially masked by muscle activity but fast activity or sharp waves may be recorded predominantly over frontal regions.

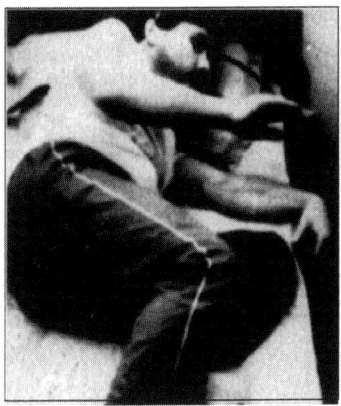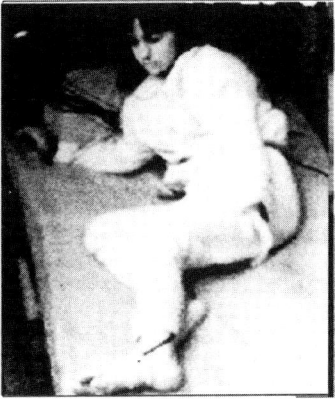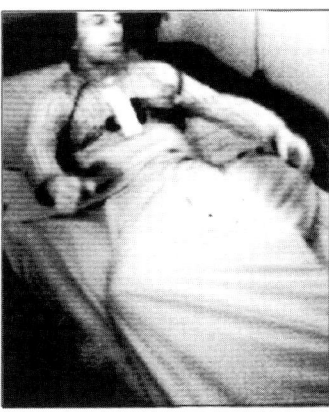

Fig. 4. Abrupt awakening from non-REM sleep in three patients. Note the dystonic posture of the hands and the surprised expression. After this very brief episode the patients returned to sleep. These episodes could recur quasi-periodically for much of non-REM sleep.

Prolonged seizures (epileptic nocturnal wandering – ENW)

These episodes are characterized by the same beginning as those described above, followed by a 1-2 minute period of semipurposeful ambulatory behaviour and complex motor activity mimicking sleepwalking (Fig. 5), a paroxysmal non-epileptic parasomnia. Video-polysomnography in four patients (Plazzi *et al.*, 1995) showed that these were stereotyped and associated with clear-cut EEG epileptiform discharge. These findings differentiate them from sleepwalking. Interictal EEG abnormalities were also present over frontal regions. All our patients with epileptic nocturnal wanderings had typical nocturnal frontal lobe seizures as well.

General clinical features of nocturnal frontal lobe epilepsy (NFLE)

NFLE affects both sexes with a slight male predominance (69 per cent). The attacks usually begin between 14 and 28 years of age, but can occur at any age. Unlike parasomnias, which tend to disappear in the second decade, NFLE seizures tend to increase in frequency. NFLE is frequently cryptogenic; in our population a known aetiology was present in 13 per cent of cases and neuroradiological studies showed abnormalities only in about one-third of patients. In most cases, ictal and interictal EEG did not show clear epileptiform abnormalities. The origin of the epileptic disturbance in the deep frontal regions makes it difficult for scalp EEG recording to detect paroxysmal abnormalities. Thus, a normal EEG does not exclude the diagnosis of NFLE and sphenoidal or supraorbital electrodes may be helpful. Carbamazepine remains the treatment of choice and is sometimes successful at very low doses taken in the evening. However, one-third of patients is resistant to all medications.

NFLE includes several distinct seizure patterns of different intensity, representing a continuum of the same epileptic condition. In our series of NFLE patients, 20 per cent had only typical frontal seizures, 9 per cent had only epileptic arousals, and no patient had only nocturnal wanderings. Six per cent had concomitant episodes of FHS, EA and ENW, and 34 per cent had both episodes of EA and FHS, sometimes during the same night (Fig. 6).

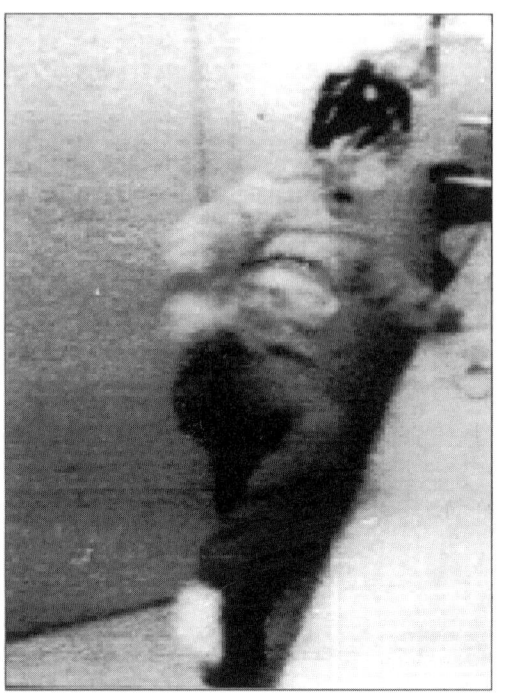 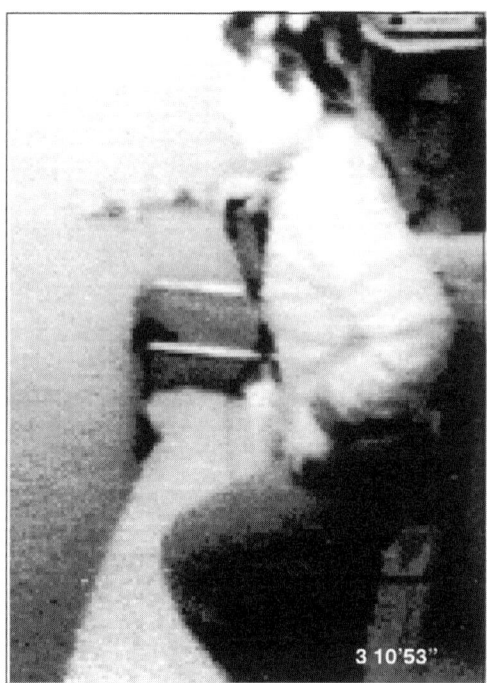

Fig. 5. Epileptic wandering in a child. Between the two photographs (about one minute) the child has jumped from the bed and moved around the room.

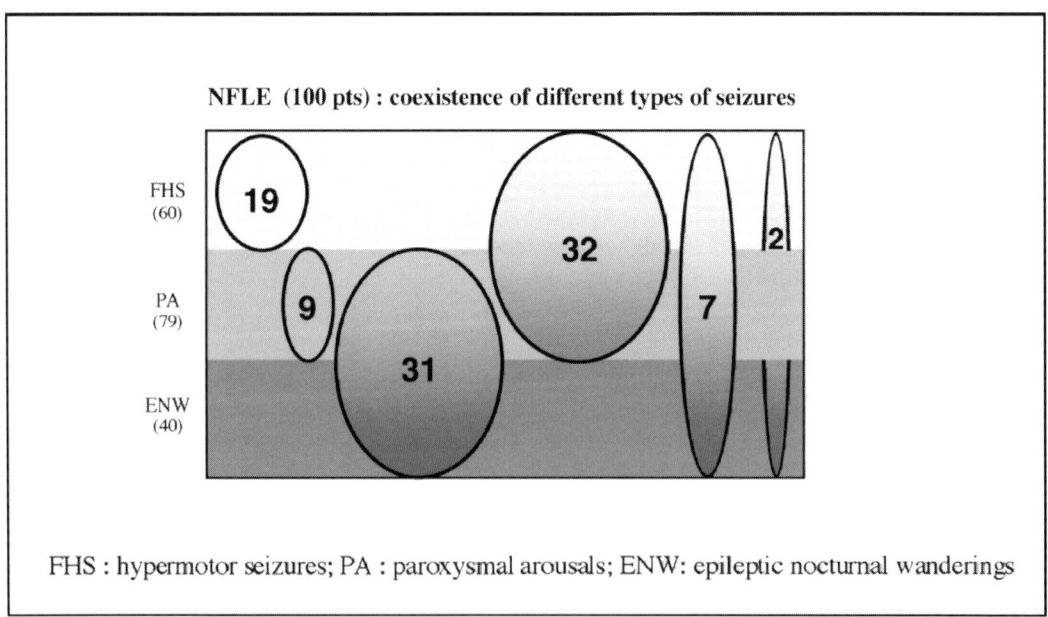

Fig. 6. Seizure types in 100 patients (Provini et al., 1999). Only a few patients have only one type of seizure; most have different seizure types, sometimes during the same night.

Acknowledgments: We thank the EEG technicians of the Department of Neurological Sciences of Bologna for technical assistance and Elena Zoni and Carlo Grassi for photographic assistance.

References

Berger, H.J.C., Berendsen-Versteeg, T.M.C. & Joosten, E.M.G. (1987): Nocturnal paroxysmal dystonia. *J. Neurol. Neurosurg. Psychiatry* **50**, 647–648.

Godbout, R., Montplaisir, J. & Rouleau, I. (1985): Hypnogenic paroxysmal dystonia: epilepsy or sleep disorder? A case report. *Clin. Electroencephalogr.* **16**, 136–142.

Lee, B.I., Lesser, R.P., Pippenger, C.E., Morris, H.H., Lüders, H., Dinner, D.S., Corrie, W.S. & Murphy, W.F. (1985): Familial paroxysmal hypnogenic dystonia. *Neurology* **35**, 1357–1360.

Lugaresi, E. & Cirignotta, F. (1981): Hypnogenic paroxysmal dystonia; epileptic seizures or a new syndrome? *Sleep* **4**, 129–138.

Lugaresi, E., Cirignotta, F. & Montagna, P. (1986): Nocturnal paroxysmal dystonia. *J. Neurol. Neurosurg. Psychiatry* **49**, 375–380.

Meierkord, H., Fish, D.R., Smith, S.J., Scott, C.A., Shorvon, S.D. & Marsden, C.D. (1993): Is nocturnal paroxysmal dystonia a form of frontal lobe epilepsy? *Mov. Disord.* **8**, 38–42.

Montagna, P., Sforza, E., Tinuper, P., Cirignotta, F. & Lugaresi, E. (1990): Paroxysmal arousal during sleep. *Neurology* **40**, 1063–1066.

Montagna, P. (1992): Nocturnal paroxysmal dystonia and nocturnal wandering. *Neurology* **42**, (Suppl. 6), 61–67.

Oldani, A., Zucconi, M., Ferini-Strambi, L., Bizzozero, D. & Smirne, S. (1996): Autosomal dominant nocturnal frontal lobe epilepsy: electroclinical picture. *Epilepsia* **37**, 964–976.

Oldani, A., Zucconi, M., Asselta, Modugno, M., Bonati, MT., Dalprà, L., Malcovati, M. Tenchini, M.L., Smirne, S. & Ferrini-Strambi L. (1998): Autosomal dominant nocturnal frontal lobe epilepsy: a video-polysomnographic and genetic appraisal of 40 patients and delineation of the epileptic syndrome. *Brain* **121**, 205–223.

Peled, R. & Lavie, P. (1986): Paroxysmal awakenings from sleep associated with excessive daytime somnolence: a form of nocturnal epilepsy. *Neurology* **36**, 95–98.

Plazzi, G., Tinuper, P., Montagna, P., Provini, F. & Lugaresi, E. (1995): Epileptic nocturnal wandering. *Sleep* **18**, 749–756.

Provini, F., Plazzi, G., Tinuper, P., Vandi, S., Lugaresi, E. & Montagna, P. (1999): Nocturnal frontal lobe epilepsy. A clinical and polygraphic overview of 100 consecutive cases. *Brain* **122**, 1017–1031.

Provini, F., Plazzi, G. & Lugaresi, E. (2000): From nocturnal paroxysmal dystonia to nocturnal frontal lobe epilepsy. *Clin. Neurophysiol.* **111**, Suppl. 2, S2–S8.

Provini, F., Montagna, P., Plazzi, G. & Lugaresi, E. (2000): Nocturnal frontal lobe epilepsy: a wide spectrum of seizures. *Mov. Disord.* **15** (6), 1264.

Scheffer, I.E., Bhatia, K.P., Lopes-Cendes, I., Fish, D.R., Marsden, C.D., Andermann, E., Andermann, F., Desbiens, R., Keene, D., Cendes, F., Manson, J.I., Constantinou, J., McIntosh, A. & Berkovic, S.F. (1995): Autosomal dominant nocturnal frontal epilepsy: a distinctive clinical disorder. *Brain* **118**, 61–73.

Sheffer, I.E. (2000): Autosomal dominant nocturnal frontal lobe epilepsy. *Epilepsia* **41**, 1059–1060.

Sforza, E., Montagna, P., Rinaldi, R., Tinuper, P., Cerullo, A., Cirignotta, F. & Lugaresi, E. (1993): Paroxysmal periodic motor attacks during sleep: clinical and polygraphic features. *Electroencephalogr. Clin. Neurophysiol.* **9**, 161–166.

Thomas, P., Picard, F., Hirsch, E., Chatel, M. & Marescaux, C. (1998): Autosomal dominant nocturnal frontal lobe epilepsy. *Rev. Neurol.* **154**, 228–235.

Tinuper, P., Cerullo, A., Cirignotta, F., Cortelli, P., Lugaresi, E. & Montagna, P. (1990): Nocturnal paroxysmal dystonia with short-lasting attacks: three cases with evidence for an epileptic frontal lobe origin of seizures. *Epilepsia* **31**, 549–556.

Tinuper, P., Plazzi, G., Provini, F., Cerullo, A. & Lugaresi, E. (1997): The syndrome of nocturnal frontal lobe epilepsy. In: *Somatic and autonomic regulation in sleep*, eds. E. Lugaresi & P.L. Parmeggiani, pp. 125–135. Milan: Springer.

Tinuper, P. & Baruzzi, A. (1999): Seizures during sleep. In: *Epilepsy: problem solving in clinical practice*, eds. D. Schmidt & S. Schachter, pp. 5–17. London: Martin Dunitz.

Tinuper, P., Lugaresi, E., Vigevano, F. & Berkovic, S.F. (in press): Nocturnal frontal lobe epilepsy. In: *Epilepsy and movement disorders*, eds. R. Guerrini, J. Aicardi, F. Andermann & D.D. Marsden. Cambridge: Cambridge University Press.

Tinuper, P. & Lugaresi, E. (2002): The concept of paroxysmal nocturnal dystonia. In: *Sleep and epilepsy: the clinical spectrum*, eds. C. Bazil, B. Malow & M. Sammaritano. Amsterdam: Elsevier Health Sciences.

Vigevano, F. & Fusco, L. (1993): Hypnogenic tonic postural seizures in healthy children provide evidence for a partial epileptic syndrome of frontal lobe origin. *Epilepsia* **39**, 110–119.

Chapter 13

Generalized epilepsies and frontal lobe epilepsies in children

Charlotte Dravet

Marseille, Rome, Pise
Personal address: 4a, avenue Toussaint-Samat, 13009 Marseille, France
charlotte.dravet@free.fr

Summary

The relationship between frontal lobe epilepsy (FLE) and the generalized epilepsies raises problems of diagnosis and treatment that have been often discussed in the literature. We consider two aspects here, the Lennox-Gastaut syndrome (LGS) and the idiopathic generalized epilepsies (IGEs) with absences. We compare the atypical absences and generalized tonic seizures of LGS to some types of seizures observed in FLE. We also present three cases in which the distinction between LGS and FLE is not clear. We discuss IGE with emphasis on the focal frontal EEG abnormalities in patients with absence epilepsy. The prognostic value of these EEG findings is not clear. We then briefly compare the epilepsies combining absences and apparently generalized tonic-clonic seizures, non-convulsive status epilepticus, and the epilepsy associated with the ring 20 chromosome syndrome.

The current classification of epilepsies and epileptic syndromes of the International League Against Epilepsy (Commission, 1989) defines the generalized epilepsies and syndromes as those epileptic disorders with generalized seizures as 'seizures in which the first clinical changes indicate initial involvement of both hemispheres. Consciousness may be impaired and this impairment may be the initial manifestation. Motor manifestations are bilateral. The ictal encephalographic patterns initially are bilateral, and presumably reflect neuronal discharge which is widespread in both hemispheres' (Commission, 1981). The main types of generalized seizures described are absence seizures, either typical or atypical, myoclonic seizures, clonic seizures, tonic seizures, tonic-clonic seizures, and atonic seizures. The generalized epilepsies are subdivided into idiopathic, symptomatic and cryptogenic types. Frontal lobe epilepsies (FLEs) are more likely than all other focal epilepsies to present with clinically generalized seizures such as 'pseudo-absences', tonic-clonic seizures without apparent focal origin (Broglin *et al.*, 1992) and tonic seizures (Chauvel *et al.*, 1992). Thus, distinguishing between FLE and generalized epilepsy may be difficult.

We consider two situations: Lennox-Gastaut syndrome (LGS) among the symptomatic or cryptogenic generalized epilepsies, and epilepsies with absences as an example of idiopathic generalized epilepsies (IGEs).

Seizures of the Lennox-Gastaut syndrome and seizures of frontal lobe epilepsy

LGS is characterized by the association of multiple seizure types (particularly atypical absences and generalized tonic seizures), EEG abnormalities including diffuse slow spike and wave complexes (SW) during wakefulness (Fig. 1), and polyspike and slow wave complexes and rapid rhythms, at 10 c/s or more, during sleep (Fig. 2); and progressive mental impairment (Beaumanoir & Dravet, 1992). Cases corresponding strictly to this definition are not very frequent and represent less than 10 per cent of the childhood epilepsies, even in specialized centres (Beaumanoir & Dravet, 1992). In practice, some patients have intractable epilepsy and several features of LGS without the complete picture, for example with tonic seizures and without atypical absences, or with slow SW on the EEGs but without the rapid rhythms during sleep, or the combination of complex partial and tonic seizures. They can be considered as atypical LGS, and may have FLE. We also know that secondary bilateral synchrony (SBS) may account for an apparent LGS in a FLE (Gastaut & Zifkin, 1988).

Case reports

1. C.F. is a girl we have observed and treated between the ages of 12 and 14. She had intractable diurnal and nocturnal seizures and learning difficulties related to slowness and memory deficit. MRI and other investigations were normal. She had diurnal complex partial seizures, beginning with conscious chest pain, followed by tachypnoea, unresponsiveness and oropharyngeal automatisms. These seizures were not frequent and were not recorded. She had no atypical absences, but had nocturnal tonic seizures (Fig. 3). Interictal EEGs showed many high-amplitude slow SW discharges, either diffuse or located in the two fronto-temporal areas and the vertex, sometimes associated with bifrontal slow waves (Figs. 4 and 5). During sleep the SW and poly-SW were increased but without the typical rapid rhythms of the LGS.

2. A.R.U. is a 7-year-old boy. His epilepsy started at 5 years with serial nocturnal axial tonic seizures. In the following months, he developed daily nocturnal and diurnal seizures: tonic seizures with head-turning to the left and rare atypical absences with a tonic component. He also had episodes of absence status with clouded consciousness and facial myoclonus. Neurological examination was normal. His intelligence was normal but attention deficits and hyperactivity led to worsening of learning problems. CT scan and MRI were normal. Single photon emission computerized tomography (SPECT) performed during sleep showed hypoperfusion in the left temporal lobe but ictal SPECT showed no abnormal perfusion in this area. Interictal EEGs showed a normal background, sometimes slower on the left, and diffuse slow SW associated with fronto-temporal spikes and SW in the left hemisphere. During sleep the abnormalities were activated and high-voltage rapid rhythms appeared (Figs. 6 and 7). Atypical absences and tonic seizures were recorded (Fig. 8) similar to those of true LGS.

3. S.G. is a right-handed man born in 1962, with no relevant personal or family history. At 10 years, he had a generalized tonic-clonic seizure and, some months later, atypical absences and tonic seizures. Some tonic seizures were preceded by conscious head and eye deviation to the right. His school performance deteriorated and at 16 ½ years, despite antiepileptic drugs, seizures increased, becoming diurnal and nocturnal. He was then referred to our centre. Clinical examination was normal but verbal expression and ideation were slow. EEGs showed diffuse slow SW, in bursts increased by hyperventilation (Fig. 9), and numerous discharges of diffuse subclinical rapid rhythms predominant in the anterior areas (Fig. 10). The CT scan showed a left frontal tumour (Fig. 11), which was removed without complication. Since surgery, he has been seizure free. Postoperative IQ was 94, with a slight frontal deficit, and EEGs showed left frontal spikes without diffuse discharges in wakefulness and sleep (Fig. 12). Medication was progressively reduced and stopped at 25 years. He

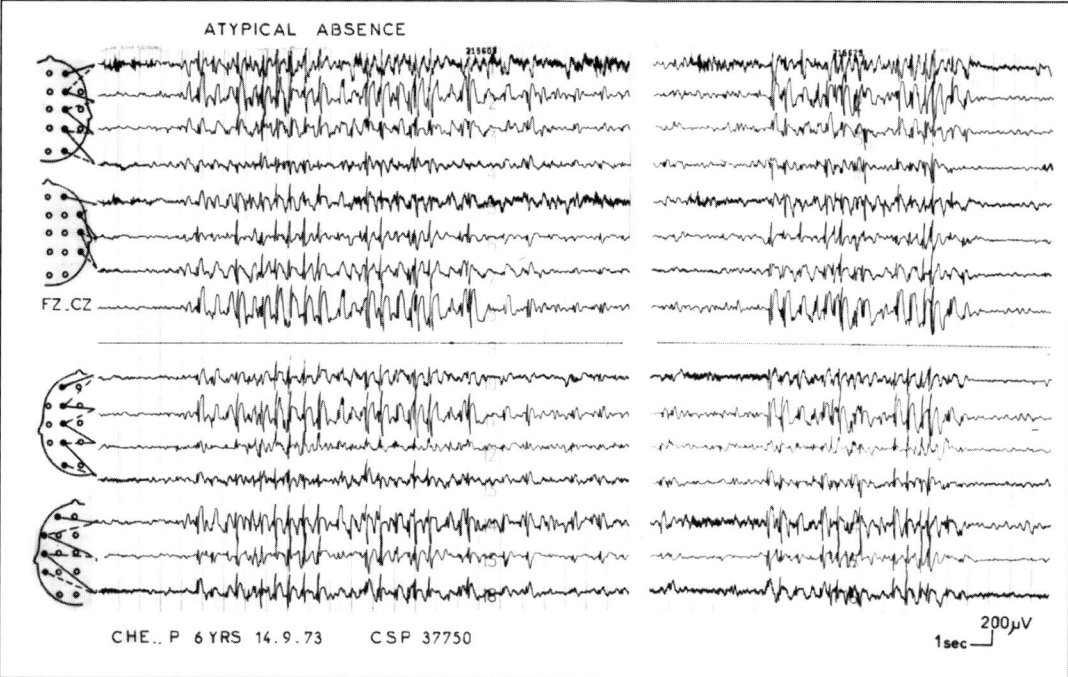

Fig. 1. Irregular slow SW in a boy of age 6 with LGS. Left: the slow SW are accompanied by an arrest of speech and drooling (atypical absence). Right: there is no apparent clinical change (interictal SW).

now has a normal profession as mechanic. Although this patient could be diagnosed as LGS, his epilepsy was clearly related to a benign frontal tumour and was cured by the lesionectomy, and probably represented SBS. However, there were no focal abnormalities over the site of the tumour in the presurgical EEGs.

There are arguments in the literature for a close relationship between the frontal lobes and LGS. In LGS the interictal diffuse EEG discharges usually predominate in the frontal areas. In some patients, depth electrode recording has shown a frontal, often bilateral, origin of the seizures (Bancaud & Talairach, 1965). The cognitive and behavioural deterioration is compatible with frontal lobe dysfunction (Kieffer-Renaux et al., 1997). The clinical appearance of the atypical absences (Broglin et al., 1992) and of the tonic seizures strongly resembles that of frontal lobe seizures.

Chauvel & Bancaud (1994) described two clinical patterns of medial intermediate frontal lobe seizures, 'frontal absences' and 'complex motor seizures'. 'Frontal absences' are characterized by speech and movement arrest, alteration of consciousness, mild gestural stereotypies, possible adversion, and rapid recovery of contact, all of these being the same as in typical and atypical absences of generalized epilepsies. 'Complex motor seizures' can present as tonic axial seizures. The authors note that 'a large proportion of syndromes described as generalized epilepsies are in fact focal seizures of frontal origin, even though the specific mechanisms of their ictal discharge synchronization are determined by subcortical, thalamic and mesencephalic networks'. Beaumanoir & Blum (2002) believe that the pathophysiological mechanisms of tonic seizures and atypical absences could depend on both the frontal lobe and subthalamic structures. However they emphasize that the generalized tonic-clonic seizures which are frequent in FLE are rare in childhood LGS.

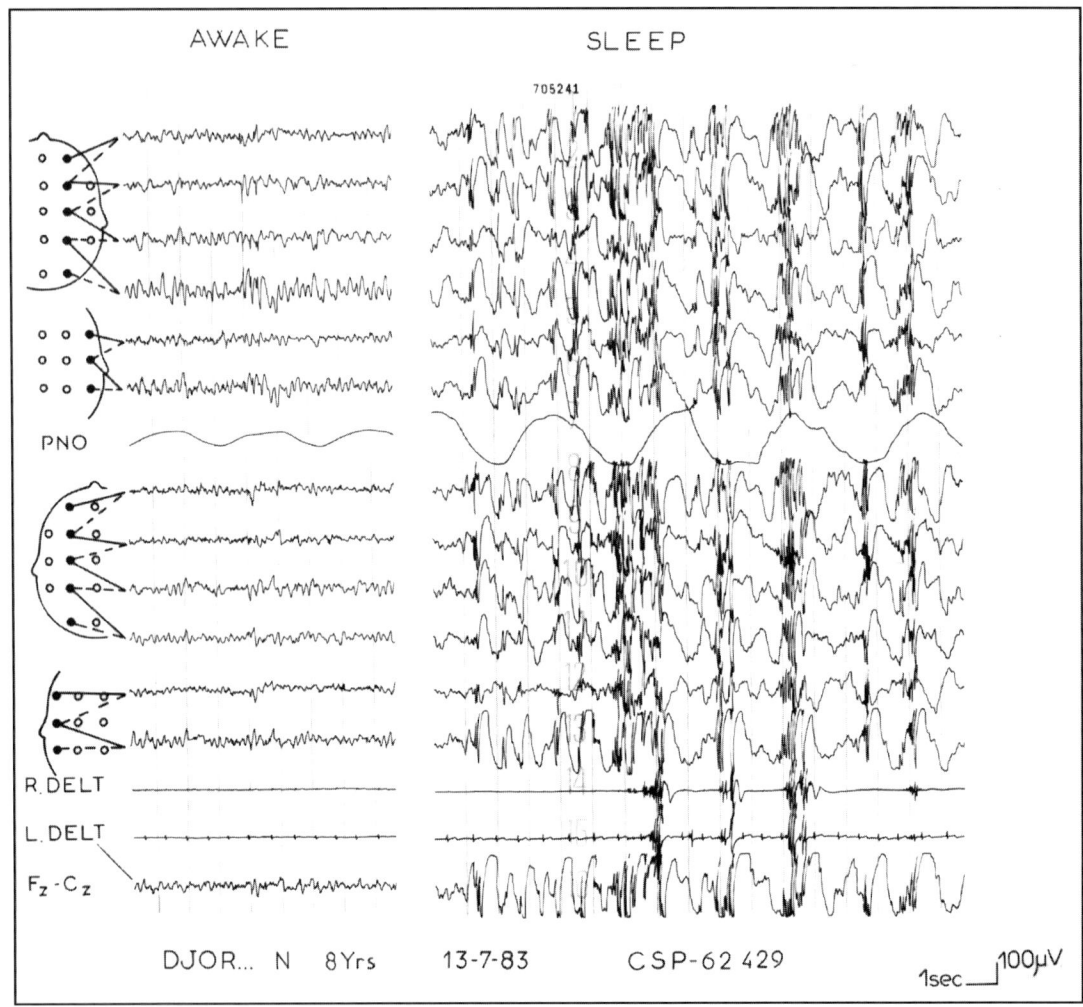

Fig. 2. Example of sleep recording in a boy of age 8 with a LGS. Left: during wake, a short burst of sharp waves in the right posterior areas. Right: during slow sleep, repeated bursts of generalized SW, poly-SW and rapid rhythms, of high amplitude, accompanied by a brief tonic contraction, mixed with a myoclonic component. R. DELT: right deltoid; L. DELT: left deltoid.

Chapter 13   Generalized epilepsies and frontal lobe epilepsies in children

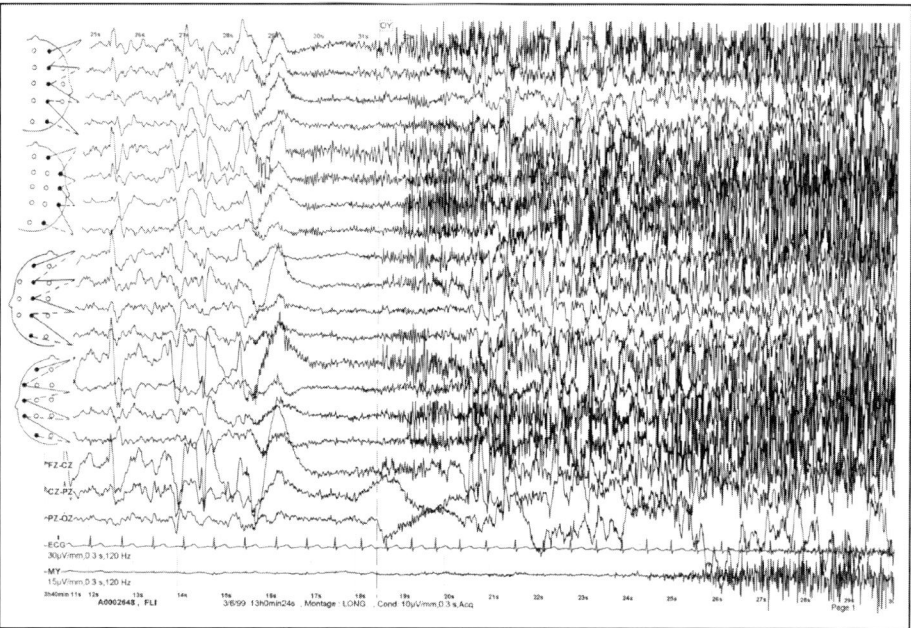

Fig. 3. A nocturnal tonic seizure recorded in a girl of age 13 (case 1, F.L.I.). After a burst of slow waves, prominent in the anterior areas, a sudden diffuse flattening with rapid rhythms is observed, of which the voltage is higher in the right frontal channel and increases progressively. Then it is difficult to differentiate EEG rhythms from muscular activities. The tonic contraction, recorded on the right deltoid (MY), starts only around 10 seconds after onset.

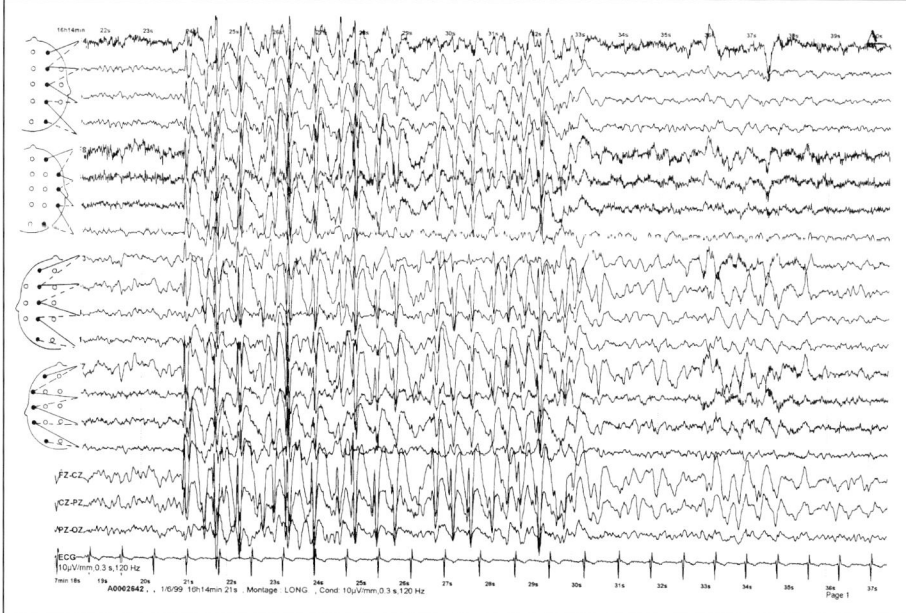

Fig. 4. In the same girl as in Fig. 3, a burst of generalized slow SW without clinical correlation, followed by slow waves in the left frontal region and in the vertex.

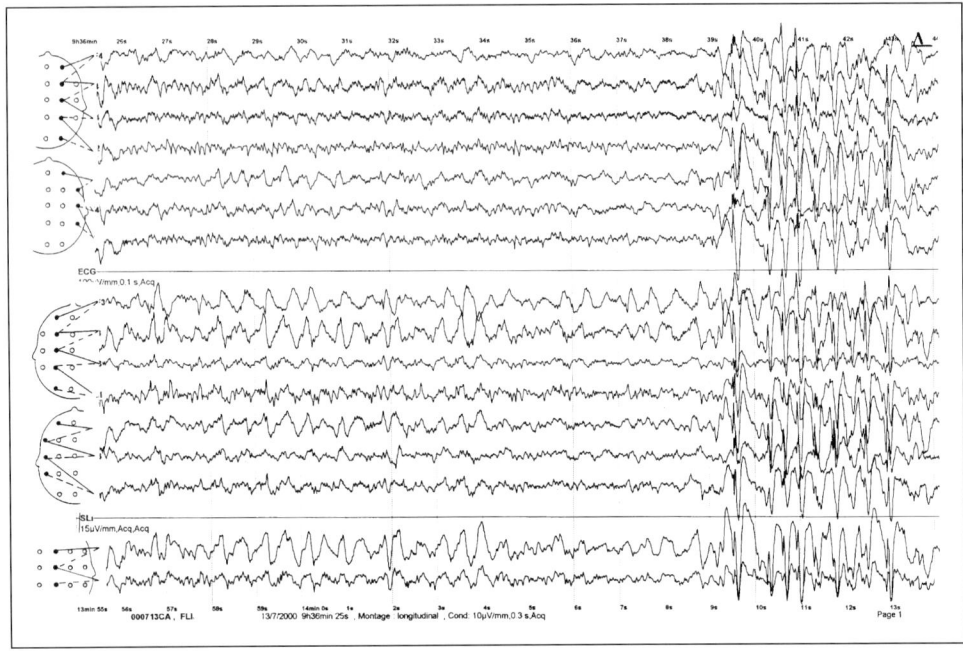

Fig. 5. In the same girl as in Figs. 3 and 4, at 14, a long discharge of slow waves in the vertex and the left frontal region, spreading to the right, precedes an apparently interictal burst of generalized slow SW.

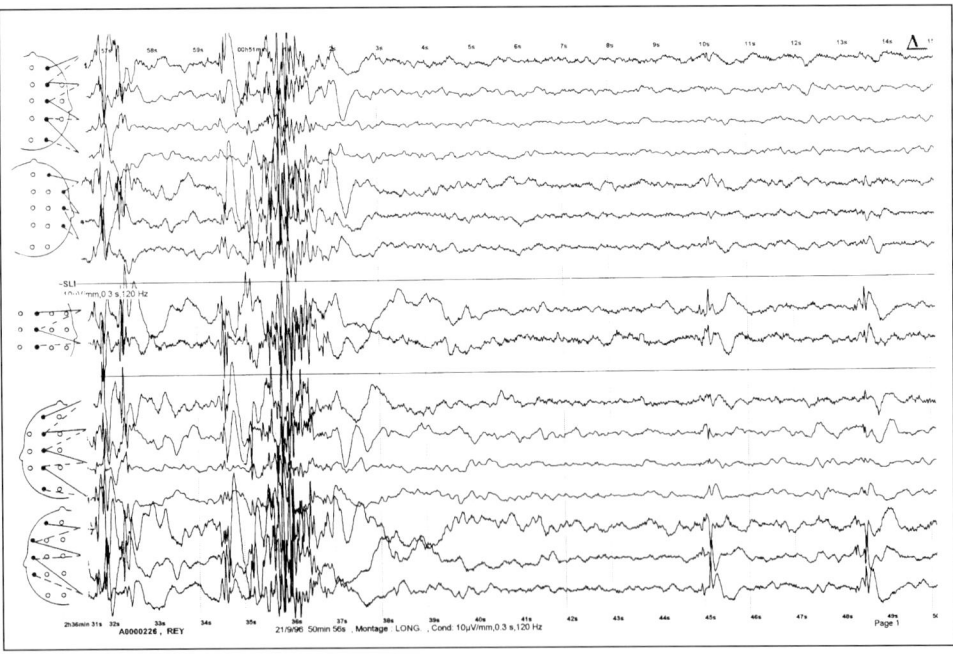

Fig. 6. Sleep EEG in a boy of age 7 (case 2, R.E.Y.). Left: short discharges of diffuse slow SW and rapid rhythms. Right: isolated SW clearly located in the left fronto-temporal region and vertex.

Chapter 13   Generalized epilepsies and frontal lobe epilepsies in children

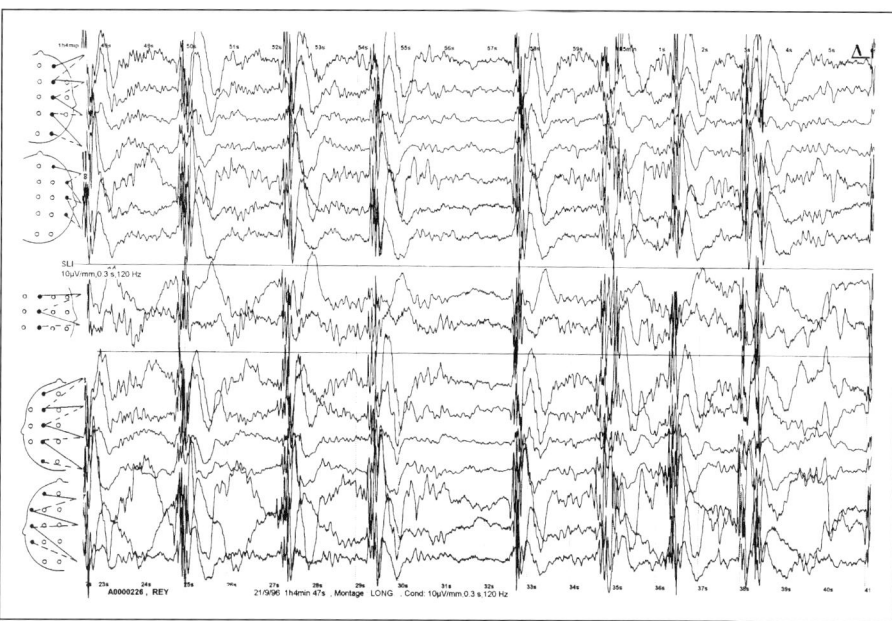

Fig. 7. Sleep recording in the same boy as in Fig. 6: generalized discharges of very high amplitude of poly-SW and rapid rhythms.

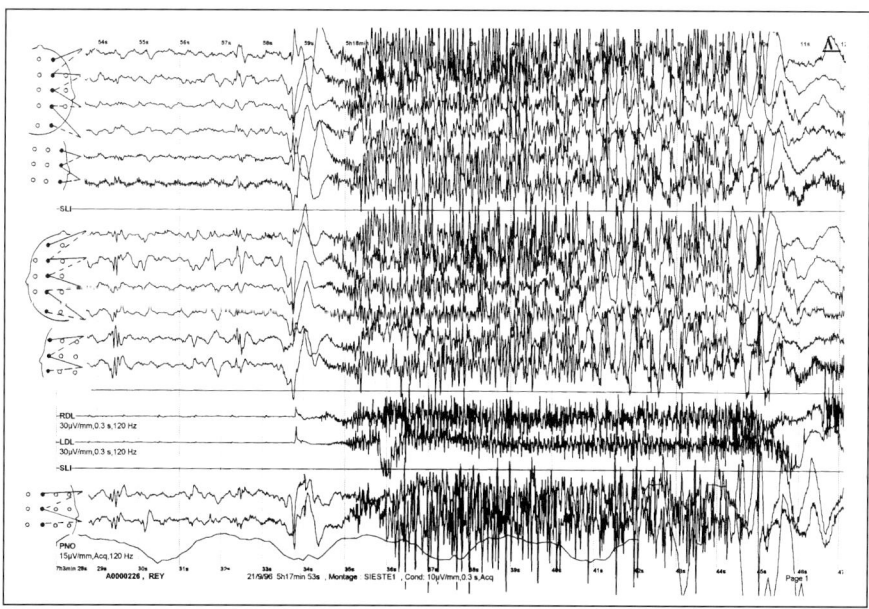

Fig. 8. In the same boy as in Figs. 6 and 7, recording of a generalized tonic seizure during sleep: onset with a high voltage slow wave, followed by a flattening with rapid rhythms of increasing voltage. The tonic contraction, recorded in the two deltoids (RDL and LDL), starts simultaneously to the flattening. The respiration (PNO) is first unchanged, then is more rapid and ample. The seizure is preceded by isolated spikes in the left fronto-temporal area.

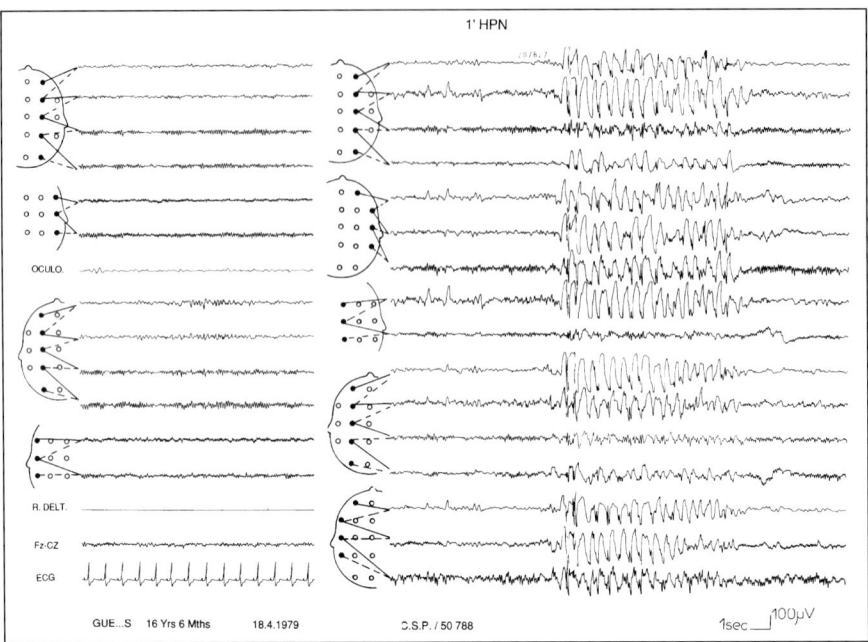

Fig. 9. Wake EEG in an adolescent of 16 ½ (case 3, G.U.E.). Left: normal background and theta waves in the left fronto-central area. Right: after one minute of hyperpnoea occurrence of a burst of subclinical generalized slow SW, preceded by right frontal and vertex isolated sharp waves.

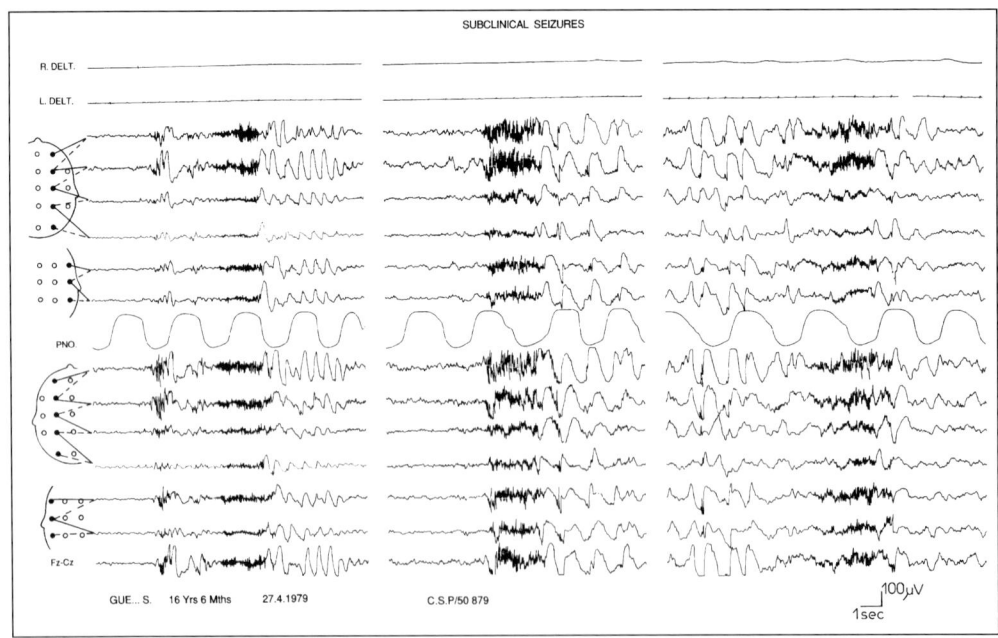

Fig. 10. In the same patient as in Fig. 9, recording of a series of brief bursts of generalized rapid rhythms, followed or preceded by slow waves and slow SW, without clinical correlate.

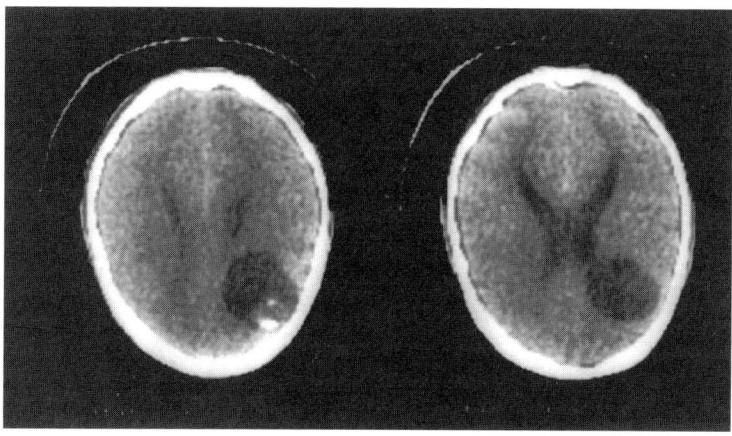

Fig. 11. The CT scan shows a left frontal cystic mass with calcification before (right) and after (left) contrast injection.

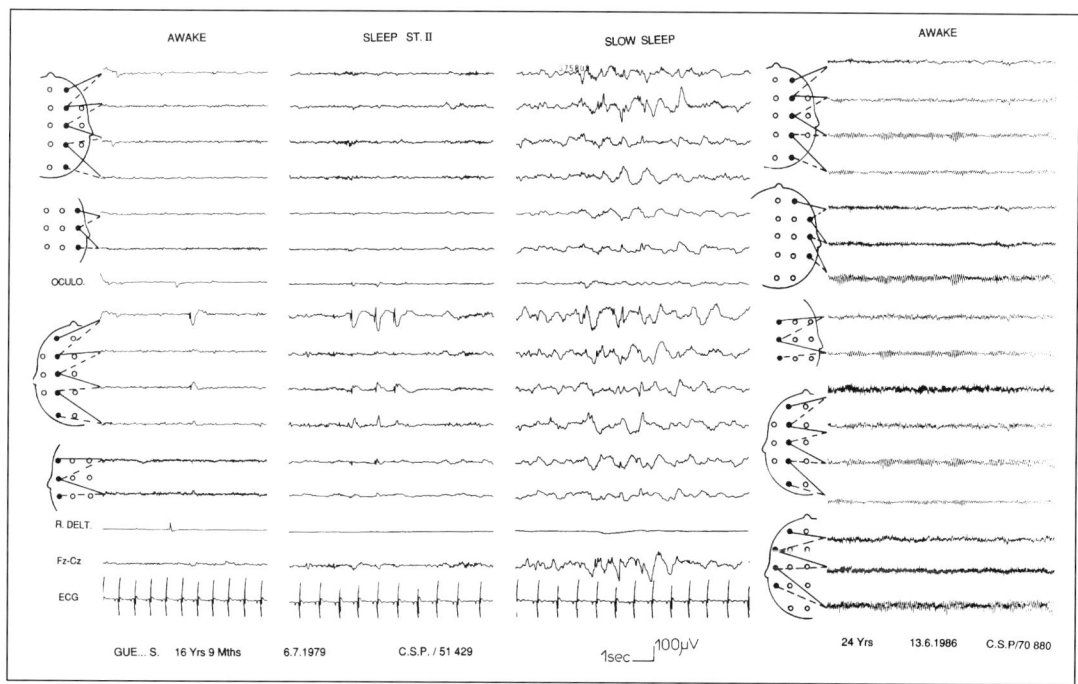

Fig. 12. Evolution after surgery. Three months later, generalized abnormalities are no longer recorded, being replaced by a left frontal spike focus, activated by sleep (the three left fragments). Seven years later the EEG is normal, without asymmetry (the right fragment).

Tassinari & Ambrosetto (1988) reported 15 adult patients with tonic seizures. Epilepsy tended to start in puberty with rare generalized convulsive seizures, usually with focal onset: complex partial seizures with simple automatisms developed later. Additional clinical features included daily drop attacks, absence-like seizures and, often, mild to moderate mental retardation. EEGs showed diffuse slow SW, activated by sleep. This electroclinical condition could be diagnosed as late-onset LGS.

However, there were several important differences from typical LGS: these patients never had tonic status epilepticus, mental retardation was less severe than in typical LGS, and EEG background rhythm was often normal. All patients had persistent focal slowing and/or sharp waves involving one or both frontal lobes. Diffuse fast discharges were often asymmetric, predominant on the side of the focal abnormalities, with contralateral predominance of polygraphic tonic EMG activity. Four patients had frontal lobe lesions (Pazzaglia *et al.*, 1985). The authors believe that this electroclinical pattern represents the evolution of a focal epilepsy involving the frontal lobe. The same pattern has been described in some patients with post-traumatic FLE (Niedermeyer *et al.*, 1970). We have also observed such patients and recorded the generalized and focal seizures (Fig. 13).

We do not have sufficient data to understand the origin and the physiopathology of LGS. However, we could think that several mechanisms must be involved, including cortical and subcortical structures, and particularly the frontal lobes.

Absence seizures and frontal lobe epilepsy

In IGE, absence seizures with or without generalized tonic-clonic seizures occur in several syndromes: absence epilepsy in childhood, absence epilepsy in adolescence, and juvenile myoclonic epilepsy. Some other generalized epilepsy syndromes with absences have been proposed, such as *absences with perioral myoclonias, eyelid myoclonias with absence.*

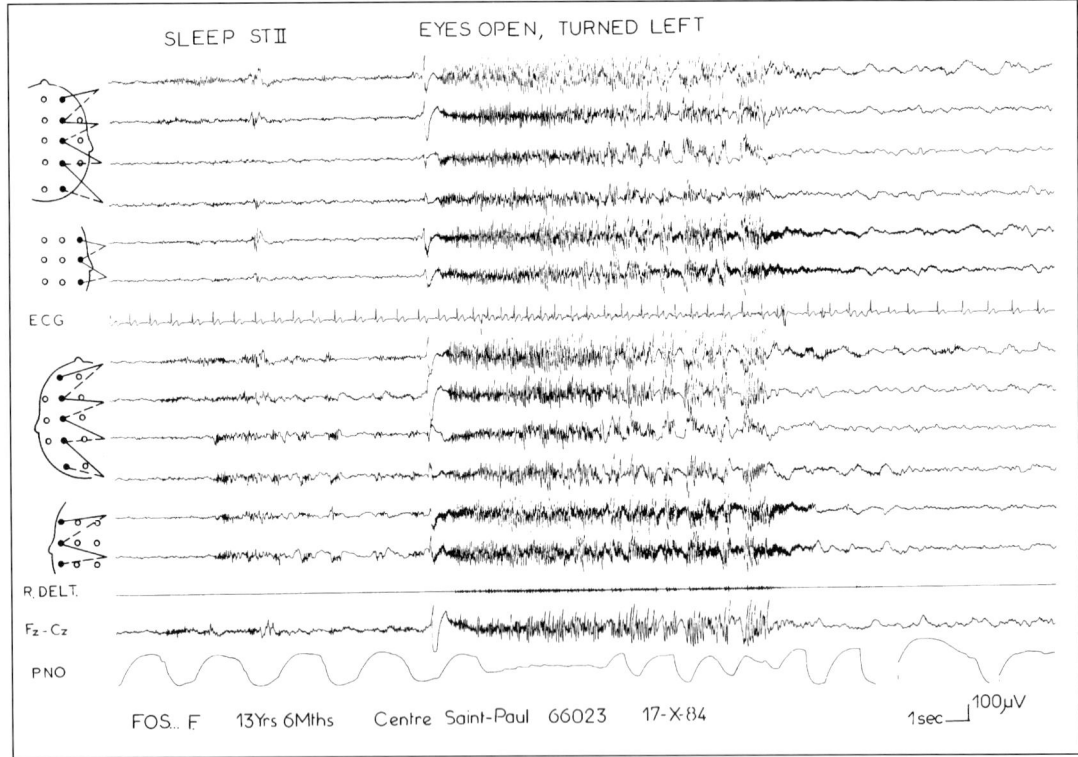

Fig. 13. Sleep recording in an adolescent of age 13½ with a late LGS. Left: subclinical burst of bilateral anterior rapid rhythms, with subsequent diffusion on the whole left hemisphere. Right: typical generalized tonic seizure with tonic contraction recorded on the right deltoid (R.DELT), tachycardia (ECG) and brief apnoea (PNO). Clinically, the patient opens his eyes and turns left.

The prognosis of these epilepsies is variable and several prognostic factors have been described. Interictal focal, mainly frontal, spikes and SW are present in the EEGs of patients with childhood *absence epilepsy* (Gabor & Ajmone Marsan, 1969; Gastaut *et al.*, 1974). Focal ictal onset in the frontal or fronto-temporal area may also be recorded (Holmes *et al.*, 1987, Loiseau, 1992). These focal frontal discharges in children with absences have been associated with cognitive and behavioural disturbances and with a poor prognosis for the absences compared to that without frontal discharges (Covanis *et al.*, 1992). A question then arises about these absences as a manifestation of FLE, which could explain their frequent intractability and poor outcome. However, others (Bartolomei *et al.*, 1997; Panayiotopoulos, 1997) did not find that these EEG patterns indicate a poor prognosis.

In some patients, actually, absences can be the expression of partial epilepsy originating in the frontal lobe, mimicking generalized epilepsy. Such absences are usually associated with other seizure types (Loiseau & Cohadon, 1970). This diagnosis is often difficult and may lead to wrong treatment (Loiseau, 1992; Broglin *et al.*, 1992). Roger & Bureau (1992) studied some diagnostic criteria distinguishing frontal lobe epilepsy from IGE. They reported six patients with severe and intractable absences and generalized tonic-clonic seizures diagnosed as IGE. FLE was diagnosed in all after video-EEG recording of several seizures and sleep EEG. They concluded that the diagnosis of IGE should be systematically questioned when seizures are refractory and especially if they become intractable, or if new seizure types appear.

Non-convulsive absence status observed mainly in the elderly can be either a generalized or a FLE (Rohr-Le Floch *et al.*, 1988; Thomas *et al.*, 1999).

A type of *absence status* occurs in patients with epilepsy and ring 20 chromosome abnormality. They develop severe epilepsy with onset in childhood, not always associated with mental retardation. Absences and generalized tonic or tonic-clonic seizures occur. Most striking are those characterized by several hours of variable impairment of consciousness, with or without perioral myoclonias (Inoue *et al.*, 1997; Canevini *et al.*, 1998; Kobayashi *et al.*, 1998; Petit *et al.*, 1999). The interictal EEGs are normal or show diffuse theta waves. The ictal EEG shows long discharges of theta waves, spikes, and SW, either generalized or over both frontal areas, with or without clinical correlation. Biraben *et al.* (2001) discuss the nosological status of this epilepsy and its pathogenesis. They hypothesize that it is due to dysfunction of the subcortical regulation of cortical electrogenesis.

References

Bancaud, J., Talairach, J., Bonis, A., Schaub, C., Szikla, G., Morel, P.O. & Bordas-Ferrer, M. (1965): *La stéréoencéphalographie dans l'épilepsie*. Paris: Masson.

Bartolomei, F., Roger, J., Bureau, M., Genton, P., Dravet, C., Viallat, D. & Gastaut, J.L. (1997): Prognostic factors for childhood and juvenile absence epilepsies. *Eur. Neurol.* **37**, 169–175.

Beaumanoir, A. & Dravet, C. (1992): The Lennox-Gastaut syndrome. In: *Epileptic syndromes in infancy, childhood and adolescence*, eds. J. Roger, M. Bureau, C. Dravet, F.E. Dreifuss, P. Wolf & A. Perret, pp. 115–132. London: John Libbey & Company.

Beaumanoir, A. & Blume, W. (2002): The Lennox-Gastaut syndrome. In: *Epileptic syndromes in infancy, childhood and adolescence*, eds. J. Roger, M. Bureau, Ch. Dravet, P. Genton, C.A. Tassinari & P. Wolf, pp. 113–135. London: John Libbey & Company.

Biraben, A., Odent, S., Lucas, J., Michez, K., Lemée, F., Henry, C., Le Berre, C., de Grissac, N., Bernard, A.M. & Scarabin, J.M. (2001): Chromosome 20 en anneau et épilepsie : diversité des crises étudiées en vidéo-EEG. Un mécanisme sous-cortical d'épileptogenèse est-il au premier plan? *Epilepsies* **13**, 9–15.

Broglin, D., Delgado-Escueta, A.V., Walsh, G.O., Bancaud, J. & Chauvel, P. (1992): Clinical approach to the patient with seizures and epilepsies of frontal origin. In: *Advances in Neurology*, eds. P. Chauvel, A.V. Delgado-Escueta, E. Halgren & J. Bancaud, vol. 57, pp. 59–88. New York: Raven Press Ltd.

Canevini, M., Sgro, V., Zuffardi, O., Canger, R., Carrozzo, R., Rossi, E., Ledbetter, D., Minicucci, F., Vignoli, A., Piazzini, A., Guidolin, L., Saltarelli, A. & Dalla Bernardina, B. (1998): Chromosome 20 ring: a chromosomal disorder associated with a particular electroclinical pattern. *Epilepsia* **39**, 942–951.

Chauvel, P., Trottier, S., Vignal, J.P. & Bancaud, J. (1992): Somatomotor seizures of frontal lobe origin. In: *Advances in neurology*, eds. P. Chauvel, A.V. Delgado-Escueta, E. Halgren & J. Bancaud, vol. 57, pp. 185–232. New York: Raven Press.

Chauvel, P. & Bancaud, J. (1994): The spectrum of frontal lobe seizures: with a note on frontal lobe syndromatology. In: *Epileptic seizures and syndromes*, ed. P. Wolf, pp. 331–334. London: John Libbey & Company.

Commission on Classification and Terminology of the International League Against Epilepsy (1981): Proposal for a revised classification of epileptic seizures. *Epilepsia* **22**, 489–501.

Commission on Classification and Terminology of the International League Against Epilepsy (1989): Proposal for a revised classification of epilepsies and epileptic syndromes. *Epilepsia* **30**, 389–399.

Covanis, A., Skiadas, K., Loli, N., Lada, C. & Theodorou, V. (1992): Absence epilepsy: early prognostic signs. *Seizure* **1**, 281–289.

Gabor, A.J. & Ajmone-Marsan, C. (1969): Coexistence of focal and bilateral diffuse paroxysmal discharges in epileptics. *Epilepsia* **10**, 453–472.

Gastaut, H. & Zifkin, B.G. (1988): Secondary bilateral synchrony and Lennox-Gastaut syndrome. In: *Neurology and neurobiology*, eds. E. Niedermeyer & R. Degen, vol. 45, The Lennox-Gastaut syndrome, pp. 221–242. New York: Alan R. Liss.

Holmes, G.H., McKeeve, A.M. & Adamson, M. (1987): Absence seizures in children: clinical and electroencephalographic features. *Ann. Neurol.* **21**, 268–273.

Inoue, Y., Fugiwara, T., Matsuda, K. et al. (1997): Ring chromosome 20 and non-convulsive status epilepticus. A new epileptic syndrome. *Brain* **120**, 939–953.

Kobayashi, K., Inagaki, M., Saski, M., Sugai, K., Ohta, S. & Hashimoto, T. (1998): Characteristic EEG findings in ring 20 chromosome as diagnostic clue. *EEG Clin. Neurophysiol.* **10**, 258–262.

Kieffer-Renaux, V., Jambaqué, I., Kaminska, A. & Dulac, O. (1997): Evolution neuropsychologique des enfants avec syndromes de Lennox-Gastaut et de Doose. *A.N.A.E.* **42**, 84–88.

Loiseau, P. (1992): Childhood absence epilepsy. In: *Epileptic syndromes in infancy, childhood and adolescence*, eds. J. Roger, M. Bureau, Ch. Dravet, F.E. Dreifuss, P. Wolf & A. Perret, pp. 135–150. London: John Libbey & Company.

Loiseau, P. & Cohadon, F. (1970): *Le petit mal et ses frontières*. Paris: Masson.

Niedermeyer, E., Walker, A.E. & Burton, C. (1970): The slow spike-wave complex as correlate of frontal and fronto-temporal post-traumatic epilepsy. *Eur. Neurol.* **3**, 330–346.

Panayiotopoulos, C.P. (1997): Absence epilepsies. In: *Epilepsy: a comprehensive textbook*, eds. J. Engel Jr & T.A. Pedley, pp. 2327–2346. Philadelphia: Lippincott-Raven Publishers.

Pazzaglia, P., D'Alessandro, R., Ambrosetto, G. & Lugaresi, E. (1985): Drop attacks: an ominous change in the evolution of partial epilepsy. *Neurology* **35**, 1725–1730.

Petit, J., Roubertie, A., Inoue, Y. & Genton, P. (1999): Non-convulsive status in the ring chromosome 20 syndrome: a video-illustration of 3 cases. *Epileptic Disord.* **1**, 237–241.

Roger, J. & Bureau, M. (1992): Distinctive characteristics of frontal lobe epilepsy *vs* idiopathic generalized epilepsy. In: *Advances in neurology*, eds. P. Chauvel, A.V. Delgado-Escueta, E. Halgren & J. Bancaud, vol. 57, pp. 399–410. New York: Raven Press.

Rohr-Le Floch, J., Gauthier, G. & Beaumanoir, A. (1988): Etats confusionnels d'origine épileptique. Intérêt de l'EEG fait en urgence. *Rev. Neurol.* **144**, 425–436.

Tassinari, C.A. & Ambrosetto, G. (1988): Tonic seizures in the Lennox-Gastaut syndrome: semiology and differential diagnosis. In: *Neurology and Neurobiology*, eds. E. Niedermeyer & R. Degen, vol. 45, The Lennox-Gastaut syndrome, pp. 109–124. New York: Alan R. Liss.

Thomas, P., Zifkin, B., Migneco, O., Lebrun, C., Darcourt, J. & Andermann, F. (1999): Non-convulsive status epilepticus of frontal origin. *Neurology* **52**, 1174–1183.

Chapter 14

Acquired epileptic frontal syndrome in children

Thierry Deonna, Anne-Lise Ziegler and Eliane Roulet-Perez

Neuropediatric Unit, Vaudois University Hospital Centre,
46, rue du Bugnon, CH-1011 Lausanne, Switzerland
Thierry.Deonna@chuv.hospvd.ch

Summary

Among children with partial epilepsy and continuous spikes and waves during slow sleep some have predominant prefrontal epileptic activity and cognitive and/or behavioural disturbances referable to dysfunction of this region. As opposed to those whose deficits predominantly involve verbal language, their disorder has been recognized more recently and not studied as extensively. Some of these children have been diagnosed with an epileptic psychosis and indeed have a particular and probably unrecognized primary direct psychiatric manifestation of epilepsy. The long-term follow-up of these children suggests that, unlike in most cases with acquired epileptic aphasia, epilepsy and focal EEG abnormalities persist and a congenital epileptogenic lesion is responsible for the syndrome in at least some cases. There are also probably minor manifestations of the syndrome presenting only insidious slowing of cognitive development with school failure and moderate hyperactivity-attention problems without loss of basic social judgement and behavioural control. Idiopathic frontal partial epilepsy with transient isolated or predominantly cognitive-psychiatric disturbances is being increasingly recognized in children, some possibly within the category of functional localization-related epilepsies of childhood.

Existence and nature of 'frontal syndrome' in children – problems

Data on the developmental consequences and long-term outcome of early frontal lobe damage in children are very limited. Early development in such children may be normal due to the late maturation of frontal structures and the nature of the cognitive functions that they subserve. Most studies describe adults with severe psychopathology and prefrontal lesions from early childhood which were thought to be the cause of their problems (Anderson *et al.*, 1999).

There are no prospective studies of children with early frontal damage followed from the onset of the lesion. It is not known to what degree plasticity may operate in these areas and how effective learning (attention, short-term memory, planning, inhibition, etc.) can take place with early damage to the prefrontal lobes. Several facets of childhood developmental disorders such as autism or attention deficit disorders are attributed to prefrontal dysfunction by analogy to what is known in adults with acquired lesions, but the evidence is still questionable.

For all these reasons, one must however be cautious in drawing conclusions from adults with various forms of frontal syndrome. With respect to frontal epilepsies, one must determine the degree to which the constellation of behavioural-cognitive disorder observed in older children with partial epilepsies can be due to disturbance of existing prefrontal functions which are affected transiently or chronically by the epileptic process.

Frontal epilepsies with ictal or post-ictal cognitive-behavioural disturbances in children

There are very limited data even in adults on transient ictal or post-ictal cognitive-behavioural manifestations with partial epilepsy and a prefrontal epileptic focus. Thomas *et al.* (1999) published adult cases of non-convulsive status epilepticus of frontal origin. They distinguished two groups, one with mainly affective or cognitive symptomatology: 'mood disturbances with affective disinhibition or affective indifference and associated subtle impairment of cognitive functions without overt confusion', and another with confusional state, major behavioural disturbances, impaired responsiveness and post-ictal amnesia.

There are only isolated case studies of children reported whose epileptic dysfunction manifested itself mainly or exclusively in the cognitive and psychiatric sphere and which could be related to a frontal dysfunction during the acute phase (Jambaqué *et al.*, 1989; Camps *et al.*, 2001). Not surprisingly, epilepsy is not the first diagnosis considered when only behavioural or cognitive deficits are present. 'Frontal behaviours' and signs of 'executive dysfunction' were reported with usually complete recovery and no residual cognitive or psychiatric symptomatology. Purely behavioural disturbances (hyperactivity, aggressivity, risky conducts, lack of interest for school) were observed during the acute phase with preservation of a normal IQ (Camps *et al.*, 2001) showing that the behavioural symptoms can be dissociated from purely cognitive ones, at least to some extent. Of course IQ measures are poor indicators of frontal dysfunction and more specific tests or questionnaires have to be used.

All these behavioural abnormalities taken in isolation are non-specific and can be viewed as reactive to an adverse life situation or of purely emotional origin. Minor behavioural dysfunctions can be related mainly to disinhibition without loss of social judgement or high-level cognitive capacity, as can be seen in 'developmental' attention deficit disorder with hyperactivity (ADD-H). Children with frontal epilepsy are potentially very interesting models to study the possible similarities between temporary prefrontal dysfunction and some well-known chronic childhood behavioural or psychopathological syndromes.

An important question is whether children with frontal epilepsy due to a small congenital prefrontal lesion will show behavioural and cognitive symptoms in the inter-ictal phase which are different from those seen with brain damage in other locations or in other types of childhood epilepsy. Lassonde *et al.* (2000) found lower scores in tests of executive function in frontal epilepsy. However, differences were minor and none of the children had major behavioural problems such as those seen in frontal epilepsy with continuous spike and wave activity in slow wave sleep (CSWS) (see below). Considering the suspected importance of frontal involvement in several childhood psychiatric syndromes, these results suggest that in most of these epileptic children, the dysfunction remains limited around the epileptogenic zone or that there is significant plasticity in cases of early frontal damage, but detailed data are very rare.

The 'acquired epileptic frontal syndrome' in children with epilepsy and CSWS

Several distinct neuropsychological syndromes are now recognized in children with partial epilepsy and CSWS (Deonna, 1997). It is generally accepted that the type of acquired disturbance is directly related to the site and function of the cortical area involved in the epileptic process, CSWS being only a marker of the severity of the epileptic dysfunction at a given time. The age at onset, level of maturation and functional maturation of the involved epileptic zone (or zones), its spread within the hemisphere or contralaterally, and the duration and intensity of the epileptic disorder and its response to treatment will determine the severity and nature of the neuropsychological dysfunction. The best-known example is acquired epileptic aphasia (Landau-Kleffner syndrome – LKS) which in its most classic form is a pure verbal auditory agnosia; other central perceptual disorders such as acquired visuospatial disorder, visual agnosia, or motor-perceptual disorders such as apraxia have been much less frequently described.

Children who present not only with a language disorder but also with mental deterioration and/or behavioural abnormalities are referred to as the 'syndrome of partial epilepsy with CSWS' or 'CSWS syndrome' because historically these children were described emphasizing the sleep EEG characteristics and because their neuropsychological characteristics were much less clear-cut and more difficult to describe than the striking EEG abnormalities. This terminology has created confusion, and differentiation from acquired epileptic aphasia (AEA) is debated (see below).

In 1993, we reported four boys followed for several years with a cryptogenic partial epilepsy, a frontal epileptic focus and CSWS (Roulet et al., 1993). All had repeated cognitive and psychological evaluations and overnight EEG recordings. We found cognitive and behavioural regression followed by a variable degree of recovery in all cases, which paralleled the severity of the epilepsy measured by the intensity of epileptic activity in the sleep EEG. The neuropsychological and behavioural regression, while very severe, was different from simple global dementia. The behavioural symptoms did not correspond to a psychological reaction to the cognitive loss or to any known psychopathological syndrome. The relative severity and interplay between behavioural and cognitive symptoms varied greatly during the course of the illness. The unique clinical and EEG profile of these children suggested a frontal dysfunction which we termed 'acquired epileptic frontal syndrome' (AEFS). Given the multiple functions of the prefrontal lobes in cognition and emotions and their increasingly important role as the child grows older, one should expect a complex mixture of cognitive and psychiatric problems which is difficult to describe and analyse. These four children are probably rather exceptional because (i) they were normal up to an age when much normal development has already occurred; (ii) they became very severely affected; (iii) they were followed long enough and in detail; (iv) they improved enough with medication to allow longitudinal study of cognitive, linguistic and behavioural disturbances.

We feel that they probably represent a severe and relatively pure example of an epileptic dysfunction of the prefrontal regions within the context of this epileptic syndrome. Our experience since then and reported data suggest that non-specific behavioural symptoms such as hyperactivity, attention disorder, and school decline can occur as minor manifestations of a prefrontal epileptic dysfunction, but this is very difficult to prove because these same symptoms can also be due to drug effects, depression, or other disorders.

There are also cases with specific linguistic, behavioural and general cognitive regression in various combinations or successively. This may occur in most cases, but we suspect that these are not reported because the tendency of neurologists and neuropsychologists is to diagnose and report specific neuropsychological syndromes.

Our children had a predominant or exclusive frontal epileptogenic focus (three right, one left) throughout the course of the disease. We could not localize the EEG abnormalities more precisely within the different prefrontal areas. We occasionally recorded electrical focal frontal seizures with intermittent rapid rhythms superimposed on the background of CSWS without clinical manifestation, indicating that the frontal motor areas were not involved in the epileptic process. We did not record such discharges in other locations.

Having outlined the characteristics of our original series, we would place the problem in a more general context with the following questions.

Questions

(1) What are the precise neuropsychological and behavioural characteristics of the cases reported by Roulet *et al.* (1993) and what is the evidence for a specific acquired epileptic frontal syndrome in this original series and in other reported cases?

(2) What is the relationship between AEFS and acquired epileptic aphasia (AEA)?

(3) Is the close aetiological relationship with the benign partial epilepsies of childhood, suspected in AEA, also valid for AEFS?

(4) May some instances of autistic regression be manifestations of a very early onset of AEFS?

Characteristics of AEFS with CSWS in children

It is difficult to convey the unique, disturbing and catastrophic clinical picture of these children at their worst, which we have not encountered in any other situation in paediatric neurology. Interestingly, all professionals involved with these children in special schools admitted that they had not encountered this clinical pattern before, although there were some elements in common with many of the mentally retarded and psychotic children they knew.

Table 1 shows the main behavioural characteristics and cognitive deficiencies seen in these children at their worst. The division between cognitive and behavioural features is somewhat arbitrary, but it is helpful to group some individual features which we feel did not occur together by chance. Also and more importantly, the different behavioural and cognitive problems did not start, worsen, and improve simultaneously. For example, one child started with an insidious mental regression without major behavioural change and only later became markedly disturbed, but another presented with predominantly a behaviour problem which only later appeared to be followed by a marked cognitive regression. The rapidity of all these changes was also very variable occurring over a few days or weeks to several months.

Table 1. Major cognitive and behavioural characteristics of children with acquired epileptic frontal syndrome and CSWS

Behavioural (at worst)	Cognitive*
Inattention, hyperactivity	Orientation in time
Impulsivity, aggressivity	Reasoning
Mood swings, disinhibition	Thought formulation
Loss of sense of danger	Memorizing strategy
Perseveration, mouthing objects	
Reduced play	No new learning

* Language form, rote memory, visuo-perceptual and constructional abilities relatively spared.

The cognitive deficits of these children are difficult to measure because of their severe behavioural problems. We performed repeated evaluations starting at the most basic levels and taking advantage of the periods when their behaviour improved. The strange impression we had of these children probably stems from the many dissociations between their cognitive abilities and their behaviour: a very low level of reasoning, absence of any planned activity and of new learning despite good preservation of language form, rote memory and some visuospatial abilities; coupled with preserved basic social skills (eye contact, social smile, greeting formulas, handshake) yet otherwise aberrant behaviour and discourse. These features were at once suggestive but different from those seen in children with autistic disorders, in whom non-verbal communication is also affected. Roulet et al. (1993) clearly showed that the general cognitive decline documented on successive standardized tests (Fig. 1) was not a general global slowness affecting all domains, but had remarkable 'peaks and troughs' also resembling what occurs in high-functioning autistic children. The lowest results on the Wechsler intelligence scale (WISC) were obtained on subtests requiring reasoning (similarities, picture arrangement, arithmetic) whereas some visuospatial items (puzzles, cubes) which could be solved by purely visual inspection or by trial and error were preserved. Interestingly, when the children improved, all scores improved, but the same large discrepancies persisted between different domains (Fig. 2).

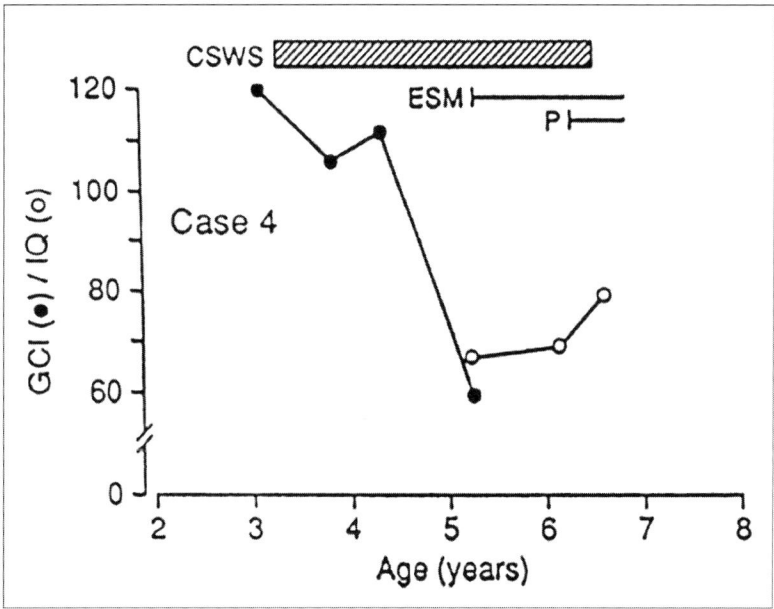

Fig. 1. Cognitive regression in acquired epileptic frontal syndrome and CSWS documented by serial cognitive measurements with stabilization and improvement in the course of the disease (case 4 of Roulet et al., 1993). GCI = General cognitive index of McCarthy; IQ = WISC III; ESM = ethosuximide; P = prednisone.

The absence of visible motor or sensory symptoms and the preservation of many capacities such as language and some social and visuospatial skills were in sharp contrast with the disorientation in time, inability to carry out simple arithmetic reasoning, and the absence of any sustained activity with no apparent distress or frustration and no insight into their errors. Before giving them specific tasks or even when witnessing the very poor results and absence of apparent effort, the examiner

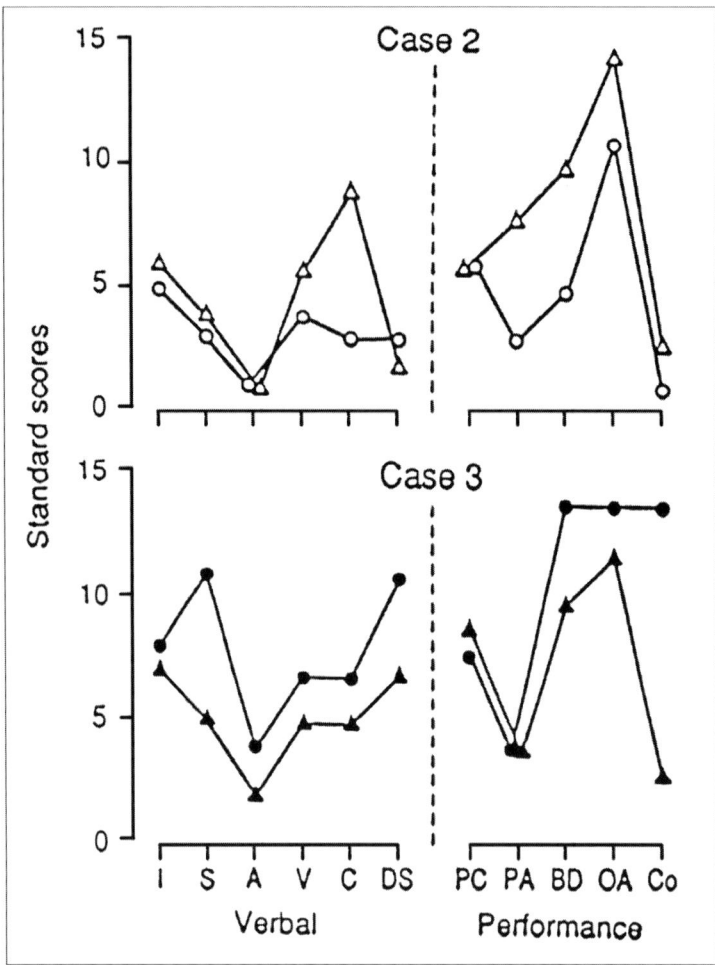

Fig. 2. Details of subtest results (WISC-R) in two children with acquired epileptic frontal syndrome and CSWS obtained in case 2 at 8 years 4 months (○) and 9 years 5 months (△), and in case 3 at 7 years 8 months (▲) and 9 years 7 months (●). I = information; S = similarities; A = arithmetic; V = vocabulary; C = comprehension; DS = digit span; PC = picture completion; PA = picture arrangement; BD = block design; OA = object assembly; Co = coding.

might believe that they were careless or provocative in their attitude. The knowledge that these children were normal before the onset of their disease added to everybody's perplexity.

The dissociation of cognitive and behavioural deterioration in time and severity, the rapidity of onset, and improvement in the same child in the course of the syndrome suggest that these two facets of the disorder, although they coexisted at one or several points, were not the consequence of each other, i.e. the behavioural disorder was not an emotional reaction to a loss of cognitive capacities and the cognitive decline was not due to oppositional conduct or lack of motivation. This became clear when a child improved markedly in behaviour, was very cooperative and willing to do cognitive tasks, but still had severe cognitive difficulties.

These associations and dissociations suggest a variable severity and timing of the involvement of different prefrontal structures in the epileptic process.

Another important characteristic of these children was their language disorder. Language was surprisingly normal in its structure (form), with severe aberrations of its use (pragmatics). Echolalia, repetitive questioning, irrelevant answers, and digressions were very striking. These language characteristics are typical of children with so-called 'semantic-pragmatic disorder', a variety of developmental language disorder described by Bishop (1999), which she has renamed 'pragmatic language impairment' and which is often combined with non-linguistic features of an autistic disorder. Our patients are interesting because they mimic some of the characteristics of developmental language disorders. One very crucial question is whether an epileptogenic pathology starting at a very early age could mimic developmental cases of autism or even more severe cases of autistic regression (see below).

Adult follow-up of our cases of AEFS

We were able to obtain information on all the cases of Roulet *et al.* (1993) about 10 years later. In August 2000, they were respectively 22, 18, 19 and 16 years old. Two have had no more seizures while being off antiepileptic drugs and two still have seizures and take antiepileptic medication. One (case 3) started having convulsions during sleep from the age of 2 ½ years. Behavioural deterioration was first noted from the age of 5 years and CSWS was present from the first sleep EEG at 5 years 8 months. During childhood he had persistent predominantly nocturnal seizures with generalized and partial seizures of frontal type. He had intractable complex partial seizures and was investigated at age 15 years for possible surgery. The MRI of the brain showed no lesion. Several generalized and partial seizures were recorded. EEG, SPECT and PET suggested a right frontal onset. Depth electrode monitoring was suggested but refused by the family. At age 15 years, his verbal IQ was 79 and his performance IQ was 91. He had difficulties in planning (Tower of London, Rey's complex figure) and identifying categories (Wisconsin card sorting). His concepts of time and number, and abstract thinking were limited. He was well-mannered but over-friendly and naïve with perseverative thoughts and unusual subjects of interest. These cognitive and behavioural features were very suggestive of a residual frontal syndrome.

Other reported cases of partial epilepsy with CSWS of frontal origin (?)

There have been several studies of children with epilepsy and CSWS. It is increasingly recognized that rather than specific neuropsychological syndromes, more global learning and behavioural problems can be the main or only manifestations. In group studies of these children, 'behaviour disturbances' and 'frontal symptoms' are often mentioned as the main or only deficit without detailed analysis (Bulteau *et al.*, 1997; Bureau, 1995; Veggiotti *et al.*, 1999). We are also aware of several remarkably dramatic examples which were not published, often because insufficient data could be obtained or because interested professionals were involved too late in the development of the disease to make the study totally convincing.

Here is a very striking illustration of this situation, studied by Peyre & Rousselle (1998):

This girl was totally normal until age 7 years when she became hyperactive, inattentive, aggressive and uninhibited. She was treated in a child psychiatric department and was excluded from school because of the severe behaviour disturbance. At 8 years she had a waking EEG for suspected absences, showing bilateral generalized spike and wave activity. At that time she was confused, disoriented in time and space, and had perseverations and hyperphagia. She was described as untestable. Valproate was given without improvement and stopped. At 9 years, when first seen by Dr. Rousselle, her first sleep EEG showed CSWS and bifrontal spike and wave activity. At 10 years prednisone was administered for 6 months with disappearance of CSWS and some clinical improvement, but with reappearance of CSWS after steroids were stopped. At 11 years, she was given ethosuximide with disappearence of CSWS and major improvement which was continuing at the age of 13 years. This case illustrates many common and difficult problems with this disorder. The child first presented with purely behavioural symptoms without clinical seizures and was thought initially to have a primary psychological problem.

Transient psychosis with epilepsy and CSWS. The 'psychiatric' face of AEFS?

Kyllerman *et al.* (1996) published a case of transient psychosis with epilepsy and CSWS. The authors describe the evolution and fluctuations of the different cognitive and psychiatric components which resemble very much what we had observed. This girl was normal until rare *Grand Mal* seizures occurred at age 6 years. A few months later, she had insidious cognitive deterioration followed by a first psychotic phase. The psychotic symptoms disappeared but the child was left with moderate mental retardation. At 8 years she had a transitory second psychotic phase but further cognitive loss was documented with inability to learn new material. During the psychotic phase, there was loss of speech, impulsivity, hyperactivity, disorientation, aggressivity, unawareness of danger, feeding disturbances and incontinence. The EEG showed a left temporoparietal focus with diffuse CSWS and frontal predominance and SPECT showed decreased perfusion in the left frontotemporal region. This observation is very similar to what we observed in the nature and change of the symptoms over time. Many of the behavioural symptoms are compatible with a massive frontal dysfunction interfering with social judgement, organization of action and control of impulses. The fact that this aspect was transitory but was preceded and followed by a fluctuating and progressive cognitive regression suggests (as in our cases) that the epileptic activity was variable in intensity and/or predominant site of involvement within the prefrontal regions. The title of the article, its publication in a psychiatric journal and the emphasis given to the behavioural manifestations have probably obscured its importance and hindered its recognition among child neurologists. The vast literature on psychiatric symptoms in epilepsy contains very few well-documented descriptions of these symptoms and their relationship to epilepsy. Acquired epileptic frontal syndrome appears to be one of the disorders in which prolonged psychiatric symptoms are a direct manifestation of epilepsy in children.

Relationship between acquired epileptic aphasia (AEA – Landau-Kleffner syndrome, LKS) and acquired epileptic frontal syndrome with CSWS

Most reported cases of LKS had pure isolated language loss (acquired verbal auditory agnosia), with normal non-verbal intelligence. Although these children had severe behavioural problems in reaction to their communicative loss, they were able to learn, retained an adapted social behaviour and were not psychotic (Deonna *et al.*, 1989). They could learn written and sign language. Some authors considered that these cases were fundamentally different from those with language regression as part of a complex cognitive and psychiatric disorder with mental retardation. It became however clear that some children developed a combination of severe cognitive and behavioural problems before, during or after an acquired aphasia, and that it was somewhat arbitrary to consider that they were fundamentally different. This occurred especially but not only in children whose syndrome started early.

Robinson *et al.* (2001) reported 18 cases of AEA. Several had severe behavioural disturbances with additional frontal foci or spread to the frontal area from the temporal regions. Five of these children had subpial transection (Irwin *et al.*, 2001). Postoperatively, the behaviour disorder rapidly and spectacularly improved, but language improved very slowly and with significant residual deficit at the time of follow-up (Irwin, 2001). This suggests that, in these cases at least, the behaviour disorder is not caused by the communicative problem and is itself part of the probably frontal brain dysfunction. One personal case with long-term follow-up illustrates this problem:

Childhood acquired epileptic aphasia, cognitive and behavioural regression with CSWS
Adult follow-up with diagnosis of frontal dysplasia

This child has been followed from 3 years to 26 years. As a young child he had major behaviour problems and a specific acquired language disorder. His behaviour was so destructive that he was institutionalized for 2 years. Behaviour, language and cognitive skills improved (Roulet *et al.*, 1991). However his epilepsy, which was not very severe in childhood and which was in remission until age 19 years, became increasingly intractable. Presurgical investigation at 25 years showed intense epileptiform activity in the left frontal and orbital frontal areas. Invasive monitoring showed that the epileptic focus was very close to Broca's area. Resection was followed by improvement in seizure frequency. Histology showed cortical dysplasia which had not been visible on MRI. This observation shows the catastrophic effects of early prolonged frontal epileptic activity on both behaviour and language in a young child. Both were affected at some time but improved at different periods during childhood with temporary remission of epilepsy. Aetiology of epilepsy was only found at surgery. This case also illustrates that some instances of apparently idiopathic partial epilepsy with CSWS can be due to an unrecognized lesion (Roulet *et al.*, 1998).

Our observation and some of the cases reported by Robinson *et al.* (2001) also show that some children have more extensive deficits, with cognitive regression and severe behavioural abnormalities. These patients, in our experience, have more extensive epileptic disturbance involving frontal regions, do not always improve at puberty, and may harbour an unidentified epileptogenic lesion. Their EEG and clinical characteristics are somewhat different from 'pure' cases of AEA, whose seizure manifestations and EEG characteristics are more like the idiopathic epilepsies of genetic origin.

Relationship with the benign partial epilepsies and 'benign partial epilepsy with frontal foci'

Several cases of AEA began with partial motor seizures and EEG features of benign partial epilepsy of childhood with Rolandic spikes (BPERS) but then developed aphasia, either spontaneously or related to medication (Prats *et al.*, 1998). For these and other reasons, we and others believe that AEA can be the extreme end of severity of these usually benign perisylvian epilepsies. Does this also apply to cases of primary frontal foci and frontal symptomatology? Case studies in children and long-term follow-up of our cases give no strong indication of this, but suggest instead that unrecognized congenital epileptogenic lesions are most often, and possibly always, present in these epilepsies.

Although the location of the epileptic focus in BPERS can change and is sometimes more anterior or posterior than the typical centro-temporal localization (Peterson, 1992; Deonna, 2000a), there has been no description of the neuropsychological disturbances which may occur when the epileptic dysfunction predominantly involves the frontal regions.

The Strasbourg group (Raffo *et al.*, 2001) described five children with idiopathic partial epilepsy and rare polymorphic seizures compatible with a frontal origin. Their EEGs showed clusters of frontal slow spike and wave activity on a slow background, with rare but more typical centro-temporal spikes increased during sleep, but without CSWS. The centro-temporal foci sometimes appeared later in the course of the disease. These children had transient behavioural and cognitive disturbances during the active phase with good outcome and no cognitive sequelae. Detailed neuropsychological description of these cases would be important. It is surprising that this has not been identified before. Beaumanoir & Nahory (1983) described 11 cases of 'benign' frontal epilepsy in children without note of cognitive problems, but there have been no similar publications. We have not seen this pattern in a recent prospective neuropsychological study of 22 children with benign localization-related epilepsy, although we did not exclude patients whose otherwise typical functional foci were not strictly localized to the centro-temporal region (Deonna *et al.*, 2000).

We retrospectively diagnosed an 8-year-old boy with idiopathic frontal epilepsy and EEG abnormalities similar to those described by Beaumanoir and the Strasbourg group, who responded immediately to antiepileptic treatment. Only at the first follow-up visit did we learn that during the four months prior to the onset of epilepsy, his behaviour had deteriorated so much that his mother was treated for a depression. Behavioural problems disappeared as soon as the epilepsy was treated. It is very likely that these symptoms were a direct manifestation of his epilepsy before obvious seizures led to diagnosis. Behavioural disturbances preceding the onset of Rolandic epilepsy were observed in the original reports of this syndrome (Loiseau et al., 1967; Beaussart, 1972) and in some cases a time-limited moderate frontal dysfunction was possibly responsible. Behaviour disturbance pre-dating epilepsy in children has been discussed by Austin et al. (2001) who postulated that this may be due to transient cognitive impairment with subclinical seizures. These may be the persistent manifestations of focal epilepsy in the prefrontal areas, for which there are no obvious manifestations suggestive of epilepsy.

The history of childhood epilepsy and epileptic syndromes has taught us that excluding complex or atypical cases from any study may give a biased idea of reality. The cases reported by the Strasbourg group did not have predominant centro-temporal foci; they have slow EEG background activity and are abnormal neurologically, and would have been excluded from most studies on benign partial epilepsies of childhood with Rolandic spikes.

Partial epilepsy of frontal origin in very young children. Can it be a cause of disintegrative disorder, autistic regression and regressive pervasive developmental disorders?

In our original cases, epilepsy started in children who had already reached some major social, emotional and cognitive milestones. They had all been normal and behavioural regression was very evident. Despite this, they were difficult to study; if the epilepsy starts in the first 2 years, it will be even more difficult to distinguish the effect of the underlying brain pathology from that of the epileptic disorder itself.

The severely disturbed behaviour seen in our patients in the social and communicative spheres were not fundamentally autistic in the strict sense. This led to the suspicion that epilepsy could be directly responsible for some instances of so-called disintegrative disorder or autistic regression, whether or not the children had been recognized with clinical epilepsy. Other children initially diagnosed within the autistic spectrum were later recognized to have an early form of LKS.

Such cases have led to a flurry of EEG studies including sleep studies in these children, but the CSWS pattern seems rather rare in these situations (Tuchman, 1997). Lewine et al. (1999) studied 50 children diagnosed as 'regressive autistic spectrum disorders' aged 4 to 13 years with MEG-EEG during sleep: 68 per cent had perisylvian and multifocal (including frontal) epileptiform abnormalities on the EEG but only one had the CSWS pattern. This is all the more important because this was a very selected group: 15 of the 50 had had definite seizures and the others were suspected of having seizures or a variant of LKS. This does not mean that epilepsy does not play a role in some cases, but the epileptic mechanisms, mode of spread and loci of dysfunction might be different from the more typical acquired epileptic aphasia or AEFS with CSWS. Such regressions are seen in some very young children with complex partial seizures or epileptic spasms of frontal origin who can present with various combinations of cognitive delay, aberrant language, and autistic symptoms occasionally with peculiar epileptic stereotypies (Deonna et al., 1995). Marked cognitive and behavioural improvement may occur with antiepileptic treatment. Prefrontal dysplasia can sometimes be found on MRI (Fohlen et al., 2000; Deonna et al., 2001).

Conclusions

Among children with partial epilepsy and CSWS some have predominant prefrontal epileptic activity and cognitive and/or behavioural disturbances referable to dysfunction of this region. As opposed to those whose deficits involve predominantly verbal language, their disorder has been recognized more recently and not studied as extensively. The symptoms are initially non-specific and the often severe behavioural disturbances make precise evaluation of cognitive regression difficult. Recognition of the epileptic nature of psychiatric problems is crucial, especially for treatment. Some of these children have been diagnosed with epileptic psychosis and indeed have a particular and probably unrecognized primary direct psychiatric manifestation of epilepsy. There is not always a clear boundary between these cases and those with purely linguistic problems such as acquired epileptic aphasia. In the course of their epileptic syndrome, the linguistic or cognitive/behavioural dimension can vary depending on the extension of the focal epileptic zone or the presence of several epileptic foci variably active at different times. Also, there are minor manifestations of the syndrome with only insidious slowing of cognitive development, deterioration of school performance, and limited hyperactivity-attention problems without loss of basic social judgement and behavioural control (Deonna et al., 1997).

This type of epilepsy does not seem to be a frequent cause of clinical situations labelled as disintegrative psychosis or autistic regression. However, there are rare reports of children with early language regression and autistic features with epileptic origin (Uldall et al., 2000).

Long-term follow-up of our children shows that, unlike in most acquired epileptic aphasias, which are considered idiopathic, epilepsy and focal EEG abnormalities can persist in these patients and a congenital epileptogenic lesion is present in at least some cases. CSWS is now more often recognized in congenital lesional epilepsies of various types. The pattern seems to be aetiologically non-specific; additional factors such as a genetic epileptic predisposition may play a role.

The role of a thalamic lesion in contributing to the development of this epileptic syndrome has also been recently suggested from isolated case studies and experimental literature (Monteiro et al., 2001).

The relationship between partial epilepsies with CSWS and functional partial epilepsies such as benign Rolandic epilepsy appears quite strong in cases of acquired epileptic aphasia and other manifestations of perisylvian dysfunction; this does not appear to be so with children with acquired epileptic frontal syndrome, but more data are needed.

The key feature of the clinical syndrome is dissociation: (i) dissociation between different aspects of cerebral activity: the child can lose cognitive functions while retaining normal behaviour, or behaviour can become severely disturbed with preservation of cognitive functions; (ii) dissociations within a single sphere: the structural aspects of language can be preserved while its use is very aberrant; (iii) dissociation in time: the natural course is unpredictable and variable in the speed of onset and recovery of the various symptoms and signs.

Further study of cases with acquired epileptic frontal syndrome with CSWS and more generally the study of the transient epileptic cognitive and behavioural manifestations of frontal origin in children are most important. The description and understanding of their clinical manifestations involve core issues and border zones between child neurology and psychiatry. They are very difficult to study because, in addition to the nature of the problems, evaluation requires cooperation between several non-medical disciplines on single case studies as well as availability of competent people and adequate tools.

References

Anderson, S.W., Bechara, A., Damasio, H., Tranel, D. & Damasio, A.R. (1999): Impairment of social and moral behaviour related to early damage in human prefrontal cortex. *Nature Neurosci.* **11**, 1032–1037.

Austin, J.K., Harezlak, J., Dunn, D.W., Huster, G.A., Rose, D.F. & Ambrosius, W.T. (2001): Behaviour problems in children before first recognized seizures. *Paediatrics* **107**, 115–122.

Beaumanoir, A. & Nahory, A. (1983): Les épilepsies bénignes partielles: 11 cas d'épilepsie partielle frontale à évolution favorable. *Rev. EEG Neurophysiol.* **13**, 207–211.

Beaussart, M. (1972): Benign epilepsy of children with Rolandic (centro-temporal) paroxysmal foci. A clinical entity. Study of 221 cases. *Epilepsia* **13**, 795–811.

Bishop, D. (2000): Pragmatic language impairment: a correlate of SLI, a distinct subgroup, or part of the autistic continuum? In: *Speech and language impairments in children. Causes, characteristics, intervention and outcome*, eds. D.V.M. Bishop & L.B. Leonard, pp. 99–113. Hove: Psychology Press.

Bulteau, C., Jambaqué, I., Kieffer, V. & Dulac, O. (1997): Aspects neuropsychologiques du syndrome de pointes ondes continues pendant le sommeil lent. *A.N.A.E.* **41**, 5–9.

Bureau, M. (1995): 'Continuous spikes and waves during slow sleep' (CSWS): definition of the syndrome. In: *Continuous spikes and waves during slow sleep. Electrical status epilepticus during slow sleep. Acquired epileptic aphasia and related conditions*, eds. A. Beaumanoir, M. Bureau, T. Deonna, L. Mira & C.A. Tassinari, pp. 17–26. Mariani Foundation Paediatric Neurology Series 1, vol. 3. London: John Libbey & Company.

Camps, R., Hugonenq, C., Livet, M.O. & Mancini, J. (2001): Syndrome dysexécutif et trouble des conduites transitoires chez un enfant de 10 ans présentant une épilepsie frontale. *XIe Réunion de la Société Française de Neurologie Pédiatrique*, Clermont-Ferrand, 25-27 January 2001 (abstract).

Deonna, T. (2000): Acquired epileptic aphasia (AEA) or Landau-Kleffner syndrome: from childhood to adulthood. In: *Speech and language impairments in children. Causes, characteristics, intervention and outcome*, eds. D.V.M. Bishop & L.B. Leonard, pp. 261–272. Hove: Psychology Press.

Deonna, T., Peter, C., & Ziegler, A.L. (1989): Adult follow-up of the acquired aphasia-epilepsy syndrome in childhood. Report of 7 cases. *Neuropaediatrics* **20**, 132–138.

Deonna, T., Ziegler, A.L., Maeder, M.I., Ansermet, F. & Roulet, E. (1995): Reversible behavioural autistic-like regression: a manifestation of a special (new?) epileptic syndrome in a 28-month-old child. A 2-year longitudinal study. *Neurocase* **1**, 91–99.

Deonna, T., Davidoff, V., Maeder, M.I., Zesiger, P. & Marcoz, J.P. (1997): The spectrum of acquired cognitive disturbances in children with partial epilepsy and continuous spike-waves during sleep. *Eur. J. Paediatr. Neurol.* **1**, 19–29.

Deonna, T., Zesiger, P., Davidoff, V., Maeder, M., Mayor, C. & Roulet, E. (2000): Benign partial epilepsy of childhood: a neuropsychological and EEG study of cognitive function. *Dev. Med. Child Neurol.* **42**, 595–603.

Deonna, T., Fohlen, M., Jalin, C., Delalande, O., & Ziegler, A.L. (2001): Epileptic stereotypies in children. In: *Epilepsy and movement disorders*, eds. R. Guerrini, J. Aicardi, F. Andermann & M. Hallett. Cambridge: Cambridge University Press.

Fohlen, M., Jalin, C. & Delalande, O. (2003): Electroclinical semeiology of frontal lobe seizures in infants and children: contribution of intracranial video EEG recording. In: *Frontal seizures and epilepsies in children*, eds. A. Beaumanoir, F. Andermann, P. Chauvel, L. Mira & B. Zifkin, pp. 187–194. Mariani Foundation Paediatric Neurology Series, vol. 11. Paris, London: John Libbey Eurotext.

Irwin, K., Birch, V., Lees, J., Polkey, C., Alarcon, G., Binnie, C., Smedley, M., Baird, G. & Robinson, R.O. (2001): Multiple subpial transection in Landau-Kleffner syndrome. *Dev. Med. Child Neurol.* **43**, 248–252.

Jambaqué, I. & Dulac, O. (1989): Syndrome frontal réversible et épilepsie chez un enfant de 8 ans. *Arch. Fr. Pédiatr.* **46**, 525–529.

Kyllerman, M., Nyden, A., Praquin, N., Rasmussen, P., Wetterquist, A.K. & Hedström, A. (1996): Transient psychosis in a girl with epilepsy and continuous spikes and waves during slow sleep (CSWS). *Eur. Child Adol. Psychiatry* **5**, 216–221.

Lassonde, M., Hernandez, M.T. & Sauerwein, H. (2003): Neuropsychology of frontal lobe epilepsy in children. In: *Frontal seizures and epilepsies in children*, eds. A. Beaumanoir, F. Andermann, P. Chauvel, L. Mira & B. Zifkin, pp. 147–158. Mariani Foundation Paediatric Neurology Series, vol. 11. Paris, London: John Libbey Eurotext.

Lewine, J.D., Andrews, R., Chez, M., Patil, A.A., Devinsky, O., Smith, M., Kanner, A., Davis, J.T., Funke, M., Chong, B., Provencal, S., Weisend, M., Lee, R.R. & Orrison, W.W. Jr. (1999): Magnetoencephalographic patterns of epileptiform activity in children with regressive autism spectrum disorders. *Paediatrics* **104**, 405–418.

Loiseau, P., Cohadon, F. & Mortureux, Y. (1967): A propos d'une forme singulière d'épilepsie de l'enfant. *Rev. Neurol.* **116**, 244–248.

Monteiro, J.P., Roulet Perez, E., Davidoff, V. & Deonna, T. (2001): Primary neonatal thalamic haemorrhage and epilepsy with continuous spike-waves during sleep: a longitudinal follow-up of a possible significant relation. *Eur. J. Paediatr. Neurol.* **5**, 41–47.

Petersen, J. (1992): Atypical EEG abnormalities in children with benign partial (Rolandic) epilepsy. *Acta Neurol. Scand.* (Suppl.) **6**, 45–48.

Peyre, M.P. (1998): Syndrome frontal révélateur d'une épilepsie partielle idiopathique avec POCS. Thèse, Lyon.

Prats, J.M., Garaizar, C., Garcia-Nieto, M.L. & Madoz, P. (1998): Antiepileptic drugs and atypical evolution of idiopathic partial epilepsy. *Pediatr. Neurology* **18**, 402–406.

Raffo E., De Saint-Martin, A., Carcangiu, R., Seegmuller, C., Marescaux, C. & Hirsch, E. (2001): Epilepsie idiopathique à paroxysmes frontaux: à propos de 5 observations. *XIe Réunion de la Société Française de Neurologie Pédiatrique*, Clermont-Ferrand, 25-27 January 2001 (abstract).

Robinson, R.O., Baird, G., Robinson, G. & Simonoff, E. (2001): Landau-Kleffner syndrome: course and correlates with outcome. *Dev. Med. Child Neurol.* **43**, 243–247.

Roulet, E., Deonna, T., Gaillard, F., Peter-Favre, C. & Despland, P.A. (1991): Acquired aphasia, dementia and behaviour disorder with epilepsy and continuous spike and waves during sleep in a child. *Epilepsia* **32**, 495–503.

Roulet Perez, E., Davidoff, V., Despland, P.A. & Deonna, T. (1993): Mental and behavioural deterioration of children with epilepsy and CSWS: acquired epileptic frontal syndrome. *Dev. Med. Child Neurol.* **35**, 661–674.

Roulet Perez, E., Seek, M., Mayer, E., Despland, P.A., De Tribolet, N. & Deonna, T. (1998): Childhood epilepsy with neuropsychological regression and continuous spike-waves during sleep: epilepsy surgery in a young adult. *Eur. J. Paediatr. Neurol.* **2**, 303–311.

Thomas, P., Zifkin, B., Migneco, O., Lebrun, C., Darcourt, J. & Andermann, F. (1999): Nonconvulsive status epilepticus of frontal origin. *Neurology* **52**, 1174–1183.

Tuchman, R.F. & Rapin, I. (1997): Regression in pervasive developmental disorders: seizures and epileptiform electroencephalogram correlates. *Paediatrics* **99**, 560–566.

Uldall, P., Sahlholdt, L. & Alving, J. (2000): Landau-Kleffner syndrome with onset at 18 months and an initial diagnosis of pervasive developmental disorder. *Eur. J. Paediatr. Neurol.* **4**, 81–86.

Veggiotti, P., Beccaria, F., Guerrini, R., Capovilla, G. & Lanzi, G. (1999): Continuous spike-and-wave activity during slow-wave sleep: syndrome or EEG pattern? *Epilepsia* **40** (11), 1593–1601.

Chapter 15

Neuropsychology of frontal lobe epilepsy in children

Maryse Lassonde, Hannelore C. Sauerwein and Maria-Teresa Hernandez

Experimental Neuropsychology Research Group, Department of Psychology, University of Montreal, C.P. 6128, succ. Centre-Ville, H3C 3JF Montreal, Canada
Maryse.Lassonde@UMontreal.CA

Summary

Neuropsychological studies in adult patients with frontal lobe epilepsy have revealed specific patterns of dysfunction. However, very few studies have assessed the impact of frontal lobe seizures in children. In this chapter, we attempt to provide a neuropsychological description of children suffering from frontal lobe epilepsy based on single case studies reported in the adult literature and a group study that was conducted at our centre. In the latter, we compared school-age children with frontal lobe epilepsy (FLE) to children with temporal lobe epilepsy (TLE) and generalized absence seizures (GEA). The children were submitted to a battery of neuropsychological tests that had been shown to be sensitive to frontal dysfunction in adult patients. Norms for these tests were obtained from 200 school-children 7–16 years old. In keeping with the cases described in the literature, FLE children had more difficulties than the children with other types of epilepsy on tasks assessing attention, programming of complex motor sequences, visuo-spatial organization, verbal fluency, mental flexibility, response inhibition and planning ability. They were also more susceptible to interference on verbal and visual memory tasks. These problems were more marked in the group 8–12 years old. Finally, FLE children had more attention problems, thought problems and social problems according to parents' and teacher's ratings. The implications of these findings for the cognitive and behavioural rehabilitation of these children are discussed.

The frontal lobes are known to subserve a variety of motor and higher-order cognitive functions involved in the organization and self-regulation of behaviour (Botez, 1987; Damasio & Anderson, 1986; Luria, 1969; Milner, 1982; Shue & Douglas, 1992). Evidence suggests that insult to the frontal lobes, especially the prefrontal regions, results in deficits in 'executive functions' and adaptive behaviour. The term 'executive functions' has been defined as the ability 'to maintain an appropriate problem-solving set for the attainment of future goals' (Welsh & Pennington, 1988). Executive functions include planning, organized search, concept formation, working memory, hypothesis testing, abstract reasoning, self-monitoring of behaviour, impulse control and attention control (Botez, 1987; Luria, 1969; Milner, 1963, 1964; Petrides, 1993a, 1993b). In addition, the frontal lobes guide and coordinate motor programs and play a role in memory and learning (Botez, 1987; Lepage *et al.*, 1999; Luria, 1969).

Frontal lobe lesions in adults have been found to affect the ability to initiate, modulate and inhibit ongoing mental activity (Duncan, 1986), to engage in goal-directed behaviour and to interact adequately on the social level (Grattan & Eslinger, 1992). Given the protracted development of the frontal lobes, it can be expected that some of these impairments are variably present in children suffering from frontal lobe epilepsy (FLE). The nature and extent of the deficits would not only depend on the site of the lesion (unilateral left or right, bilateral) but also on the child's age and personality development at the time of the insult. This has important implications for the child's rehabilitation which should be constantly adapted to the changing pattern of behavioural and cognitive limitations imposed by the illness at a given stage in development.

In this chapter, we attempt to provide a neuropsychological description of children with frontal lobe epilepsy based on single studies reported in the literature and a group study that was conducted at our centre. In addition, we describe several neuropsychological tests, adapted from batteries used to evaluate frontal lobe functioning in adult patients, that have proven to be useful in the assessment of children.

Functions of prefrontal cortex: evidence from studies in adult patients

Studies of frontal lobe lesions in adults indicate that the prefrontal cortex is not unitary in function (Damasio & Anderson, 1993; Fuster, 1997; Luria, 1969, Shue & Douglas, 1992). Thus, insult to the medial and orbito-frontal regions has been associated with emotional disturbances including lack of spontaneity and emotional indifference, or conversely, euphoria, impulsiveness and lack of inhibition, all of which may result in inappropriate social behaviour (Botez, 1987). In contrast, dorsolateral lesions have been found to produce deficits in attentional processes, working memory, and cognitive functions such as memory, learning and visuo-spatial functions (Fuster, 1997; Goldman-Rakic & Friedman, 1991; Petrides *et al.*, 1993a).

Patients with frontal lobe damage are often rigid in their thinking and unable to adapt their behaviour to new situations. This rigidity can be observed in motor acts as well as in verbal and cognitive behaviour. For instance, patients have difficulties performing rapid alternating movements (Luria, 1969). Once started, they cannot easily inhibit an activity, a verbal response, or an idea when it is no longer appropriate. It has also been suggested that due to their poor attention control, patients with frontal lobe dysfunction have difficulties keeping all the necessary information 'on line' when executing a new task, whereas patients with lesions of the temporal lobe seem to have difficulties storing the information (Luria, 1969). Some of the cognitive and behavioural consequences of frontal lobe lesions seen in these patients can also be demonstrated in non-human primates having undergone ablation of this area (Goldman-Rakic & Friedman, 1991).

Finally, the left-right asymmetry found in posterior association cortex also applies to frontal lobe functions. There is evidence that the left frontal lobe is primarily involved in language-related activities whereas the right frontal lobe subserves essentially non-verbal (visual and visuo-spatial) functions (Bazin *et al.*, 2000; Benton, 1968; Marlowe, 1992; Milner, 1971).

Maturational aspects of frontal lobe function: evidence from studies in healthy children

Frontal lobe development continues into the second decade. An initial growth spurt from birth to the second year is followed by slowing of the growth rate between the fourth and seventh year. Frontal lobe development includes significant increases in the size and complexity of nerve cells, progressive myelination which continues until puberty, increased cortical fissure development required for refined control of behaviour, and notable changes in synaptic density (Dempster,

1993). Synaptic density is highest during the first two years after which synaptic elimination occurs throughout childhood and adolescence (Dempster, 1993). In parallel, the frontal lobes develop rich connections with posterior and subcortical regions of the brain (Fuster, 1997; Luria, 1973).

There is evidence that the structural and physiological changes occurring during frontal lobe development coincide with an increasing efficiency in information synthesis and activity modulation (Dempster, 1993). According to developmental studies, this integrative capacity is accelerated between 8 and 12 years (Chelune & Baer, 1986; Welsh & Pennington, 1988). The performance of children below the age of 8 years resembles that of adult patients with frontal lesions in several aspects (Chelune & Baer, 1986; Passler *et al.*, 1985). Functional maturation of the frontal lobes is reached when the children are able to self-regulate their behaviour, presumably around puberty (Welsh *et al.*, 1991).

Several studies have evaluated the emergence of frontal lobe functions in children at different age levels. In most cases, the tests of frontal functions in these studies are adaptations of those designed for adults (Levin *et al.*, 1991; Welsh & Pennington, 1988). In a study by Levin *et al.* (1991), children aged 7 to 15 years were given the Wisconsin card sorting test (WCST), the Verbal and the Design fluency test, the children's version of the California verbal learning test (CVLT), a word memory and learning test, a Go–No go task, the Tower of London and the Delayed Alternation Task. Children from 7 to 12 years of age showed an increase in mental flexibility, whereas the 13–15 years old showed an increased efficiency on tasks assessing verbal learning and memory, planning ability and speed of execution. No age differences were observed on the Delayed alternation test and on the verbal fluency test. Interestingly, a recent fMRI study, comparing children between 10 and 13 years to adults (mean age 28.7 years) (Gaillard *et al.*, 2000), concluded that children and adults activate similar left frontal regions during verbal fluency tasks. However, the children showed more widespread activation, including activation of right hemisphere structures, which was taken to reflect the developmental aspect of ongoing neuronal organization.

In another developmental study, Welsh *et al.* (1991) compared adults (mean age: 22 yrs) and children aged 3 to 12 years to determine when children attain adult-like performance in different frontal lobe functions. The subjects were submitted to a battery including a motor planning task, a visual search task, the Verbal fluency test, the WCST, the Tower of Hanoi, the Matching familiar figures test, and a picture-recognition task. In addition, their cognitive level was assessed on the Iowa test of basic abilities. The earliest skill that was mastered was picture-recognition memory which attained adult-level performance at age 4. By the age of 6, the children were competent at visual search and simple planning tasks, whereas conceptual shift and accurate performance on matching tasks were not achieved before the age of 10 years. It seemed that efficiency in motor sequencing, verbal fluency and more complex planning tasks continues to develop beyond the age of 12 since the 12-year-olds in the study failed to attain adult-level performance on these tasks.

Neuropsychological findings in children with frontal lobe lesions

There is a wealth of literature documenting the impact of neurological disease on frontal lobe functions in children. For instance, impairments in executive functions have been reported in closed head injury (Levin *et al.*, 1994, 1996), meningitis (Taylor *et al.*, 1992), foetal alcohol syndrome (Streissguth *et al.*, 1994) and exposure to environmental toxins (Needleman, 1982), to name but a few. Some of the deficits can be directly related to frontal lobe dysfunction. Using functional imaging to study executive functions in head-injured children, Levin *et al.* (1994) observed that frontal lobe damage, but not extrafrontal damage, was associated with impaired performance on the Tower of London, a task that measures planning ability and response inhibition.

Studying four children with frontal lobe injury, Mateer & Williams (1991) found cognitive and behavioural changes marked by impaired attention, irritability and social problems in the absence of apparent intellectual, linguistic or perceptual deficits. Neuropsychological assessment on the revised Wechsler intelligence scale for children (WISC-R) in the post-acute stage revealed a full-scale IQ within the average range. However, the children were impaired on two subtests measuring attention (Arithmetic and digit span). Attention deficits were also evident on other tasks, such as the Trail making test parts A and B, and two cancellation tasks. Two children had deficits on tasks assessing visuo-spatial organization skills (Block design) and planning ability (Mazes). Two other children had academic difficulties in reading, spelling, reading comprehension and arithmetic. All four children had impaired reading speed and paragraph copy on the Diagnostic reading aptitude and Achievement tests, and in the word reading condition of the Stroop test. One child showed reduced verbal fluency on an animal naming test.

Performance on verbal memory tasks, including paragraph recall and sentence memory of the Detroit test of learning aptitude was severely impaired in one case, whereas memory for form and location (Tactual performance test of the Halstead Reitan test battery) and spatial memory (subtest of the Kaufman assessment battery for children) were preserved.

On the behavioural level, all the children were prone to mood swings, irritability and impulsiveness, and they were impaired with respect to social skills, coping strategies and daily living skills.

Neuropsychological findings in frontal lobe epilepsy: studies in adults

Epilepsy is associated with abnormal brain activity which may adversely affect functions subserved by the region involved (Jambaqué & Dulac, 1989; Seidenberg, 1989). Several studies suggest that focal epilepsy mimics the effects of focal lesions by producing different cognitive consequences depending on the area involved in the production of the seizures (Helmstaedter *et al.*, 1996).

Much of the data on dysfunction in frontal lobe epilepsy is derived from the preoperative work-up and postoperative follow-up of patients with focal cortical resections. Depending on the affected area(s), these patients present deficits on tasks involving spatial and non-spatial processing, sensory delay (Milner, 1964; Stuss & Benson, 1986), associative learning (Petrides, 1985), attention (Helmstaedter *et al.*, 1996; Shue & Douglas, 1992), working memory (Swartz *et al.*, 1996) and monitoring of a sequence of events (Frisk & Milner, 1999; Milner, 1963, 1982). Furthermore, compared to patients with temporal lobe epilepsy (TLE), FLE patients have been found to be significantly impaired on tasks requiring motor programming and coordination, response maintenance and response inhibition (Helmstaedter *et al.*, 1996). Similarly, comparison between non-resected FLE and TLE patients has revealed difficulties in motor programming on Luria's motor sequencing task, as well as impairments in response maintenance and response inhibition on the Stroop test, and deficits in concept formation and planning behaviour on the WCST (Helmstaedter *et al.*, 1996; Milner, 1964; Shue & Douglas, 1992). Interestingly, some of the deficits can also be demonstrated in cases of so-called benign forms of FLE (Devinsky *et al.*, 1997).

Neuropsychological consequences of frontal lobe epilepsy in children

Single case studies

Although epilepsy is one of the most prevalent neurological disorders in childhood, very few researchers have studied the impact of FLE on cognition and behaviour in children with FLE. Most of our knowledge about the neuropsychological consequences of FLE in children is based on a few single case reports. Boone *et al.* (1988) reported a frontal syndrome with a focus in the left frontal lobe in a 13-year-old girl. The patient had a frontal syndrome characterized by sudden behavioural changes including sexual disinhibition, diminished concern for personal hygiene and a tendency to physical and verbal aggression. Neuropsychological testing revealed impaired performance on tasks requiring motor speed (Finger tapping test or FTT), attention (Digit span of the WISC-R), alternation between two concepts (Trail making test, part B), planning ability (Mazes of the WISC-R) and response inhibition (Stroop test). Motor performance on the FTT was depressed for each hand, particularly the left. Attention was also impaired. In contrast, no deficits were observed on tests of abstract reasoning, conceptual shift (WCST) and sequential organization of visual information (Picture arrangement of the WISC-R). Similarly, visual perceptual organization (Hooper visual organization test), basic language skills (Reitan indiana aphasia screening exam) and fund of general knowledge (Information subtest of the WISC-R) were within the normal range. Visuo-motor integration and constructional skills were also preserved although impulsive responses were noted on Beery's developmental test of visual motor integration. Performance on Rey's auditory verbal learning test was normal, whereas overall performance on the Wechsler memory scale was impaired. Her handwriting was uneven, with large overlapping letters. The frontal symptoms and her scores improved when the seizures were controlled by medication.

A frontal syndrome was also observed by Jambaqué and Dulac (1989) in an 8-year-old boy with a focus in the right fronto-temporal region. Like the patient reported by Boone *et al.* (1988), the child had difficulties controlling his temper and showed marked personality and affective changes. Initial testing on the WISC-R revealed a global IQ in the high average range with the highest score on Block design, measuring visuo-spatial abilities, and the lowest score on the subtests Coding and Mazes, assessing performance speed and planning ability. He also had a marked attention deficit. The child was hyperactive and had difficulties inhibiting motor responses. His ability to reproduce a sequence of hand movements was also impaired. Manual dexterity was also affected as shown by a deterioration of his handwriting. Verbal fluency was reduced although language functions were within the normal range. As in the case reported by Boone *et al.* (1988), seizure control resulted in an improvement in most functions.

Group study

To our knowledge, no group studies have been reported to date. In the following section, we describe the performance of FLE children and children with other types of epilepsy on a selection of neuropsychological tests considered to be most sensitive to frontal lobe dysfunction (Hernandez *et al.*, 2002; Hernandez *et al.*, in preparation). The FLE group consisted of 16 children (four girls and 12 boys). The performance of this group was compared to that of a group of eight children (four girls and four boys) with temporal lobe epilepsy (TLE) and a third group of eight children (four girls and four boys) with generalized epilepsy and typical absences as the principal seizure type (GEA). Half of the FLE patients were chosen from the patient pool of the Hôpital Saint-Vincent-de-Paul in Paris. The other half of the FLE children and all the TLE and GEA children were selected from the Hôpital Sainte-Justine in Montreal. The case histories were obtained from the children's medical files. Additional information was obtained from the parents in a semi-structured interview. Parents gave their informed consent for the participation of their children in the study.

To be included in the study the children had to have an IQ in the normal range (> 85) and a principal diagnosis of frontal, temporal or generalized epilepsy according to their clinical history and EEG records. Children with concomitant CNS pathology (e.g. hemiplegia, tumours, head injury), brain surgery and/or psychiatric problems were excluded. The three groups were matched with respect to global IQ, assessed on the WISC-III (Wechsler, 1991), chronological age, age at seizure onset and duration of epilepsy. Half of the patients in the FLE and TLE groups had bilateral foci. The other half had a unilateral focus, 25 per cent in the right and 25 per cent in the left hemisphere. A structural lesion (cortical dysplasia) was present in three FLE and two TLE patients. All but two children were on medication; in six FLE children and four TLE children the seizures were controlled with a single drug whereas 10 FLE and three TLE children received more than one drug. None of the children had any seizure for at least two months prior to testing.

The children performed a battery of tests designed to assess motor programming, executive functions, attention and working memory. Normative data were obtained from an unselected group of 200 healthy french-speaking children, aged 8 to 16.5 years (Lussier, 1992; Lussier *et al.*, 1998), except for the Purdue pegboard test and the WCST for which norms for children are provided in the test manual. Parents were also asked to rate the behaviour and social competence of their child on the Achenbach child behaviour checklist (Achenbach & Edelbrock, 1993).

Intelligence

The effect of frontal lobe lesions on intelligence is the subject of ongoing debate. There is reasonable agreement in the literature that the global score on psychometric tests is preserved (Damasio & Anderson, 1993). Like adult frontal patients (Milner, 1963, 1964), FLE children (Boone *et al.*, 1988; Jambaqué & Dulac, 1989) and children with frontal lobe injury (Mateer & Williams, 1991) are reported to have normal psychometric intelligence on the Wechsler intelligence scale. However, they may score lower on a number of selective subtests measuring attention and concentration (Digit span and arithmetic), visuo-motor processing speed (Coding) and planning ability (Mazes) (Jambaqué & Dulac, 1989). Unlike adult patients, who perform poorly on the Block-Design subtest (Milner, 1963, 1964), FLE children do not seem to have difficulties on this test (Boone *et al.*, 1988; Jambaqué & Dulac, 1989).

Consistently with the literature, the FLE children in our sample were not impaired in general intelligence, verbal reasoning, or non-verbal reasoning abilities, but scored lower than both TLE and GEA children in processing speed and planning ability on the Coding and symbol search subtests and the Mazes. Similar deficits have been reported for adult patients on the Porteus Maze (Botez, 1987) and the stylus maze (Milner, 1964). Taken together, these results suggest that planning and processing speed are selectively affected in FLE.

Motor coordination

Motor coordination tasks, such as the Purdue pegboard test (Lezak, 1983) and Thurstone's uni- and bimanual performance test (Lezak, 1983), are commonly used in the pre- and post-surgical neuropsychological assessment of epileptic children and adults (see Lassonde & Sauerwein, 1996). The former requires the placement of pegs in rows of holes laid out vertically on a board. The test is alternately performed with the preferred hand, the non-preferred and with both hands simultaneously. The score is the number of pegs placed in 30 and 60 seconds. In Thurstone's uni- and bimanual performance test, the child has to use a stylus to touch a metal plate divided into four sections in a prescribed order, clockwise or counterclockwise. The task requires rapid sequential movements with each hand in the unimanual condition and asynchronous simultaneous movements with both hands in the bimanual condition. The score is the number of correct contacts without a break in sequence in 30 seconds.

The FLE children were impaired with the non-dominant hand and in the bimanual condition compared to TLE and GEA children. This was especially true for the younger FLE children (aged 8–12 years), who experienced greater difficulties on the more complex Uni- and bimanual performance test, whereas the younger TLE and GEA children did not differ from the older ones (aged 9–16 years). The results suggest that FLE interferes with the execution of complex motor activity, involving primarily bimanual operations and the coordination of the non-dominant hand, most probably because the latter hand is less frequently engaged in skilled activities than is the dominant hand. The findings further indicate that the development of these functions is delayed in children with FLE.

Motor programming and mental flexibility

Difficulties on tasks requiring rapid alternation of movements and conceptual shift are common clinical features in adults with frontal lobe lesions (Luria, 1969) and FLE (Helmstaedter *et al.*, 1996). Typically, the patients display perseverative behaviour on tasks requiring alternating sequential hand movements (fist-palm-side) or alternating graphic sequences, reproduction of rhythmic structures, inverse tapping (one tap for every two taps of the experimenter and vice versa), alternating graphic sequence (Peña-Casanova, 1990) and reciprocal coordination tasks (palm-fist alternation) (Luria, 1969).

Compared to TLE and GEA children, fewer FLE children obtained perfect scores on the sequencing tests. In addition, the FLE children were generally slower and more rigid in their movements and had greater difficulties maintaining a smooth flow of movements. Some of these problems have also been reported for the 8-year-old boy with FLE evaluated by Jambaqué and Dulac (1989). He had difficulties reproducing asymmetrical motor sequences and performing an inverse tapping task. He was also unable to reproduce rhythmic sequences of increasing length that were tapped on the table by the experimenter. This rigidity reflects the inability, commonly observed in adults with frontal lobe dysfunction, to inhibit ongoing motor activity and to adjust movements to the changing pattern of the task.

Concept formation and conceptual shift

The Wisconsin card sorting test (WCST) (Lezak, 1983) is a cognitive measure of mental flexibility. This test also assesses strategy search and concept formation ability. The child is given a pack of cards and has to match them one by one with four target cards. The cards have to be sorted first by colour, then by form and finally by number. The child has to detect the sorting principle on his own by responding to feedback (right or wrong) of the examiner. As soon as one concept is acquired, as shown by 10 consecutive correct responses, the response category is changed without informing the child, who must adapt the responses accordingly. The measures include the number of categories successfully completed (from zero to six), the number of perseverative responses (i.e. a response that would have been correct for the preceding concept but is no longer valid) and the number of perseverative errors (i.e. persistent responses to the previous category despite negative feedback).

The WCST is sensitive to perseveration and assesses the ability to effect conceptual shift (Roberts & Pennington, 1996). The subject has to inhibit an activity that occurs or interferes with an upcoming solution to a problem. Adults with frontal lobe lesions have been shown to make significantly more perseverative errors and produce fewer conceptual shifts than non-frontal controls (Milner, 1963, 1964). When this test is given to children, the performance of normal 6-year-olds is similar to that of frontal lobe damaged adults (Chelune & Baer, 1986). However, older children are able to inhibit inappropriate responses.

We found no differences between FLE, TLE and GEA children on any of the measures. Similarly, the performance of the 13-year-old FLE girl in the case study discussed above (Boone et al., 1988) was comparable to that of normal 13-year-old children. It is possible that there is fractionation within executive skills, with some of the functions being more affected than others in FLE due to differences in underlying pathology, aetiology or localization of the lesion.

Verbal search

The Thurstone word fluency test (Lezak, 1983; Milner, 1964) is used routinely to assess systematic and spontaneous verbal search, a function considered to be mediated by the frontal lobes. In the phonetic or morphological condition of this test, the subject has to generate as many words as possible beginning with a specific letter within a limited period of time. In the semantic condition, he/she is asked to produce words belonging to a specific semantic category (given names, names of fruits, vegetables and animals).

The FLE children studied by our group generated significantly fewer words than the GEA children in the phonemic condition and fewer category-specific names than the TLE subjects in the semantic condition. Again, this effect was mainly attributable to the poorer performance of the younger FLE children. Similar results have been reported by Jambaqué & Dulac (1989) whose 8-year-old patient showed reduced verbal fluency whereas the 13-year-old girl studied by Boone et al. (1988) was not impaired in this function. Although a developmental trend has been demonstrated for this test (Welsh & Pennington, 1988; Welsh et al., 1991), the results cannot entirely be attributed to maturational factors since the younger TLE and GEA children in our study did not differ from the older ones. It is more likely that FLE children had difficulties initiating an effective verbal search, which is characteristic of adults with frontal lobe lesions who are given this kind of task (Lezak, 1983; Milner, 1964).

Attention and working memory

Attention control is considered an important function of the prefrontal cortex (Fuster, 1997). Deficits in FLE children have been reported in Digit span (Boone et al., 1988) as well as on the Continuous performance test (CPT) (Jambaqué & Dulac, 1989). The latter has proved to be most useful in the evaluation of sustained auditory and visual attention (Rosvolt et al., 1956). Preliminary results of our study (Hernandez et al., in preparation) suggest that FLE children are more impaired than TLE and GEA children on these attention tasks.

The Self-ordered pointing test (Petrides & Milner, 1982) was designed to assess the production and application of memory strategies through visual association. The subject has to point to one of six to 10 abstract designs on consecutively presented cards without pointing twice to the same design. After completing the test, a recognition condition is administered where the subject is asked to find the designs pointed to previously among an array of abstract patterns. Petrides & Milner (1982) found impairments on this task in their patients with frontal lesions, especially those with left frontal lesions. Difficulties on this kind of test have been related to deficits in working memory and lack of self-monitoring strategies (Petrides et al., 1993b). Working memory refers to the attention-demanding activity to momentarily keep 'on line' all the information necessary for the successful execution of a mental task. PET studies indicate that the mid-dorsolateral frontal cortex (Brodmann's areas 46 and 9) is critically involved in this kind of activity (Petrides et al., 1993a).

Unlike in adult patients, no differences were observed between our FLE, TLE and GEA subjects on the self-ordered pointing test. All three groups had more difficulties than healthy controls on the pointing task, but not on the recognition task. This suggests that working memory may be affected in various types of epilepsy. This test may therefore not be sensitive enough to differentiate frontal epilepsy from other epilepsy types.

Visual memory and visuo-spatial organization

The Rey-Osterrieth figure (Lezak, 1983) measures planning ability as well as visuo-spatial organization and memory. The test consists of a complex geometric design that has to be reproduced first from a model and immediately thereafter from memory. Difficulties in reproduction and immediate recall of this figure have been occasionally reported for adults with frontal lobe dysfunction (Kaplan, 1983). The deficits seen in these patients have been attributed primarily to difficulties in visuo-spatial organization. By contrast, patients with TLE appear to be impaired on the memory part of this task, which is in line with the memory deficits commonly reported in children with TLE (Seidenberg, 1989). This pattern also emerged in our group study (Hernandez *et al.*, in preparation).

Planning ability

Adult patients with frontal lobe lesions, including FLE, consistently show difficulties on tests requiring anticipation, planning and speed of execution (Shallice, 1982). The Tower of London is the test most frequently used to measure these functions in both children and adults (Levin *et al.*, 1994, 1996; Shallice, 1982). The material consists of three coloured spheres (blue, green and red) which are stacked on three pegs of different lengths (one peg which can hold three, one which can hold two and one which can only hold one sphere). Always starting from the same configuration, the subject is asked to match 12 models of increasing difficulty, using a specified, limited number of moves. A maximum of six trials is allowed for each model. The planning time, execution time and total time are recorded. Additional measures include the number of models correctly completed on the first trial, the number of trials taken to copy a model correctly and the total number of trials taken by the child to complete all 12 models.

To our knowledge, there are no studies that have employed this test in FLE children. However, children with FLE have shown impairments on other measures of planning skills such as the Mazes subtest of the WISC (Boone *et al.*, 1988; Jambaqué & Dulac, 1989). The FLE children tested by our group were impaired with respect to both planning time and execution time. They took less time to anticipate and plan their moves but required significantly more time to complete the models than did TLE and GEA children. This test may therefore be an important instrument to measure frontal lobe dysfunction and to differentiate FLE children from children with other types of epilepsy.

Affective and social behaviour

Although the frontal lobes are associated with the control and self-regulation of cognitive, affective and social behaviour, the assessment of emotional and social adaptation in FLE children has been largely ignored by researchers and treatment providers. This is the more surprising since the children are acquiring skills for future psychosocial adjustment (Seidenberg, 1989) and are thus particularly vulnerable to the negative impact of their epilepsy. Several studies have shown that insult to the frontal lobes during childhood can have long-term consequences for cognitive and behavioural adaptation (Marlowe, 1992; Grattan & Ettlinger, 1992). Neuropsychological assessment of FLE children should therefore include other sources of information such as behaviour questionnaires, school records, interviews with parents and teachers, and observation of the child in different social settings, to identify possible changes in behaviour patterns. In our study, the parents of FLE children tended to report more problems (attention, thought, social) on the Achenbach child behaviour check list (Achenbach & Edelbrock, 1993) than the parents of the other two epilepsy groups.

Conclusions

FLE children present many deficits commonly seen in adults with frontal lobe epilepsy. Specifically, FLE children showed difficulties on tasks assessing attention, programming of complex motor sequences, mental flexibility, verbal search, visuo-spatial organization, response inhibition and planning ability. Some of the impairments were more marked in children below the age of 13, suggesting that the epilepsy may delay the emergence of these skills.

In keeping with previous findings, intellectual functions were not selectively impaired. Attentional capacities were impaired in FLE children, whereas visual working memory was not selectively affected in the FLE group. All three groups had some difficulties on the Self-ordering pointing task compared to healthy children, which suggests that this attention-demanding function is impaired in many types of epilepsy.

As for concept formation and mental flexibility, the WCST failed to discriminate between the three groups, possibly because not all FLE children in our study showed the characteristic pattern due to differences in the underlying pathology and aetiology.

Finally, a specific behaviour profile of FLE was obtained using parents' ratings, showing that FLE children had more attention problems, thought problems and social problems than the other two epilepsy groups, which may have serious consequences for their social adjustment.

The effects of age, sex, age at seizure onset, side of lesion and anticonvulsant medication on frontal lobe functioning remain to be explored. In addition, more research is necessary to arrive at a better understanding of frontal lobe functioning in epilepsy in relation to the functioning of other parts of the brain. Longitudinal studies in larger samples and neuroimaging techniques such as fMRI, PET and SPECT may help to shed more light on the impact of FLE on executive functions and behaviour in children.

Implications for the rehabilitation of children with frontal epilepsy

The identification, understanding and treatment of specific difficulties of FLE children are important, especially since some of these problems carry over into adulthood. Rehabilitation of the FLE child requires a multidisciplinary approach, including pharmacological management, tutoring if necessary, and psychological support. Specific remediation programs for the training of executive functions (Akhutina, 1997) may be needed. Parents and teachers should be involved. FLE children require external structure. They need help in the organization and planning of their work and activities. A behavioural modification approach may be useful. Training in social skills and self-management may be necessary to help the child achieve greater autonomy and to raise self-esteem. We suggest that intervention begin as early as possible to prevent academic failure, affective disorders and maladjustment.

References

Achenbach, T.M. & Edelbrock, C. (1993): *Manual for the child behaviour check list*. Burlington VT: University of Vermont, Department of Psychiatry.

Akhutina, T.V. (1997): The remediation of executive functions in children with cognitive disorders: the Vygotsky-Luria neuropsychological approach. *J. Int. Disab. Res.* **41**, 144–151.

Bazin, B., Cohen, L., Lehericy, S., Pierrot-Deseilligny, C. & Baulac Le Bihan, D. (2000): Study of hemispheric lateralization of language regions by functional MRI. *Rev. Neurol. (Paris)* **156**, 145–148.

Benton, A.L. (1968): Differential behavioural effects of frontal lobe disease. *Neuropsychologia* **6**, 53–60.

Boone, K.B., Miller, B.L., Rosenberg, L., Durazo, A., McIntyre, H. & Weil, M. (1988): Neuropsychological and behavioural abnormalities in an adolescent with frontal lobe seizures. *Neurology* **38**, 583–586.

Botez, M.I. (1987): Les syndromes du lobe frontal. In: *Neuropsychologie clinique et neurologie du comportement*, ed. M.I. Botez, pp. 117–134. Montréal: Québec: Les Presses de l'Université de Montréal et Paris: Masson.

Chelune, G.J. & Baer, R.A. (1986): Developmental norms for the Wisconsin Card Sorting Test. *J. Clin. Exp. Neuropsychol.* **8** (3), 219–228.

Damasio, A.R. & Anderson, S.W. (1993): The frontal lobes. In: *Clinical neuropsychology*, eds. K.M. Heilman & E. Valenstein, pp. 409–460. New York: Oxford University Press.

Dempster, F.N. (1993): Resistance to interference: developmental changes in a basic processing mechanism. In: *Emerging themes in cognitive development foundations*, eds. M.L. Howe & R. Pasnak, vol. 1, pp. 3–27. New York: Springer-Verlag.

Devinsky, O., Gershengorn, J., Brown, E., Perrine, K., Vazquez, B. & Luciano, D. (1997): Frontal functions in juvenile myoclonic epilepsy. *Neuropsychiatry, Neuropsychol. Behav. Neurol.* **10** (4), 243–246.

Douglas, V.I. (1983): Attentional and cognitive problems. In: *Developmental neuropsychiatry*, ed. M. Rutter, pp. 280–329. New York: Guilford.

Duncan, J. (1986): Disorganization of behaviour after frontal lobe damage. *Cogn. Neuropsychol.* **3**, 271–290.

Frisk, V. & Milner, B. (1990): The relationship of working memory to the immediate recall of stories following unilateral temporal or frontal lobectomy. *Neuropsychologia* **28**, 121–135.

Fuster, J.M. (1997): Human neuropsychology. In: *The prefrontal cortex*, ed. J.M. Fuster, pp. 150–184. New York: Lippincott-Raven.

Gaillard, W.D., Hertz-Pannier, L., Mott, S.H., Barnett, A.S., Le Bihan, D. & Theodore, W.H. (2000): fMRI of verbal fluency in children and adults. *Neurology* **54**, 180–187.

Goldman-Rakic, P.S. & Friedman, H.R. (1991): The circuitry of working memory revealed by anatomy and metabolic imaging. In: *Frontal lobes function and dysfunction*, eds. H.S. Levin, H.M. Eisenberg & A.L. Benton, pp. 72–91. New York: Oxford University Press.

Grattan, R.M. & Eslinger, P.J. (1992): Long-term psychological consequences of childhood frontal lobe lesion in patient D.T. *Brain Cogn.* **20**, 185–195.

Helmstaedter, C., Kemper, B. & Elger, C.E. (1996): Neuropsychological aspects of frontal lobe epilepsy. *Neuropsychologia* **34** (5), 399–406.

Hernandez, M.T., Sauerwein, H.C., Jambaque, I., De Guise, E., Lussier, F., Lortie, A., Dulac, O. & Lassonde, M. (2002): Deficits in executive functions and motor coordination in children with frontal lobe epilepsy. *Neuropsychologia* **40**, 384–400.

Hernandez, M.T., Sauerwein, H.C., Jambaqué, I., De Guise, E., Lussier, F., Lortie, A., Dulac, O. & Lassonde, M. (in preparation): Learning, attention, memory and social adjustment in children with frontal lobe epilepsy.

Jambaqué, I. & Dulac, O. (1989): Syndrome frontal réversible et épilepsie chez un enfant de 8 ans. *Arch. Fr. Pediatr.* **46**, 525–529.

Kaplan, E. (1983): A process approach to neuropsychological assessment. In: *The assessment of aphasia and related disorders*, eds. H. Goodglass & E. Kaplan, pp. 125–167. Philadelphia: Lea and Febiger.

Lassonde, M. & Sauerwein, H.C. (1996): Tests spécifiques dans l'évaluation neuropsychologique pré- et post-chirurgicale de l'enfant atteint d'épilepsie. *A.N.A.E.*, Numéro Hors-Série, 43–48.

Lepage, M., Beaudoin, G., Boulet, C., O'Brien, I., Marcantoni, W., Bourgoin, P. & Richer, F. (1999): Frontal cortex and the programming of repetitive tapping movements in man: lesion effects and functional neuroimaging. *Brain Res.* **8**, 17–25.

Levin, H.S., Culhane, K.A., Hartmann, J., Evankovich, K., Mattson, A.J., Harward, H., Ringholz, G., Ewing-Cobs, L. & Fletcher, J.M. (1991): Developmental changes in performance on tests of purported frontal lobe functioning. *Dev. Neuropsychol.* **7** (3), 377–395.

Levin, H.S., Fletcher, J.M., Kufera, J.A., Haward, H., Lilly, M.A., Mendelsohn, D.B., Bruce, D. & Eisenberg, H.M. (1996): Dimension of cognition measured by the Tower of London and other cognitive tasks in head-injured children and adolescents. *Dev. Neuropsychol.* **12**, 17–34.

Levin, H.S., Mendelsohn, D.B., Lilly, M.A. & Fletcher, J.M. (1994): Tower of London performance in relation to magnetic resonance imaging following closed head injury in children. *Neuropsychology* **8**, 171–179.

Lezak, M.D. (1983): *Neuropsychological assessment*. New York: Oxford University Press.

Luria, A.R. (1969): Frontal lobe syndromes. In: *Handbook of clinical neurology*, eds. P.J. Vinken, G.W. Bruyn & A. Biemond, vol. 2, pp. 725–757. Amsterdam, Holland: North-Holland Publishing Company.

Luria, A.R. (1973): *The working brain: an introduction to neuropsychology*. New York: Basic Books.

Lussier, F. (1992): Dysfonctionnement frontal chez des patients atteints du Syndrome de Gilles de la Tourette. Unpublished doctoral dissertation. Montréal: Université de Montréal.

Lussier, F., Guérin, F., Dufresne A. & Lassonde, M. (1998): Étude normative développementale des fonctions exécutives: la tour de Londres. *A.N.A.E.* **47**, 42–52.

Marlowe, W. (1992): The impact of right prefrontal lesion on the developing brain. *Brain Cogn.* **20**, 205–213.

Mateer, C.A. & Williams, D. (1991): Effects of frontal lobe injury in childhood. *Dev. Neuropsychol.* **7** (2), 359–376.

Milner, B. (1963): Effects of different brain lesions on card sorting. *Arch. Neurol.* **9**, 90–100.

Milner, B. (1964): Some effects of frontal lobectomy in man. In: *The frontal granular cortex and behaviour*, eds. J.M. Warren & K. Akert, pp. 313–334. New York: McGraw Hill.

Milner, B. (1971): Interhemispheric differences in the localization of psychological processes in man. *Br. Med. J.* **27** (3), 272–277.

Milner, B. (1982): Some cognitive effects of frontal lobe lesions in man. *Philos. Trans. R. Soc. Lond. Sci.* **298**, 211–226.

Needleman, H.L. (1982): The neuropsychiatric implications of low level exposure to lead. *Psychol. Med.* **12**, 461–463.

Passler, M.A., Isaac, W. & Hynd, G.W. (1985): Neuropsychological development of behaviour attributed to frontal lobe performance in children. *Dev. Neuropsychol.* **1** (4), 349–370.

Peña-Casanova, J. (1990): Programa integrado de exploracion Neuropsicologica-Test Barcelona Manual. Barcelona: Masson.

Petrides, M. (1985): Deficits on conditional associative-learning tasks after frontal- and temporal-lobe lesions in man. *Neuropsychologia* **23** (5), 601–614.

Petrides, M. & Milner, B. (1982): Deficits on subject-ordered tasks after frontal and temporal lobe lesions in man. *Neuropsychologia* **20**, 249–262.

Petrides, M., Alivisatos, B., Evans, A.C. & Meyer, E. (1993a): Dissociation of human mid-dorsal from posterior dorsolateral frontal cortex in memory processing. *Proc. Natl. Acad. Sci. USA* **90**, 873–877.

Petrides, M., Alivisatos, B., Meyer, E. & Evans, A.C. (1993b): Functional activation of human frontal cortex during the performance of verbal working memory tasks. *Proc. Natl. Acad. Sci. USA* **90**, 878–882.

Roberts, R.J. & Pennington, B.F. (1996): An interactive framework for examining prefrontal cognitive processes. *Dev. Neuropsychol.* **12** (1), 105–126.

Rosvold, H.E., Mirsky, A.F., Sarason, I., Bransome, E.D. Jr. & Beck, L.H. (1956): A continuous performance test of brain damage. *J. Consult. Psychol.* **20**, 343–350.

Seidenberg, M. (1989): Neuropsychological functioning of children with epilepsy. In: *Neuropsychological, psychosocial and intervention aspect of childhood epilepsies*, eds. B.P. Herman & M. Seidenberg, pp. 71–82. New York: John Wiley and Sons.

Shallice, T. (1982): Specific impairments of planning. *Philos. Trans. R. Soc. Lond. Sci.* **298**, 199–209.

Shue, M.L. & Douglas, V.I. (1992): Attention deficit hyperactivity disorder and the frontal lobe syndrome. *Brain Cogn.* **20**, 104–124.

Streissguth, A., Sampson, P.D., Carmichael, O.H., Bookstein, F.L., Barr, H.M., Scott, M., Feldman, J. & Mirsky, A.F. (1994): Maternal drinking during pregnancy. Attention and short-term memory performance in 14-year offspring: a longitudinal prospective study. *Alcohol. Clin. Exp. Res.* **18**, 202–218.

Stuss, D.T. & Benson, D.F. (1986): *The frontal lobes*. New York: Academic Press.

Swartz, B.E., Halgren, E., Simpkins, F., Fuster, J., Mandelkern, M., Krisdakumtorn, T., Gee, M., Brown, C., Ropchan, J.R. & Blahd, W.H. (1996): Primary or working memory in frontal lobe epilepsy: an FDG-PET study of dysfunctional zones. *Neurology* **46**, 737–747.

Taylor, H.G., Barry, C.T. & Shatschneider, C. (1992): School-age consequences of *Haemophilus influenzae* type b meningitis. *J. Clin. Psychol.* **22**, 196–206.

Wechsler, D. (1991): *Wechsler Intelligence Scale for Children-Third Edition*. New York: Psychological Corporation and Harcourt Brace Jovanovich.

Welsh, M.C. & Pennington, B.F. (1988): Assessing frontal lobe functioning in children: views from developmental psychology. *Dev. Neuropsychol.* **4** (3), 199–230.

Welsh, M.C., Pennington, B.F. & Groisser, D.B. (1991): A normative-developmental study of executive function: a window on prefrontal function in children. *Dev. Neuropsychol.* **7**, 131–149.

Chapter 16

Functional imaging of frontal lobe epilepsies

John S. Duncan

*National Society for Epilepsy, University College London & National Hospital for Neurology & Neurosurgery,
Chalfont St Peter, Buckinghamshire, SL9 0LR, UK*
j.duncan@ion.ucl.ac.uk

Summary

Optimal magnetic resonance imaging (MRI) can reveal structural pathology underlying frontal lobe epilepsy in up to 75 per cent of potential candidates for surgical treatment. Functional imaging has a role in defining the source of the epilepsy, particularly in those in whom the MRI is unremarkable or unclear. Inter-ictal magnetic resonance spectroscopic imaging and positron emission tomography with ^{18}F-fluorodeoxyglucose or ^{11}C-flumazenil may define areas of functional abnormality. A combination of ictal and inter-ictal single photon emission computerized tomography scans may indicate the parts involved in seizure generation. Functional MRI shows promise as a non-invasive method to identify the cerebral generators of inter-ictal epileptic activity. Functional MRI also has a role in identifying the parts of the brain involved in cognitive tasks, such as language. It is possible that in the future batteries of cognitive activation paradigms will help to direct safer surgical therapy.

In the last decade, much progress has been made in the structural and functional imaging of the brain in epilepsy. The correlation of structure with function is essential in the understanding of transient disorders of brain function, which often have a structural basis.

The investigation and treatment of patients with epilepsy has been revolutionized in the last decade with the advent of magnetic resonance imaging (MRI). The best results are obtained using T2-weighted and high-resolution T1-weighted volumetric techniques with thin partitions, covering the whole brain and allowing viewing of the structures in two orthogonal planes. Interpretation needs to analyse the cortical grey matter, the grey-white boundary, white matter and ventricles. It is often difficult to be certain whether subtle abnormalities of sulcal morphology are outside the normal range. Analysis of MRIs of young children needs to take into account the normal development of myelination and the indistinct grey-white matter boundary on T2-weighted images in children aged less than 2 years.

Malformations of cortical development (MCD) are commonly identified as causes of frontal lobe epilepsy. These abnormalities are increasingly being recognized in patients with seizure disorders previously regarded as cryptogenic, and these data may lead to a reclassification of a patient's epilepsy syndrome from cryptogenic and generalized to symptomatic and localization-related. The range of MCD identified with MRI includes schizencephaly, agyria, diffuse and focal macrogyria, focal polymicrogyria, minor gyral abnormalities, subependymal grey matter heterotopias, bilateral subcortical laminar heterotopia, tuberous sclerosis, focal cortical dysplasia and dysembryoplastic neuroepithelial tumours (DNTs).

Focal cortical dysplasia may result in refractory partial seizures. The possibility of surgical treatment means that its identification with MRI has important consequences (Palmini *et al.*, 1991a; Kuzniecky, 1995). Macrogyria, microgyria and other disorders of gyrus formation may be apparent (Guerrini *et al.*, 1992). A focal area of polymicrogyria, for example, may not be evident on sagittal, coronal or axial scans and only be evident on a reformatted tangential slice that cuts across the affected area, or on a three-dimensional reconstruction of the surface of the brain (Barkovich *et al.*, 1995). Quantitative analysis of the relative volumes of grey and white matter in a cerebral hemisphere that appears macroscopically normal, in patients with apparently localized neuronal migration defect, may reveal widespread abnormalities (Sisodiya *et al.*, 1995) implying that the migration disorder is more extensive. These findings are in agreement with the poor likelihood of a focal cortical resection rendering a patient with a malformation of cortical development seizure-free, and with the contention that even high-resolution contemporary MRI only reveals the 'tip of the iceberg' of abnormal cortical development.

The complete removal of discrete epileptogenic neocortical lesions, identified with MRI, is highly successful in controlling seizures (Williamson *et al.*, 1992; Kuzniecky *et al.*, 1993a). If no lesion is identifiable on a high-quality MRI, or if there is incomplete removal of a lesion, such as in multilobar gliosis, the chance of relieving seizures is not good (Cascino *et al.*, 1992). Functional imaging and invasive EEG recordings may still be needed if no lesion is evident on a high-quality MRI, if there is dual pathology, or if the clinical and EEG features are discordant with the MRI.

Functional magnetic resonance imaging

Ictal and inter-ictal epileptiform activity

Functional MRI (fMRI) can detect ictal changes in cerebral blood flow (Jackson *et al.*, 1994; Detre *et al.*, 1995; Warach *et al.*, 1996). Activation of the thalamus with activation of the motor cortex has been shown in a patient with frequent partial seizures, indicating activation of a neural network (Detre *et al.*, 1996). Limitations of the method include movement artefact, although this may be compensated for by image coregistration, and the fact that it is impracticable for a patient to lie for hours in an MRI scanner awaiting the onset of a seizure.

The development of safe and reliable EEG recording from subjects having undergone fMRI studies has been a major step forward in the fMRI of inter-ictal epileptiform activity (Ives *et al.*, 1993; Lemieux *et al.*, 1997; Allen *et al.*, 1998). Focal increases in cerebral blood delivery have been identified in patients with frequent inter-ictal spikes (Krakow *et al.*, 1999a, b; Symms *et al.*, 1999). The time course of the increase was similar to that seen in cognitive activation tasks, with maxima at 4–6 seconds. EEG-triggered fMRI and 3D-EEG source localization have been used together. In a patient with frontal lobe seizures fMRI showed multiple areas of activation; 3D EEG source localization identified the same areas and suggested a left frontal onset (Seeck *et al.*, 1998). A potential development will be to use the fMRI data to constrain the solutions of dipole modelling of the source of inter-ictal epileptiform activity, and to simplify the 'inverse problem'.

Clinically, these methods will aid EEG interpretation and understanding of the pathophysiological basis of epileptic activity. Their application, utility and limitations in defining the irritative zone of the cortex that generates inter-ictal spikes, and its relationship with the epileptogenic zone that gives

Localization and lateralization of cognitive function

Another important use of fMRI in epilepsy is to delineate areas of brain that are responsible for specific functions, such as the primary sensory and motor cortex, and to identify their anatomical relation to areas of planned neurosurgical resection (Morris *et al.*, 1994; Hammeke *et al.*, 1994; Puce *et al.*, 1995; Rao *et al.*, 1995). In patients with cerebral lesions, the localization of cognitive activation may differ from the pattern in normal subjects (Alsop *et al.*, 1996). These data may be helpful in planning neocortical resections of epileptic foci, to minimize the risk of causing a fixed deficit.

Lateralization of language function may also be accomplished using fMRI (Binder *et al.*, 1995; Desmond *et al.*, 1995). There was a strong correlation between language lateralization measured with the carotid amytal test, and using fMRI with a single-word semantic decision task (Binder *et al.*, 1996), and other fMRI language studies have generally concurred with carotid amytal testing (Desmond *et al.*, 1995; Benson *et al.*, 1999). This technique has also been performed in children and adolescents (Hertz-Pannier *et al.*, 1997). Comparison of fMRI and carotid amytal testing has shown that the duration of speech arrest during the latter is not a reliable measure of language dominance (Benbadis *et al.*, 1998). Functional MRI results, however, do not always accord with the carotid amytal data (Worthington *et al.*, 1997). There is discrepancy in approximately one in 10 persons. Artefacts and technical difficulties may adversely affect both methods. Further, identification of the areas of brain involved in language is not the same as determining if someone can speak when half of the brain is anaesthetized.

Activation patterns related to verb generation, object naming and reading have been compared, and only verb generation gave reliable lateralization compared with carotid amytal and cortical stimulation testing (Benson *et al.*, 1999). Studies in which word generation is compared with the resting state usually show activation of anterior language areas. Comparisons of semantic tasks with non-linguistic control tasks show more widespread activation in the dominant hemisphere (Binder *et al.*, 1997).

As well as predicting the lateralization of language function, fMRI may localize cerebral areas involved in language. In the future, these data may assist in planning surgical resections in the language-dominant hemisphere. There are, however, important caveats. Absence of activation on one language task does not guarantee that that part of the brain is inert. Conversely, an area that is activated may have only a peripheral and non-essential role in verbal communication. Although interpretation of activation studies of primary motor and somatosensory cortex may be straightforward, the integration of cognitive activation data into surgical decision-making needs to be cautious, particularly for more sophisticated paradigms. There are two principal caveats: first, if a cerebral area does not activate on a specific task, this does not imply that it may be removed with impunity; secondly, the activation of a particular cerebral area with a specific task does not necessarily imply that surgery to that area would cause a clinically significant fixed deficit.

Magnetic resonance spectroscopy

Proton spectroscopy

The metabolites which are detectable using proton magnetic resonance spectroscopy (MRS) depend on the conditions used for the acquisition. Some molecules, for example gamma-aminobutyric acid

(GABA), glutamate, glutamine and lactate, give rise to MR signals that exhibit spin-spin coupling, which results in the signals changing with time. As a result, the detection of their resonance is dependent on the echo time used. In epilepsy studies *in vivo*, the principal signals of interest have been those from N-acetyl aspartate (NAA), creatine + phosphocreatine (Cr), choline-containing compounds (Cho), and lactate (Lac). There is evidence that NAA is located primarily within neurons and precursor cells and a reduction of NAA signal is usually regarded as indicating loss or dysfunction of neurons. Cr and Cho are found in neurons and in glial cells.

A ^{1}H MRSI study reported reduced NAA in frontal lobes ipsilateral to frontal lobe epileptic foci (Garcia *et al.*, 1995) and the decrease in NAA was inversely related to seizure frequency in patients with frontal lobe epilepsy, suggesting that a higher seizure frequency is associated with more neuronal dysfunction or loss (Garcia *et al.*, 1997). In patients with extratemporal epilepsy, NAA/Cho ratios and Cr were reduced over a wide area, particularly at the site of seizure onset (Stanley *et al.*, 1998).

Reduced NAA/Cho and NAA/Cr ratios have been shown in focal cortical dysplasia (Kuzniecky *et al.*, 1997). In two children with hemimegalencephaly, the white matter of the affected hemisphere had markedly reduced concentrations of NAA and glutamate, with mild abnormalities in the contralateral hemisphere, and with less marked changes in the grey matter. NAA/Cr has been reported to be reduced in hamartomas compared to normal hypothalami (Tasch *et al.*, 1998). In a magnetic resonance spectroscopic imaging (MRSI) study of cerebral malformations, there was a decrease of NAA in heterotopias, and abnormalities were also noted in brain that appeared normal on MRI (Li *et al.*, 1998). Interpretation of these studies, however, is difficult without correction being made for partial volume effects.

Quantitative MRSI at short echo time has shown heterogenous findings in patents with MCD. The most common finding has been reduced NAA, but increases are also found, and abnormalities are noted in areas that appear normal on structural MRI (Woermann *et al.*, 2001).

^{31}P spectroscopy

Cerebral metabolites detectable with 31P MRS include adenosine triphosphate (ATP), phosphomonoesters (PME), phosphodiesters (PDE), phosphocreatine (PCr), and inorganic phosphate (P_i). At neutral pH, P_i exists principally as HPO_4 and H_2PO_4. The chemical shift of ^{31}P in these two molecules differs by approximately 2.4 ppm, but rapid exchange between the two forms results in only a single MR spectral peak being detected. The resonance frequency of the peak is dependent on the pH of the tissue; this is reflected in the effective chemical shift of P_i and thus pH is measurable *in vivo*. In eight patients with frontal lobe epilepsy, increased pH in all eight and decreased PME in seven patients were found in the epileptogenic frontal lobes, but no alteration in P_i levels were detected (Garcia *et al.*, 1994). If confirmed, the neurobiological significance of an increase in pH associated with a seizure focus is not clear. Seizures have been shown to produce acidosis. Hugg *et al.* (1992) postulated that an increase in pH might be the consequence of an adaptation in brain buffering in response to repeated acidotic episodes associated with seizures, but there is no direct evidence for this. It is not clear whether ^{31}P MRS provides useful lateralizing and localizing data beyond that available from optimal MRI, and comparative studies using suboptimal MRI should be treated with caution.

Over the last decade MRS has advanced as a non-invasive tool for investigating cerebral metabolism. The rapid developments now being made in MR hardware and software may enable parametric imaging of the cerebral concentrations of these compounds, and this may have important consequences for the non-invasive investigation and the medical and surgical treatment of patients with epilepsy.

Single photon emission computerized tomography

Single photon emission computerized tomography (SPECT) is principally used, in the investigation of the epilepsies, to image the distribution of cerebral blood flow (CBF). In addition, there have been a few studies of specific receptors in the brain.

Inter-ictal SPECT studies

It was established in the 1980s that the marker of an epileptic focus studied inter-ictally in adults and children with SPECT is a region of reduced CBF, but it was soon noted that the results were not always reliable (Stefan *et al.*, 1987; Dietrich *et al.*, 1991). Focal abnormalities of regional CBF have been visualized with SPECT in patients with infantile spasms (Chiron *et al.*, 1993), Landau-Kleffner syndrome (O'Tuama *et al.*, 1992), continuous spike and wave activity during slow-wave sleep (Gaggero *et al.*, 1995), Lennox-Gastaut syndrome (Heiskala *et al.*, 1993), and tuberous sclerosis (Tamaki *et al.*, 1991). Lobar localization (e.g. frontal *vs* temporal) has been difficult with, in one large representative series, correct localization in only 38 per cent in inter-ictal studies of patients with unilateral temporal lobe EEG foci (Rowe *et al.*, 1991).

Localization with inter-ictal SPECT is more difficult in patients with extratemporal epilepsy (Marks *et al.*, 1992; Dasheiff, 1992). In a blinded comparative study, inter-ictal SPECT was less effective at lateralizing the focus of temporal lobe epilepsy than MRI, with correct lateralization in 45 per cent compared to 86 per cent. Furthermore, agreement of MRI and EEG data was a good predictor of a satisfactory result from surgical treatment, whereas SPECT was not and was prone to give an incorrect result in patients whose MRI was not lateralizing (Jack *et al.*, 1994). In consequence, inter-ictal SPECT has little place in the routine investigation of patients with epilepsy.

Inter-ictal ^{99m}Tc-hexamethyl-propyleneamine oxime (HMPAO) SPECT has been shown to have inferior resolution and reliability for identifying a focal deficit compared to ^{18}fluorodeoxyglucose (^{18}FDG) positron emission tomography (PET) in the evaluation of patients with partial seizures (Leiderman *et al.*, 1992; Nagata *et al.*, 1995; Mastin *et al.*, 1996).

Ictal and post-ictal SPECT studies

It was established over a decade ago that the increase in CBF associated with a seizure may be detected using SPECT (Bonte *et al.*, 1983; Lee *et al.*, 1986). This may provide useful localizing information in patients with partial seizures. It has also been suggested that a focal increase of blood flow may occur before seizure activity is detected on a scalp EEG (Baumgartner *et al.*, 1998). An injection of ^{99m}Tc-HMPAO at the time of seizure results in an image of the distribution of CBF 1 to 2 minutes after tracer administration, which is then stable for several hours so that the patient may be imaged when the seizure is over. The general pattern is of localized ictal hyperperfusion, with surrounding hypoperfusion, followed by accentuated hypoperfusion in the region of the focus, which gradually returns to the inter-ictal state. Combined data from inter-ictal and ictal SPECT scans give much more data than inter-ictal scans alone and may be useful in the evaluation of extra-temporal epilepsy. In complex partial seizure disorders, the epileptic focus has been identified in 69–93 per cent of ictal SPECT studies (Lee *et al.*, 1988; Stefan *et al.*, 1990; Shen *et al.*, 1990; Marks *et al.*, 1992; Harvey *et al.*, 1993; Duncan *et al.*, 1993b; Markand *et al.*, 1994).

In extra-temporal seizures, ictal SPECT studies localized the focus in 92 per cent, compared to 46 per cent for post-ictal studies, and inter-ictal SPECT was of little value (Newton *et al.*, 1995). Ictal ^{99m}Tc-HMPAO scans may be useful in the evaluation of patients with extra-temporal seizures and unremarkable MRI (Marks *et al.*, 1992; Harvey *et al.*, 1993; Duncan *et al.*, 1997). Asymmetric tonic posturing, contralateral head and eye deviation and unilateral clonic jerking were associated with an ictal increase in CBF in the frontocentral, medial frontal or dorsolateral areas (Harvey et al., 1993b). Varying patterns have been seen in patients with autosomal dominant frontal lobe epilepsy (Hayman et al., 1997).

Ictal SPECT with injection 2 to 5 seconds after seizure onset showed two patterns in supplementary sensorimotor area (SSMA) seizures; one was involvement of the ipsilateral SSMA, the dorsal premotor and the motor cortex, and the second pattern was of bilateral asymmetric medial frontal increased blood flow, reflecting propagation of seizure activity (Laich et al., 1997). Injection of tracer at onset of the seizure is important in the evaluation of brief extra-temporal seizures. In another series of SSMA seizures, in which tracer was injected up to 30 seconds after seizure onset, findings were less clear-cut (Ebner et al., 1996).

Post-ictal SPECT has shown a focal increase in CBF in areas of focal cortical dysplasia (Otsubo et al., 1993) and a focal ictal CBF rise has been demonstrated in patients with malformations of cortical development and non-localizing ictal scalp EEG, and used to identify surgically resectable epileptic tissue (Kuzniecky et al., 1993b). A focal increase in CBF may be seen in epilepsia partialis continua, even when the EEG does not show focal epileptic activity (Katz et al., 1990).

The coregistration of post-ictal SPECT images with a patient's MRI improves anatomical determination of abnormalities of CBF (Hogan et al., 1997). A greater advance, however, has been the coregistration of inter-ictal with ictal or post-ictal SPECT images, to result in an 'ictal difference image' that may be coregistered with an individual's MRI. This technique enhances objectivity and accuracy of data interpretation (Zubal et al., 1995; O'Brien et al., 1998; O'Brien et al., 1999).

Ictal ^{99m}Tc-HMPAO scans must always be interpreted with caution. Simultaneous video-EEG is essential to determine the relationship between onset of a seizure and tracer delivery; without this there is the risk of confusing ictal and post-ictal data. A further problem is that spread to other areas of the brain may occur within seconds of seizure onset and so an image of cerebral blood flow distribution 1 to 2 minutes after the onset of a seizure may indicate other than the site of onset. Ictal and post-ictal SPECT studies carried out in patients with intracranial EEG have shown that the former generally accurately reflect the site of seizure activity (Spanaki et al., 1999).

Until recently, ^{99m}Tc-HMPAO had to be constituted immediately prior to injection, resulting in a delay of up to 1 minute. A preparation has now been developed which is stabilized with cobalt chloride. This allows the labelled tracer to be prepared in advance and injected into a patient at any time over the subsequent 6 hours. The advantage of this development is that the interval between seizure onset and tracer delivery to the brain can be significantly reduced.

An alternative is to use ready constituted ^{99m}Tc-ECD, or bicisate, which is stable for several hours, may be injected within two to twenty seconds of seizure onset and demonstrates a focal increase in CBF (Grunwald et al., 1994; Packard et al., 1996; Lancman et al., 1997). The interval between seizure onset and injection may also be shortened by the use of an automated injection device that may be activated by the patient when they detect the beginning of a seizure (Sepkuty et al., 1998). Extra-temporal seizures may be very brief, increasing the need for injection of blood flow tracer as soon as possible after the start of a seizure. With the inevitable interval between injection and fixation of the tracer in the brain, however, it may not be possible to obtain true ictal studies.

When compared against EEG data, ictal SPECT and inter-ictal PET had lower sensitivity and higher specificity for extra-temporal than for temporal seizures (Spencer, 1994).

Iomazenil

^{123}I-Iomazenil is a derivative of the central benzodiazepine receptor antagonist flumazenil. Early studies with ^{123}I-Iomazenil showed a reduction in binding in region of the epileptic focus (Van Huffelen *et al.*, 1990; Bartenstein *et al.*, 1991), with generally concordant results with ictal EEG recordings. Similar results have been reported elsewhere (Cordes *et al.*, 1992; Duncan *et al.*, 1993a). Studies with higher resolution cameras and optimal scan orientation have suggested that the area of reduced specific binding of ^{123}I-Iomazenil is more restricted than the defect of blood flow and of greater sensitivity for the localization of an epileptogenic focus (Johnson *et al.*, 1992; Venz *et al.*, 1994; Tanaka *et al.*, 1997). Reduced binding of ^{123}I-Iomazenil has been found in a focal area of MCD, in which reduced CBF was not detectable, implying that the former may have greater sensitivity for detecting areas of cortical abnormality (Bartenstein *et al.*, 1992). In a comparison with flumazenil and FDG-PET, ^{123}I-Iomazenil SPECT was inaccurate at localizing epileptic foci (Lamusuo *et al.*, 1997).

An advantage of SPECT over PET is that SPECT is much less expensive and the equipment is more widespread. A further advantage is the ability to obtain images representative of CBF at the time of seizures. These data need careful and cautious interpretation and are non-quantitative. If further SPECT tracers that probe the integrity of specific receptors and neurotransmitters are developed, the technique may have further applications in the investigation and management of the epilepsies.

Positron emission tomography

Cerebral blood flow and glucose metabolism

Positron emission tomography (PET) may be used to map cerebral blood flow, using ^{15}O-labelled high-quality water, and regional cerebral glucose metabolism using ^{18}FDG. PET produces quantitative data with superior spatial resolution to SPECT. Clinical and research PET data should always be interpreted in the light of high-quality anatomical MRI, providing a structural-functional correlation. Computer programs to coregister MRI and PET datasets on a pixel-by-pixel basis have been fundamental in making these correlations (Woods *et al.*, 1993). Statistical parametric mapping has been shown to be useful in the evaluation of ^{18}FDG-PET scans for clinical purposes, with the advantages of allowing a rapid and objective evaluation (Wong *et al.*, 1996; Signorini *et al.*, 1999).

An epileptogenic focus, studied inter-ictally, is associated with an area of reduced glucose metabolism and reduced blood flow that is usually considerably larger than the pathological abnormality (Engel *et al.*, 1982; Franck *et al.*, 1986). ^{18}FDG-PET scans provide superior resolution and greater reliability for identifying a focal deficit than do PET scans using ^{15}O-water or SPECT scans of cerebral blood flow (Leiderman *et al.*, 1994), and there may be focal uncoupling of glucose metabolism and blood-brain barrier transport or blood flow. The most likely reason for the large region of reduced blood flow and metabolism around an epileptogenic focus is inhibition or deafferentation of neurons. Comparison of ^{18}FDG-PET scans with ^{11}C-flumazenil scans (Savic *et al.*, 1993) indicates that neuronal loss is confined to a more restricted area than the region of reduced metabolism.

Partial seizures are associated with an ictal increase in regional cerebral glucose metabolism and blood flow in the region of the epileptogenic focus, and often a suppression elsewhere (Engel *et al.*, 1983; Chugani *et al.*, 1994). In general, ictal PET scans can only be obtained fortuitously, because of the 2-minute half-life of ^{15}O and the fact that cerebral uptake of ^{18}FDG occurs over 40 minutes after injection, so that cerebral glucose utilization data will reflect an amalgam of the ictal and post-ictal conditions.

^{18}FDG-PET shows hypometabolism in about 60 per cent of patients with frontal lobe epilepsy. In 90 per cent of those with a hypometabolic area, structural imaging shows a relevant underlying abnormality. In common with temporal lobe epilepsy, the area of reduced metabolism in frontal lobe epilepsy may be much larger than the pathological abnormality. In contrast, however, the hypometabolic area may be restricted to the underlying lesion (Henry et al., 1991; Engel et al., 1995). There have been three main patterns of hypometabolism described in patients with frontal lobe epilepsy: no abnormality, a discrete focal area of hypometabolism, and diffuse widespread hypometabolism.

An uncommon finding has been the patient with a multilobar or extensive structural lesion and a small area of hypometabolism (Swartz et al., 1989). It has been the general experience that the epileptic focus is contained within the hypometabolic area, if one exists (Theodore et al., 1986; Swartz et al., 1989; Henry et al., 1991; Sadzot et al., 1992). Quantitative analysis of ^{18}FDG-PET scans was found to enhance sensitivity and accuracy of determination over visual assessment (Swartz et al., 1995). Analysis of groups of patients with neocortical seizures showed that those with unilateral clonic seizures had principally contralateral peri-Rolandic hypometabolism and a lesser degree of contralateral frontomesial hypometabolism. Those with focal tonic seizures had hypometabolism within the frontomesial and peri-Rolandic regions that was unilateral in all patients with lateralized tonic seizures. Patients with versive seizures had mainly contralateral hypometabolism without a consistent pattern. Patients in all groups had bilateral hypometabolism of the thalamus and cerebellum (Schlaug et al., 1997). These patterns imply the cerebral areas involved in particular features of seizures and seizure spread.

Published clinical series indicate that ^{18}FDG-PET does not appear to provide additional clinically useful information in the majority of patients with frontal lobe epilepsy. Status epilepticus arising from the motor cortex has been associated with hypermetabolism, and also with hypometabolism (Franck et al., 1986; Engel et al., 1983; Hajek et al., 1991). Scans performed with $H_2^{15}O$ have shown increased blood flow and oxygen consumption and reduced oxygen extraction fraction in the frontal lobe in patients with epilepsia partialis continua (Franck et al., 1986). A rare finding, in patients with frontal epilepsy of early childhood onset, has been an inter-ictal focal increase in metabolism (Chugani et al., 1993).

Dysfunctional working memory in patients with frontal lobe epilepsy has been associated with an impaired task-related metabolic response (Swartz et al., 1996). In view of the limitations of PET activation studies, however, functional MRI investigations will be the method of choice to resolve the functional anatomy of cognitive deficits.

Focal cortical hypometabolism is commonly seen in patients with tuberous sclerosis (Szelies et al., 1983; Pawlik et al., 1990). Glucose metabolism has been detected using ^{18}FDG-PET in the layers of ectopic neurons in band heterotopia (Miura et al., 1993; De Volder et al., 1994) and in heterotopic nodules and displaced grey matter (Bairamian et al., 1985; Falconer et al., 1990), implying synaptic activity. In 15 out of 17 patients with MCD, both MRI and ^{18}FDG-PET identified ectopic grey matter, and hypometabolism concurred with MRI findings of abnormal cortex. Analysis was by visual inspection and ^{18}FDG-PET did not identify abnormalities that were not evident on MRI, although in some cases the area of hypometabolism was more extensive than the MRI lesion (Lee et al., 1994). Abnormalities of glucose metabolism, identified with ^{18}FDG-PET in the contralateral hemisphere in patients with hemimegalencephaly, have been associated with a worse prognosis following surgery (Rintahaka et al., 1993). In perisylvian dysgenesis there was a heterogeneous pattern, with areas of relatively normal metabolism and of reduction in areas of polymicrogyria and in nearby cortex that appeared normal on MRI (Van Bogaert et al., 1998).

Activation studies

Cognitive activation tasks involving motor learning, visual attention and other tasks, using $H_2^{15}O$ PET in patients with MCD have shown that malformed cortex may participate in higher cerebral functions, but also showed widespread atypical cortical organization, indicating that there may be extensive disorganization of normal structure-function correlates in these patients, that would have implications for the planning of any surgical resection (Richardson et al., 1998a; Muller et al., 1998). Cognitive activation tasks in those with epilepsy will increasingly be carried out using fMRI rather than $H_2^{15}O$ PET.

In conclusion, studies with ^{18}FDG-PET have defined the major cerebral metabolic associations and consequences of epilepsy but the data are non-specific with regard to aetiology, and abnormalities are more widespread than the pathological lesions. The role of ^{18}FDG-PET in the clinical evaluation of patients has been reduced by the advances made in MRI over the last 5 years. Activation studies with $H_2^{15}O$ are useful for determining the functional anatomy of cerebral processes in both healthy and pathological brains, but these studies are now increasingly performed with functional MRI.

Specific ligands

Positron emission tomography may be used to demonstrate the binding of specific ligands. The technique is costly and scarce, but gives quantitative data with superior spatial resolution to SPECT.

Central benzodiazepine receptors

The most important inhibitory transmitter in the central nervous system, gamma-aminobutyric acid (GABA), acts at the $GABA_A$-central benzodiazepine receptor (cBZR) complex to increase chloride conductance and thereby to hyperpolarize the resting membrane potential (Meldrum et al., 1989). Flumazenil is a specific, reversibly bound antagonist at the alpha-subunit types 1, 2, 3 and 5 of the cBZR (Olsen et al., 1990), and ^{11}C-flumazenil is a PET ligand that acts as a useful marker of the $GABA_A$-cBZR complex in vivo (Mazière et al., 1984; Samson et al., 1985).

The binding of ^{11}C-flumazenil to central benzodiazepine receptors in epileptogenic foci was initially found to be reduced by an average of 30 per cent, with no change in the affinity of the ligand for the receptor (Savic et al., 1988). Comparative studies with ^{18}FDG-PET scans have shown the area of reduced ^{11}C-flumazenil binding to be more restricted than that of reduced glucose metabolism (Savic et al., 1993).

A pixel-based analysis identifies areas of brain where there is a focal increase or decrease of receptor binding. The method does not quantify the changes and does not differentiate between abnormalities that are the result of changes in the amount of grey matter or of receptor density. Quantification of PET data requires a volume-of-interest based approach, and in view of the size of the hippocampus and the limited spatial resolution of PET, correction for partial volume effect (Meltzer et al., 1996; Labbe et al., 1998).

It seems most likely that cBZR changes reflect localized neuronal and synaptic loss in the epileptogenic zone and that the more extensive hypometabolism is a result of diaschisis (Feeney & Baron, 1986). In clinical terms, ^{11}C-flumazenil PET may be superior to ^{18}FDG for the localization of the source of the seizure.

Malformations of cortical development commonly underlie partial seizures, are of heterogenous appearance and may not be detectable on MRI (Desbiens et al., 1993). A statistical parametric mapping analysis of cBZR visualized with ^{11}C-flumazenil PET and coregistered with high quality MRI in 12 patients with partial seizures and MCD found areas of abnormal cerebral cBZR binding in 10. The abnormal regions were frequently more extensive than the abnormality seen with MRI, and were also noted in distant sites at which the cortex appeared unremarkable on MRI (Richardson et al., 1996). In contrast to studies with ^{18}FDG, in which reduced metabolism may be the result of diaschisis, reduced ^{11}C-flumazenil binding implies neuronal deficits. A further novel finding of this investigation was of areas of increased binding to cBZR in many patients with MCD, which has not been found in patients with epilepsy caused by other pathologies. Possible explanations of this finding include increased neuron density, the presence of ectopic neurons bearing cBZR and of an increased number of available receptors, that may reflect abnormal neurons or a response to the abnormal circuitry implicit in MCD, with a change in available receptor numbers and/or affinity.

A subsequent voxel-based comparison of the binding of flumazenil to cBZR with the distribution of cortical grey matter in 10 patients with MCD showed that some regions with abnormal ^{11}C-flumazenil binding were accounted for by abnormalities of the cortical grey matter volume. In other areas, there was disproportionate ^{11}C-flumazenil binding compared to the local grey matter, including areas where analysis of the PET data alone did not reveal an abnormality, implying abnormal receptor density per neuron or a change in affinity (Richardson et al., 1997a). These results underline the importance of interpreting PET data in the light of high-resolution structural imaging. These findings may also be of clinical importance in the evaluation of patients with MCD for possible surgical treatment. Further studies need to be done to determine whether the finding of widespread abnormalities of cBZR is an adverse prognostic factor for surgical outcome in patients in whom MRI and other investigatory data implicate a single restricted focus.

The utility of ^{11}C-flumazenil PET in the clinical investigation of patients with refractory partial seizures and unremarkable high quality MRI is currently under investigation. Six patients with frontal lobe epilepsy were shown to have a reduction in BZR binding with ^{11}C-flumazenil PET, consistent with clinical and EEG data (Savic et al., 1995). In two of four patients who also had ^{18}FDG scans, the focus was characterized by a region of reduced metabolism that was more extensive than the reduction in cBZR. The MRI was unremarkable in five, implying superior sensitivity of the PET technique over the MRI. Comparisons of this nature, however, clearly depend on the relative sophistication of the instruments and methods used.

In 18 patients with refractory extra-temporal partial seizures and unremarkable high resolution MRI, ^{11}C-flumazenil PET showed focal decreases in six and focal increases in binding in 10 (Richardson et al., 1998b). The clinical significance of these findings is not yet clear.

In six patients with partial seizures as a result of acquired lesions, however, only decreases in flumazenil binding were seen. The implication of these data is that focally increased ^{11}C-flumazenil binding is a marker of MCD and may indicate occult MCD in patients who are MRI-negative. At present there is no correlative neuropathological material available to confirm or refute this.

Analysis of groups of patients who have similar forms of epilepsy is also of interest. In a group of 10 patients with frontal lobe epilepsy, there was an increase in flumazenil binding in the putamen, particularly ipsilateral to the seizure focus, and in related motor areas. Further, the extent of the increase was inversely related to the seizure frequency, suggesting the possibility that increased inhibition in the basal ganglia may modulate neocortical seizure threshold (Richardson et al., 1997b). In this study there was no correlation between extent of abnormality of neocortical flumazenil binding and seizure frequency. In contrast, Savic et al. (1996) reported in 19 patients with partial seizures and normal MRI that the severity of cBZR reduction, in regions of interest that were placed visually on the PET images, correlated with seizure frequency. Further, in those patients with daily seizures cBZRs were also reduced in the primary projection areas of the focus.

In a clinical series of 100 patients with partial seizures having pre-surgical evaluation, 50 per cent of those with extra-temporal seizures, and 81 per cent of abnormalities on ^{11}C-flumazenil PET scans were concordant with abnormalities on MRI. In patients with cryptogenic frontal lobe epilepsy, ^{11}C-flumazenil PET gave evidence of lateralization and localization of seizure onset in 55 per cent (Ryvlin et al., 1998).

In conclusion, ^{11}C-flumazenil PET scan data are good markers for neuronal integrity in hippocampus and neocortex and may also identify ectopic neurons in MCD. There may also be abnormalities of cBZR availability on neurons but definitive correlative in vitro studies have not yet been completed. The future clinical role of ^{11}C-flumazenil PET is likely to be in the pre-surgical evaluation of those patients in whom MRI is not definitive and in those with evidence of MCD.

Serotoninergic neurons

Increased concentrations of serotonin and serotonin immunoreactivity have been reported in resected human epileptic cortex. Alpha-[11C] methyl-L-tryptophan ([11C]AMT) is a marker for serotonin synthesis. In children with tuberous sclerosis, uptake was increased in some tubers that appeared to be the sites of seizure onset. Other tubers showed decreased uptake. In contrast, FDG-PET showed hypometabolism in all tubers. This study suggests that [11C]AMT PET may be useful to detect epileptogenic foci in patients with tuberous sclerosis and possibly other forms of cerebral malformation (Chugani et al., 1998).

Peripheral benzodiazepine receptors

The peripheral benzodiazepine receptor ligand ^{11}C-PK11195 labels macrophages and activated microglia, and thus is a marker of inflammatory responses in the brain. Increased binding has been demonstrated in Rasmussen's encephalitis, reflecting the inflammatory nature of the condition, and is in contrast to hippocampal sclerosis in which there is no increased binding (Banati et al., 1999).

In conclusion, PET studies are useful for investigating neurochemical abnormalities associated with the epilepsies, both static inter-ictal disturbances and dynamic changes in ligand-receptor interaction that may occur at the time of seizures. The development of further ligands in the coming years, particularly tracers that are specific for excitatory aminoacid receptors, subtypes of the opioid receptors, and the $GABA_B$ receptor, are necessary to understand further the processes that give rise to and respond to the various forms of the epilepsies. All functional data needs to be interpreted in the light of the structure of the brain. Coregistration with high-quality MRI is now readily achievable and essential. It will also be important to carry out parallel studies with in vitro autoradiography and quantitative neuropathological studies on surgical specimens and *post mortem* material.

References

Allen, P.J., Polizzi, G., Krakow, K., Fish, D.R. & Lemieux, L. (1998): Identification of EEG events in the MR scanner: the problem of pulse artifact and a method for its subtraction. *Neuroimage* **8**, 229–239.

Alsop, D.C., Detre, J.A., D'Esposito, M., Howard, R.S., Maldjian, J.A., Grossman, M., Listerud, J., Flamm, E.S., Judy, K.D. & Atlas, S.W. (1996): Functional activation during an auditory comprehension task in patients with temporal lobe lesions. *Neuroimage* **4**, 55–59.

Bairamian, D., Di Chiro, G., Theodore, W.H. et al. (1985): MR imaging and positron emission tomography of cortical heterotopia. *Comput. Assist. Tomography* **9**, 1137–1139.

Banati, R.B., Goerres, G.W., Myers, R., Gunn, R.N., Turkheimer, F.E., Kreutzberg, G.W., Brooks, D.J., Jones T. & Duncan, J.S. (1999): [11C](R)-PK11195 positron emission tomography imaging of activated microglia in vivo in Rasmussen's encephalitis. *Neurology* **53**, 2199–2203.

Barkovich, A.J., Rowley, H.A. & Andermann, F. (1995): MR in partial epilepsy: value of high-resolution volumetric techniques. *Am. J. Neuroradiol.* **16**, 339–343.

Bartenstein, P., Ludolph, A., Schober, O. *et al.* (1991): Benzodiazepine receptors and cerebral blood flow in partial epilepsy. *Eur. J. Nucl. Med.* **18**, 111–118.

Bartenstein, P., Lehmenkuhler, C., Sciuk, J. & Schuierer, G. (1992): Cortical dysplasia as an epileptogenic focus: reduced binding of 123I-iomazenil with barely perceptible 99mTc-HMPAO SPECT. *Nuklearmedizin* **31**, 142–144.

Baumgartner, C., Serles, W., Leutmezer, F., Pataraia, E., Aull, S., Czech, T., Pietrzyk, U., Relic, A. & Podreka, I. (1998): Preictal SPECT in temporal lobe epilepsy: regional cerebral blood flow is increased prior to electroencephalography-seizure onset. *J. Nucl. Med.* **39**, 978–982.

Benbadis, S.R., Binder, J.R., Swanson, S.J., Fischer, M., Hammeke, T.A., Morris, G.L., Frost, J.A. & Springer, J.A. (1998): Is speech arrest during Wada testing a valid method for determining hemispheric representation of language? *Brain Lang.* **65**, 441–446.

Benson, R.R., Fitzgerald, D.B., LeSueur, L.L., Kennedy, D.N., Kwong, K.K., Buchbinder, B.R. *et al.* (1999): Language dominance determined by whole brain functional MRI in patients with brain lesions. *Neurology* **52**, 798–809.

Binder, J.R., Rao, S.M., Hammeke, T.A., Frost, J.A., Bandettini, P.A., Jesmanowicz, A. & Hyde, J.S. (1995): Lateralized human brain language systems demonstrated by task subtraction functional magnetic resonance imaging. *Arch. Neurol.* **52**, 593–601.

Binder, J.R., Frost, J.A., Hammeke, T.A., Cox, R.W., Rao, S.M. & Prieto, S.M. (1997): Human brain language areas identified by functional magnetic resonance imaging. *J. Neurosci.* **17**, 353–362.

Bonte, F.J., Stokely, E.M., Devous, M.D. Sr & Homan, R.W. (1983): Single-photon tomographic study of regional cerebral blood flow in epilepsy. A preliminary report. *Arch. Neurol.* **40**, 267–270.

Cascino, G.D., Jack, C.R. Jr, Parisi, J.E. *et al.* (1992): MRI in the presurgical evaluation of patients with frontal lobe epilepsy and children with temporal lobe epilepsy: pathologic correlation and prognostic importance. *Epilepsy Res.* **11**, 51–59.

Chiron, C., Dulac, O., Bulteau, C., Nuttin, C., Depas, G., Raynaud, C. & Syrota, A. (1993): Study of regional cerebral blood flow in West syndrome. *Epilepsia* **34**, 707–715.

Chugani, H.T., Shewmon, D.A., Khanna, S. & Phelps, M.E. (1993): Interictal and postictal focal hypermetabolism on positron emission tomography. *Pediatr. Neurol.* **9**, 10–15.

Chugani, H.T., Rintahaka, P.J. & Shewmon, D.A. (1994): Ictal patterns of cerebral glucose utilization in children with epilepsy. *Epilepsia* **35**, 813–822.

Chugani, D.C., Chugani, H.T., Muzik, O., Shah, J.R., Shah, A.K., Canady, A., Mangner, T.J. & Chakraborty, P.K. (1998): Imaging epileptogenic tubers in children with tuberous sclerosis complex using alpha-[11C]methyl-L-tryptophan positron emission tomography. *Ann. Neurol.* **44**, 858–866.

Cordes, M., Henkes, H., Ferstl, F., Schmitz, B., Hierholzer, J., Schmidt, D. & Felix, R. (1992): Evaluation of focal epilepsy: a SPECT scanning comparison of ^{123}-I-iomazenil vs HMPAO. *Am. J. Neuroradiol.* **13**, 249–253.

Dashieff, R.M. (1992): A review of interictal cerebral blood flow in the evaluation of patients for epilepsy surgery. *Seizure* **1**, 117–125.

De Volder, A.G., Gadisseux, J.F., Michel, C.J., Maloteaux, J.M., Bol, A.C., Grandin, C.B., Duprez, T.P. & Evrard, P. (1994): Brain glucose utilization in band heterotopia: synaptic activity of 'double cortex'. *Pediatr. Neurol.* **11**, 290–294.

Desbiens, R., Berkovic, S.F., Dubeau, F., Andermann, F., Laxer, K.D., Harvey, S., Leproux, F., Melanson, D., Robitaille, Y., Kalnins, R. *et al.* (1993): Life-threatening focal status epilepticus due to occult cortical dysplasia. *Arch. Neurol.* **50**, 695–700.

Desmond, J.E., Sum, J.M., Wagner, A.D. *et al.* (1995): Functional MRI measurement of language lateralization in Wada-tested patients. *Brain* **118**, 1411–1419.

Detre, J.A., Sirven, J.I., Alsop, D.C., O'Connor, M.J. & French, J.A. (1995): Localization of subclinical ictal activity by functional magnetic resonance imaging: correlation with invasive monitoring. *Ann. Neurol.* **38**, 618–624.

Detre, J.A., Alsop, D.C., Aguirre, G.K. & Sperling, M.R. (1996): Coupling of cortical and thalamic ictal activity in human partial epilepsy: demonstration by functional magnetic resonance imaging. *Epilepsia* **37**, 657–661.

Dietrich, M.E., Bergen, D., Smith, M.C., Fariello, R. & Ali, A. (1991): Correlation of abnormalities of interictal n-isopropyl-p-iodoamphetamine single-photon emission tomography with focus of seizure onset in complex partial seizure disorders. *Epilepsia* **32**, 187–194.

Duncan, S., Gillen, G.J. & Brodie, M.J. (1993a): Lack of effect of concomitant clobazam on interictal ^{123}I-iomazenil SPECT. *Epilepsy Res.* **15**, 61–66.

Duncan, R., Patterson, J., Roberts, R., Hadley, D.M. & Bone, I. (1993b): Ictal/postictal SPECT in the pre-surgical localisation of complex partial seizures. *J. Neurol. Neurosurg. Psychiatr.* **56**, 141–148.

Duncan, R., Patterson, J., Hadley, D. & Roberts, R. (1997): Ictal regional cerebral blood flow in frontal lobe seizures. *Seizure* **6**, 393–401.

Ebner, A., Buschsieweke, U., Tuxhorn, I., Witte, O.W. & Seitz, R.J. (1996): Supplementary sensorimotor area seizure and ictal single-photon emission tomography. *Adv. Neurol.* **70**, 363–368.

Engel, J., Kuhl, D.E., Phelps, M.E. & Mazziotta, J.C. (1982): Interictal cerebral glucose metabolism in partial epilepsy and its relation to EEG changes. *Ann. Neurol.* **12**, 510–517.

Engel, J., Kuhl, D.E., Phelps, M.E., Rausch, R. & Nuwer, M. (1983): Local cerebral metabolism during partial seizures. *Neurology* **33**, 400–413.

Engel, J., Henry, T.R. & Swartz, B.E. (1995): Positron emission tomography in frontal lobe epilepsy. *Epilepsy and the functional anatomy of the frontal lobe*, eds. H.H. Jasper, S. Riggio, P.S. Goldman-Rakic, pp. 223–238. New York: Raven Press.

Falconer, J., Wada, J.A., Martin, W. & Li, D. (1990): PET, CT, and MRI imaging of neuronal migration anomalies in epileptic patients. *Can. J. Neurol. Sci.* **17**, 35–39.

Feeney, D.M. & Baron, J.C. (1986): Diaschisis. *Stroke* **17**, 817–830.

Franck, G., Sadzot, B., Salmon, E., Depresseux, J.C., Grisar, T., Peters, J.M., Guillaume, M., Quaglia, L., Delfiore, G. & Lamotte, D. (1986): Regional cerebral blood flow and metabolic rates in human focal epilepsy and status epilepticus. *Advances in Neurology*, eds. A.V. Delgado-Escueta, A.A. Ward, D.M. Woodbury, R.J. Porter, vol. 44, pp. 935–948. New York: Raven Press.

Gaggero, R., Caputo, M., Fiorio, P., Pessagno, A., Baglietto, M.G., Muttini, P. & De Negri, M. (1995): SPECT and epilepsy with continuous spike-waves during slow-wave sleep. *Childs Nerv. Syst.* **11**, 154–160.

Garcia, P.A., Laxer, K.D., Van der Grond, J., Hugg, J.W., Matson, G.B. & Weiner, M.W. (1994): Phosphorus magnetic resonance spectroscopic imaging in patients with frontal lobe epilepsy. *Ann. Neurol.* **35**, 217–221.

Garcia, P.A., Laxer, K.D., Van der Grond, J., Hugg, J.W., Matson, G.B. & Weiner, M.W. (1995): Proton magnetic resonance spectroscopic imaging in patients with frontal lobe epilepsy. *Ann. Neurol.* **37**, 279–281.

Garcia, P.A., Laxer, K.D., Van der Grond, J., Hugg, J.W., Matson, G.B. & Weiner, M.W. (1997): Correlation of seizure frequency with N-acetyl-aspartate levels determined by 1H magnetic resonance spectroscopic imaging. *Magn. Reson. Imaging* **15**, 475–478.

Grunwald, F., Menzel, C., Pavics, L., Bauer, J., Hufnagel, A., Reichmann, K., Sakowski, R., Elger, C.E. & Biersack, H.J. (1994): Ictal and interictal brain SPECT imaging in epilepsy using technetium-99m-ECD. *J. Nucl. Med.* **35**, 1896–1901.

Guerrini, R., Dravet, C., Raybaud, C. *et al.* (1992): Epilepsy and focal gyral anomalies detected by MRI: electroclinico-morphological correlations and follow-up. *Dev. Med. Child Neurol.* **34**, 706–718.

Hammeke, T.A., Yetkin, F.Z., Mueller, W.M., Morris, G.L., Haughton, V.M., Rao, S.M. & Binder, J.R. (1994): Functional magnetic resonance imaging of somatosensory stimulation. *Neurosurgery* **35**, 677–681.

Harvey, A.S., Hopkins, I.J., Bowe, J.M., Cook, D.J., Shield, L.K. & Berkovic, S.F. (1993): Frontal lobe epilepsy: clinical seizure characteristics and localization with ictal 99mTc-HMPAO SPECT. *Neurology* **43**, 1966–1980.

Hayman, M., Scheffer, I.E., Chinvarun, Y., Berlangieri, S.U. & Berkovic, S.F. (1997): Autosomal dominant nocturnal frontal lobe epilepsy: demonstration of focal frontal onset and intrafamilial variation. *Neurology* **49**, 969–975.

Heiskala, H., Launes, J., Pihko, H., Nikkinen, P. & Santavuori, P. (1993): Brain perfusion SPECT in children with frequent fits. *Brain Dev.* **15**, 214–218.

Henry, T.R., Sutherling, W.W., Engel, J. Jr., Risinger, M.W., Levesque, M.F., Mazziotta, J.C. & Phelps, M.E. (1991): Interictal cerebral metabolism in partial epilepsies of neocortical origin. *Epilepsy Res.* **10**, 174–182.

Hertz-Pannier, L., Gaillard, W.D., Mott, S.H., Cuenod, C.A., Bookheimer, S.Y., Weinstein, S., Conry, J., Papero, P.H., Schiff, S.J., Le Bihan, D. & Theodore, W.H. (1997): Noninvasive assessment of language dominance in children and adolescents with functional MRI: a preliminary study. *Neurology* **48**, 1003–1012.

Hogan, R.E., Cook, M.J., Binns, D.W., Desmond, P.M., Kilpatrick, C.J., Murrie, V.L. & Morris, K.F. (1997): Perfusion patterns in postictal 99mTc-HMPAO SPECT after coregistration with MRI in patients with mesial temporal lobe epilepsy. *J. Neurol. Neurosurg. Psychiatry* **63**, 235–239.

Hugg, J.W., Laxer, K.D., Matson, G.B., Maudsley, A.A., Husted, C.A. & Weiner, M.W. (1992): Lateralization of human focal epilepsy by 31P magnetic resonance imaging spectroscopy. *Neurology* **42**, 2011–2018.

Ives, J.R., Warach, S., Schmitt, F., Edelman, R.R. & Schomer, D.L. (1993): Monitoring the patient's EEG during echoplanar MRI. *Electroencephal. Clin. Neurophysiol.* **87**, 417–420.

Jack, C.R. Jr., Mullan, B.P., Sharbrough, F.W., Cascino, G.D., Hauser, M.F., Krecke, K.N., Luetmer, P.H., Trenerry, M.R., O'Brien, P.C. & Parisi, J.E. (1994): Intractable nonlesional epilepsy of temporal lobe origin: lateralization by interictal SPECT *vs* MRI. *Neurology* **44**, 829–836.

Jackson, G.D., Connelly, A., Cross, J.H., Gordon, I. & Gadian, D.G. (1994): Functional magnetic resonance imaging of focal seizures. *Neurology* **44**, 850–856.

Johnson, E.W., de Lanerolle, N.C., Kim, J.H., Sundaresan, S., Spencer, D.D., Mattson, R.H., Zoghbi, S.S., Baldwin, R.M., Hoffer, P.B., Seibyl, J.P. et al. (1992): 'Central' and 'peripheral' benzodiazepine receptors: opposite changes in human epileptogenic tissue. *Neurology* **42**, 811–815.

Katz, A., Bose, A., Lind, S.J. & Spencer, S.S. (1990): SPECT in patients with epilepsia partialis continua. *Neurology* **40**, 1848–1850.

Krakow, K., Wieshmann, U.C., Woermann, F.G. et al. (1999a): Multimodal MR imaging: functional, diffusion, tensor and chemical shift imaging in a patient with localisation-related epilepsy. *Epilepsia* **40**, 1459–1462.

Krakow, K., Woermann, F.G., Symms, M.R., Allen, P.J., Lemieux, L., Barker, G.J., Duncan, J.S. & Fish, D.R. (1999b): EEG-triggered functional MRI of interictal epileptiform activity in patients with partial seizures. *Brain* **122**, 1679–1688.

Kuzniecky, R. (1995): MRI in cerebral developmental malformations and epilepsy. *Magn. Reson. Imaging* **13**, 1137–1145.

Kuzniecky, R., Burgard, S., Faught, E. & Morawetz, R. & Bartolucci, A. (1993a): Predictive value of magnetic resonance imaging in temporal lobe epilepsy surgery. *Arch. Neurol.* **50**, 65–69.

Kuzniecky, R., Mountz, J.M., Wheatley, G. & Morawetz, R. (1993b): Ictal single-photon emission computed tomography demonstrates localized epileptogenesis in cortical dysplasia. *Ann. Neurol.* **34**, 627–631.

Kuzniecky, R., Hetherington, H., Pan, J., Hugg, J., Palmer, C., Gilliam, F., Faught, E. & Morawetz, R. (1997): Proton spectroscopic imaging at 4.1 tesla in patients with malformations of cortical development and epilepsy. *Neurology* **48**, 1018–1024.

Labbé, C., Koepp, M.J., Ashburner, J., Spinks, T., Richardson, M.P., Duncan, J.S. & Cunningham, V.J. (1998): Absolute PET quantification with correction for partial volume effects within cerebral structures. *Quantitative functional brain imaging with positron emission tomography*, eds. C. Carson, M. Daube-Witherspoon, P. Herscovitch, pp. 59–66. New York: Academic Press.

Laich, E., Kuzniecky, R., Mountz, J., Liu, H.G., Gilliam, F., Bebin, M., Faught, E. & Morawetz, R. (1997): Supplementary sensorimotor area epilepsy. Seizure localization, cortical propagation and subcortical activation pathways using ictal SPECT. *Brain* **120**, 855–864.

Lamusuo, S., Ruottinen, H.M., Knuuti, J., Harkonen, R., Ruotsalainen, U., Bergman, J., Haaparanta, M., Solin, O., Mervaala, E., Nousiainen, U., Jaaskelainen, S., Ylinen, A., Kalviainen, Rinne, J.K., Vapalahti, M. & Rinne, J.O. (1997): Comparison of [18F]FDG-PET, [99mTc]-HMPAO-SPECT, and [123I]-iomazenil-SPECT in localising the epileptogenic cortex. *J. Neurol. Neurosurg. Psychiatr.* **63**, 743–748.

Lancman, M.E., Morris, H.H. 3rd, Raja, S., Sullivan, M.J., Saha, G. & Go, R. (1997): Usefulness of ictal and interictal 99mTc ethyl cysteinate dimer single photon emission computed tomography in patients with refractory partial epilepsy. *Epilepsia* **38**, 466–471.

Lee, B.I., Markand, O.N., Siddiqui, A.R., Park, H.M., Mock, B., Wellman, H.H., Worth, R.M. & Edwards, M.K. (1986): Single photon emission computed tomography (SPECT) brain imaging using N,N,N'-trimethyl-N'-(2 hydroxy-3-methyl-5-123I-iodobenzyl)-1,3-propanediamine 2 HCl (HIPDM): intractable complex partial seizures. *Neurology* **36**, 1471–1477.

Lee, B.I., Markand, O.N., Wellman, H.N., Siddiqui, A.R., Park, H.M., Mock, B., Worth, R.M., Edwards, M.K. & Krepshaw, J. (1988): HIPDM-SPECT in patients with medically intractable complex partial seizures. Ictal study. *Arch. Neurol.* **45**, 397–402.

Lee, N., Radtke, R.A., Gray, L., Burger, P.C., Montine, T.J., DeLong, G.R., Lewis, D.V., Oakes, W.J., Friedman, A.H. & Hoffman, J.M. (1994): Neuronal migration disorders: positron emission tomography correlations. *Ann. Neurol.* **35**, 290–297.

Leiderman, D.B., Balish, M., Sato, S., Kufta, C., Reeves, P., Gaillard, W.D. & Theodore, W.H. (1992): Comparison of PET measurements of cerebral blood flow and glucose metabolism for the localization of human epileptic foci. *Epilepsy Res.* **13**, 153–157.

Lemieux, L., Allen, P.J., Franconi, F., Symms, M.R. & Fish, D.R. (1997): Recording of EEG during fMRI experiments: patient safety. *Magn. Res. Med.* **38**, 943–952.

Li, L.M., Cendes, F., Bastos, A.C., Andermann, F., Dubeau, F. & Arnold, D.L. (1998): Neuronal metabolic dysfunction in patients with cortical developmental malformations: a proton magnetic resonance spectroscopic imaging study. *Neurology* **50**, 755–759.

Markand, O.N., Salanova, V., Worth, R.M., Park, H.M. & Wellman, H.H. (1994): Ictal brain imaging in presurgical evaluation of patients with medically intractable complex partial seizures. *Acta Neurol. Scand.* **89**, Suppl. 152, 137–144.

Marks, D.A., Katz, A., Hoffer, P. & Spencer, S.S. (1992): Localization of extratemporal epileptic foci during ictal single photon emission computed tomography. *Ann. Neurol.* **31**, 250–255.

Mastin, S.T., Drane, W.E., Gilmore, R.L., Helveston, W.R., Quisling, R.G., Roper, S.N., Eikman, E.A. & Browd, S.R. (1996): Prospective localization of epileptogenic foci: comparison of PET and SPECT with site of surgery and clinical outcome. *Radiology* **199**, 375–380.

Mazière, M., Hantraye, P., Prenant, C., Sastre, J. & Comar, D. (1984): Synthesis of ethyl 8-fluoro-5,6-dihydro-5-[11C]methyl-6-oxo-4H-imidazol-[1,5-a][1,4]benzodiazepine-3-carboxylate (RO15,1788-11C): a specific radioligand for the *in vivo* study of central benzodiazepine receptors by positron emission tomography. *Int. J. Appl. Radiat. Isotopes* **35**, 973–976.

Meldrum, B.S. (1989): GABAergic mechanisms in the pathogenesis and treatment of epilepsy. *Br. J. Clin. Pharmacol.* **27**, Suppl. 11, 3S-11S.

Meltzer, C.C., Zubieta, J.K., Links, J.M., Brakeman, P., Stumpf, M.J. & Frost, J.J. (1996): MR-based correction for brain PET measurements for heterogeneous grey matter radioactivity distribution. *J. Cerebr. Blood Flow Metab.* **16**, 650–658.

Miura, K., Watanabe, K., Maeda, N., Matsumoto, A., Kumagai, T., Ito, K. & Kato, T. (1993): Magnetic resonance imaging and positron emission tomography of band heterotopia. *Brain Dev.* **15**, 288–290.

Morris, G.L. 3rd, Mueller, W.M., Yetkin, F.Z., Haughton, V.M., Hammeke, T.A., Swanson, S., DeYoe, E.A., Rao, S.M., Binder, J.R., Estkowski, L.D., Bandettini, P.A., Wong, E.C. & Hyde, J.S. (1994): Functional magnetic resonance imaging in partial epilepsy. *Epilepsia* **35**, 1194–1198.

Muller, R.A., Behen, M.E., Muzik, O., Rothermel, R.D., Downey, R.A., Mangner, T.J. & Chugani, H.T. (1998): Task-related activations in heterotopic brain malformations: a PET study. *Neuroreport* **9**, 2527–2533.

Nagata, T., Tanaka, F., Yonekura, Y., Ikeda, A., Nishizawa, S., Ishizu, K., Okazawa, H., Terada, K., Mikuni, N., Yamamoto, I. *et al.* (1995): Limited value of interictal brain perfusion SPECT for detection of epileptic foci: high resolution SPECT studies in comparison with FDG-PET. *Ann. Nucl. Med.* **9**, 59–63.

Newton, M.R., Berkovic, S.F., Austin, M.C., Rowe, C.C., McKay, W.J. & Bladin, P.F. (1995): SPECT in the localisation of extratemporal and temporal seizure foci. *J. Neurol. Neurosurg. Psychiatr.* **59** 26–30.

O'Brien, T.J., So, E.L., Mullan, B.P., Hauser, M.F., Brinkmann, B.H., Bohnen, N.I., Hanson, D., Cascino, G.D., Jack, C.R. Jr. & Sharbrough, F.W. (1998): Subtraction ictal SPECT co-registered to MRI improves clinical usefulness of SPECT in localizing the surgical seizure focus. *Neurology* **50**, 445–454.

O'Brien, T.J., So, E.L., Mullan, B.P., Hauser, M.F., Brinkmann, B.H., Jack, C.R. Jr., Cascino, G.D., Meyer, F.B. & Sharbrough, F.W. (1999): Subtraction SPECT co-registered to MRI improves postictal SPECT localization of seizure foci. *Neurology* **52**, 137–146.

Olsen, R.W., McCabe, R.T. & Wamsley, J.K. (1990): GABA-A receptor subtypes: autoradiographic comparison of GABA, benzodiazepine, and convulsant binding sites in the rat central nervous system. *J. Chem. Neuroanatomy* **3**, 59–76.

Otsubo, H., Hwang, P.A., Jay, V., Becker, L.E., Hoffman, H.J., Gilday, D. & Blaser, S. (1993): Focal cortical dysplasia in children with localization-related epilepsy: EEG, MRI, and SPECT findings. *Pediatr. Neurol.* **9**, 101–107.

O'Tuama, L.A., Urion, D.K., Janiek, M.J., Treves, S.T., Bjornson, B. & Moriarty, J.M. (1992): Regional cerebral perfusion in Landau-Kleffner syndrome and related childhood aphasias. *J. Nucl. Med.* **33**, 1758–1765.

Packard, A.B., Roach, P.J., Davis, R.T., Carmant, L., Davis, R., Riviello, J., Holmes, G., Barnes, P.D., O'Tuama, L.A., Bjornson, B. & Treves, S.T. (1996): Ictal and interictal technetium-99m-bicisate brain SPECT in children with refractory epilepsy. *J. Nucl. Med.* **37**, 1101–1106.

Palmini, A., Andermann, F., Olivier, A., Tampieri, D., Robitaille, Y., Andermann, E., Wright, G. (1991): Focal neuronal migration disorders and intractable partial epilepsy: a study of 30 patients. *Ann. Neurol.* **30**, 741–749.

Pawlik, G., Holthoff, V.A., Kessler, J., Rudolf, J., Hebold, I.R., Lottgen, J. & Heiss, W.D. (1990): Positron emission tomography findings relevant to neurosurgery for epilepsy. *Acta Neurochir. Suppl. (Wien)* **50**, 84–87.

Puce, A., Constable, R.T., Luby, M.L., McCarthy, G., Nobre, A.C., Spencer, D.D., Gore, J.C. & Allison, T. (1995): Functional magnetic resonance imaging of sensory and motor cortex: comparison with electrophysiological localization. *J. Neurosurg.* **83**, 262–270.

Rao, S.M., Binder, J.R., Hammeke, T.A., Bandettini, P.A., Bobholz, J.A., Frost, J.A., Myklebust, B.M., Jacobson, R.D. & Hyde, J.S. (1995): Somatotopic mapping of the human primary motor cortex with functional magnetic resonance imaging. *Neurology* **45**, 919–924.

Richardson, M.P., Koepp, M.J., Brooks, D.J., Fish, D.R. & Duncan, J.S. (1996): Benzodiazepine receptors in focal epilepsy associated with cortical dysgenesis: an ^{11}C-flumazenil PET study. *Ann. Neurol.* **40**, 188–198.

Richardson, M.P., Friston, K.J., Sisodiya, S.M., Koepp, M.J., Ashburner, J., Free, S.L., Brooks, D.J. & Duncan, J.S. (1997a): Benzodiazepine receptors in malformations of cortical development: a voxel-based comparison of structural and functional data in cortical grey matter. *Brain* **120**, 1961–1974.

Richardson, M.P., Koepp, M.J., Brooks, D.J. & Duncan, J.S. (1997b): Extratemporal localization-related epilepsy with normal MRI: abnormalities of cortical and subcortical [11C]-flumazenil binding. *Neurology* **48**, Suppl. 2, A20–A21.

Richardson, M.P., Koepp, M.J., Brooks, D.J., Coull, J.T., Grasby, P., Fish, D.R. & Duncan, J.S. (1998a): Cerebral activation in malformations of cortical development. *Brain* **121**, 1295–1304.

Richardson, M.P., Koepp, M.J., Brooks, D.J. & Duncan, J.S. (1998b): 11C-flumazenil PET in neocortical epilepsy. *Neurology* **51**, 485–492.

Rintahaka, P.J., Chugani, H.T., Messa, C. & Phelps, M.E. (1993): Hemimegalencephaly: evaluation with positron emission tomography. *Pediatr. Neurol.* **9**, 21–28.

Rowe, C.C., Berkovic, S.F., Austin, M.C., Saling, M., Kalnins, R.M., McKay, W.J. & Bladin, P.F. (1991): Visual and quantitative analysis of interictal SPECT with technetium-99m-HMPAO in temporal lobe epilepsy. *J. Nucl. Med.* **32**, 1688–1694.

Ryvlin, P., Bouvard, S., Le Bars, D., De Lamerie, G., Gregoire, M.C., Kahane, P., Froment, J.C. & Mauguière, F. (1998): Clinical utility of flumazenil-PET *vs* FDG-PET and MRI in refractory partial epilepsy. A prospective study in 100 patients. *Brain* **121**, 2067–2081.

Sadzot, B., Debets, R.M., Maquet, P., van Veelen, C.W., Salmon, E., van Emde Boas, W., Velis, D.N., van Huffelen, A.C. & Franck, G. (1992): Regional brain glucose metabolism in patients with complex partial seizures investigated by intracranial EEG. *Epilepsy Res.* **12**, 121–129.

Samson, Y., Hantraye, P., Baron, J.C., Soussaline, F., Comar, D. & Mazière, M. (1985): Kinetics and displacement of [^{11}C]RO15,1788, a benzodiazepine antagonist, studied in human brain *in vivo* by positron tomography. *Eur. J. Pharmacol.* **110**, 247–251.

Savic, I., Persson, A., Roland, P., Pauli, S., Sedvall, G. & Widen, L. (1988): *In vivo* demonstration of reduced benzodiazepine receptor binding in human epileptic foci. *Lancet* **2**, 863–866.

Savic, I., Ingvar, M. & Stone-Elander, S. (1993): Comparison of [11C]flumazenil and [18F]FDG as PET markers of epileptic foci. *J. Neurol. Neurosurg. Psychiatry* **56**, 615–621.

Savic, I., Thorell, J.O. & Roland, P. (1995): [11C]Flumazenil positron emission tomography visualizes frontal epileptogenic regions. *Epilepsia* **36**, 1225–1232.

Savic, I., Svanborg, E. & Thorell, J.O. (1996): Cortical benzodiazepine receptor changes are related to frequency of partial seizures: a positron emission tomography study. *Epilepsia* **37**, 236–244.

Schlaug, G., Antke, C., Holthausen, H., Arnold, S., Ebner, A., Tuxhorn, I., Jancke, L., Luders, H., Witte, O.W. & Seitz, R.J. (1997): Ictal motor signs and interictal regional cerebral hypometabolism. *Neurology* **49**, 341–350.

Schmitz, E.B., Costa, D.C., Jackson, G.D., Moriarty, J., Duncan, J.S., Trimble, M.R. & Ell, P.J. (1995): Optimized interictal HMPAO-SPECT in the evaluation of partial epilepsies. *Epilepsy Res.* **21**, 159–167.

Seeck, M., Lazeyras, F., Michel, C.M., Blanke, O., Gericke, C.A., Ives, J., Delavelle, J., Golay, X., Haenggeli, C.A., de Tribolet, N. & Landis, T. (1998): Non-invasive epileptic focus localization using EEG-triggered functional MRI and electromagnetic tomography. *Electroencephalogr. Clin. Neurophysiol.* **106**, 508–512.

Sepkuty, J.P., Lesser, R.P., Civelek, C.A., Cysyk, B., Webber, R. & Shipley, R. (1998): An automated injection system (with patient selection) for SPECT imaging in seizure localization. *Epilepsia* **39**, 1350–1356.

Shen, W., Lee, B.I., Park, H.M., Siddiqui, A.R., Wellman, H.H., Worth, R.M. & Markand, O.N. (1990): HIPDM-SPECT brain imaging in the presurgical evaluation of patients with intractable seizures. *J. Nucl. Med.* **31**, 1280–1284.

Signorini, M., Paulesu, E., Friston, K., Perani, D., Colleluori, A., Lucignani, G., Grassi, F., Bettinardi, V., Frackowiak, R.S.J. & Fazio, F. (1999): Rapid assessment of regional cerebral metabolic abnormalities in single subjects with quantitative and nonquantitative [18F]FDG PET: a clinical validation of statistical parametric mapping. *Neuroimage* **9**, 63–80.

Sisodiya, S.M., Free, S.L., Stevens, J.M., Fish, D.R. & Shorvon, S.D. (1995): Widespread cerebral structural changes in patients with cortical dysgenesis and epilepsy. *Brain* **118**, 1039–1050.

Spanaki, M.V., Zubal, I.G., MacMullan, J. & Spencer, S.S. (1999): Periictal SPECT localization verified by simultaneous intracranial EEG. *Epilepsia* **40**, 267–274.

Spencer, S.S. (1994): The relative contributions of MRI, SPECT, and PET imaging in epilepsy. *Epilepsia* **35**, Suppl. 6, S72–S89.

Stanley, J.A., Cendes, F., Dubeau, F., Andermann, F. & Arnold, D.L. (1998): Proton magnetic resonance spectroscopic imaging in patients with extratemporal epilepsy. *Epilepsia* **39**, 267–273.

Stefan, H., Kuhnen, C., Biersack, H.J. & Reichmann, K. (1987): Initial experience with 99m Tc-hexamethyl-propylene amine oxime (HM-PAO) single photon emission computed tomography (SPECT) in patients with focal epilepsy. *Epilepsy Res.* **1**, 134–138.

Stefan, H., Bauer, J., Feistel, H., Schulemann, H., Neubauer, U., Wenzel, B., Wolf, F., Neundorfer, B., Huk, W.J. (1990): Regional cerebral blood flow during focal seizures of temporal and frontocentral onset. *Ann. Neurology* **27**, 162–166.

Swartz, B.E., Halgren, E., Delgado-Escueta, A.V., Mandelkern, M., Gee, M., Quinones, N., Blahd, W.H. & Repchan, J. (1989): Neuroimaging in patients with seizures of probable frontal lobe origin. *Epilepsia* **30**, 547–558.

Swartz, B.E., Khonsari, A., Vrown, C., Mandelkern, M., Simpkins, F. & Krisdakumtorn, T. (1995): Improved sensitivity of 18FDG-positron emission tomography scans in frontal and 'frontal plus' epilepsy. *Epilepsia* **36**, 388–395.

Swartz, B.E., Halgren, E., Simpkins, F., Fuster, J., Mandelkern, M., Krisdakumtorn, T., Gee, M., Brown, C., Ropchan, J.R. & Blahd, W.H. (1996): Primary or working memory in frontal lobe epilepsy: an 18FDG-PET study of dysfunctional zones. *Neurology* **46**, 737–747.

Symms, M.R., Allen, P.J., Woermann, F.G., Polizzi, G., Krakow, K., Barker, G.J., Fish, D.R. & Duncan, J.S. (1999): Reproducible localisation of interictal epileptiform activity using functional MRI. *Phys. Med. Biol.* **41**, 161–168.

Szelies, B., Herholz, K., Heiss, W.D., Rackl, A., Pawlik, G., Wagner, R., Ilsen, H.W. & Wienhard, K. (1983): Hypometabolic cortical lesions in tuberous sclerosis with epilepsy: demonstration by positron emission tomography. *J. Comput. Assist. Tomogr.* **7**, 946–953.

Tamaki, K., Okuno, T., Iwasaki, Y., Yonekura, Y., Konishi, J. & Mikawa, H. (1991): Regional cerebral blood flow in relation to MRI and EEG findings in tuberous sclerosis. *Brain Dev.* **13**, 420–424.

Tanaka, F., Yonekura, Y., Ikeda, A., Terada, K., Mikuni, N., Nishizawa, S., Ishizu, K., Okazawa, H., Hattori, N., Shibasaki, H., Konishi, J. & Onishi, Y. (1997): Presurgical identification of epileptic foci with iodine-123 iomazenil SPET: comparison with brain perfusion SPET and FDG PET. *Eur. J. Nucl. Med.* **24**, 27–34.

Tasch, E., Cendes, F., Li, L.M., Dubeau, F., Montes, J., Rosenblatt, B., Andermann, F. & Arnold, D. (1998): Hypothalamic hamartomas and gelastic epilepsy: a spectroscopic study. *Neurology* **51**, 1046–1050.

Theodore, W.H., Holmes, M.D., Dorwart, R.H., Porter, R.J., Di Chiro, G., Sato, S. & Rose, D. (1986): Complex partial seizures: cerebral structure and cerebral function. *Epilepsia* **27**, 576–582.

Van Bogaert, P., David, P., Gillain, C.A., Wikler, D., Damhaut, P., Scalais, E., Nuttin, C., Wetzburger, C., Szliwowski, H.B., Metens, T. & Goldman, S. (1998): Perisylvian dysgenesis. Clinical, EEG, MRI and glucose metabolism features in 10 patients. *Brain* **121**, 2229–2238.

Venz, S., Cordes, M., Straub, H.B., Hierholzer, J., Schroder, R., Richter, W., Schmitz, B., Meencke, H. & Felix, R. (1994): Preoperative evaluation of drug resistant focal epilepsies with ^{123}I-iomazenil SPECT. Comparison with video/EEG monitoring and postoperative results. *Nuklearmedizin* **33**, 189–193.

Warach, S., Ives, J.R., Schlaug, G., Patel, M.R., Darby, D.G., Thangaraj, V., Edelman, R.R. & Schomer, D.L. (1996): EEG-triggered echo-planar functional MRI in epilepsy. *Neurology* **47**, 89–93.

Williamson, P.D., Thadani, V.M., Darcey, T.M., Spencer, D.D., Spencer, S.S., Mattson, R.H. (1992): Occipital lobe epilepsy: clinical characteristics, seizure spread patterns, and results of surgery. *Ann. Neurol.* **31**, 3–13.

Woermann, F.G., McLean, M.A., Bartlett, P. & Duncan, J.S. (2001): Quantitative short echo time proton magnetic resonance spectroscopic imaging of malformations of cortical development causing epilepsy. *Brain* **124**, 427–436.

Wong, C.Y., Geller, E.B., Chen, E.Q., MacIntyre, W.J., Morris, H.H. 3rd, Raja, S., Saha, G.B., Luders, H.O., Cook, S.A. & Go R.T. (1996): Outcome of temporal lobe epilepsy surgery predicted by statistical parametric PET imaging. *J. Nucl. Med.* **37**, 1094–1100.

Woods, R.P., Mazziotta, J.C. & Cherry, S.R. (1993): MRI-PET registration with automated algorithm. *J. Comput. Assist. Tomogr.* **17**, 536–546.

Worthington, C., Vincent, D.J., Bryant, A.E., Roberts, D.R., Vera, C.L., Ross, D.A. & George, M.S. (1997): Comparison of functional magnetic resonance imaging for language localization and intracarotid speech amytal testing in presurgical evaluation for intractable epilepsy. Preliminary results. *Stereotact. Function. Neurosurg.* **69**, 197–201.

Zubal, I.G., Spencer, S.S., Imam, K., Seibyl, J., Smith, E.O., Wisniewski, G. & Hoffer, P.B. (1995): Difference images calculated from ictal and interictal technetium-99m-HMPAO SPECT scans of epilepsy. *J. Nucl. Med.* **36**, 684–689.

Chapter 17

Magnetic resonance imaging in the diagnosis of frontal lobe epilepsy in children

Nadia Colombo, Alberto Citterio, Laura Tassi*, Stefano Francione*,
Giorgio Lo Russo* and Giuseppe Scialfa

*Neuroradiology Service, *Centro regionale per la Chirurgia dell'Epilessia 'Claudio Munari',
Ospedale Niguarda Ca' Granda, Piazza Ospedale Maggiore 3, 20162 Milan, Italy
epsur@mailserver.unimi.it*

Summary

The identification, precise electroclinical patterns and surgical treatment of frontal lobe epilepsies are a major challenge to neurologists and neurosurgeons. The anatomic complexity of the frontal lobe, extending widely over the mesial, lateral and inferior surfaces of the brain, and the multiple connections within and beyond its boundaries, account for the varied clinical presentations of frontal lobe epilepsy. Nevertheless, several investigators have recently identified clinical syndromes of frontal lobe epilepsy related to epileptic discharges from distinct regions of the frontal lobe.

Magnetic resonance imaging (MRI) is the method of choice for imaging epileptic patients, providing detailed visualization of the complex anatomy of the brain, of cortical architecture and of the different pathological conditions associated with epilepsy. CT scan is a complementary tool to better detect intralesional calcifications and skull remodelling that can contribute to diagnosis in few cases.

Unlike temporal lobe epilepsy, for which a rich literature describes the neuropathological and the corresponding neuroimaging features of the most frequent structural abnormalities, little has been published on frontal lobe epilepsy in this regard, particularly in paediatric age groups (Robitaille *et al.*, 1992; Kuzniecky & Jackson, 1995).

We report the MRI and related histopathological results in the paediatric population referred to our institution for medically refractory frontal lobe epilepsy. Despite the limited number in our series, it is worth noting that cortical tubers (CTs) of tuberous sclerosis complex and focal cortical dysplasias (FCD) of any histologic subtype were the major structural anomalies observed in surgical specimens (61 per cent).

Materials and methods

Between June 1996 and July 2000, we evaluated 24 patients (14 females, 10 males) under the age of 16 years for drug-resistant frontal lobe epilepsy at the Epilepsy Surgery Centre 'Claudio Munari' of Niguarda Hospital in Milan.

Magnetic resonance imaging (MRI) examination was performed in all patients with a 1.5 Tesla magnet (Philips ACS-NT). The following sequences were acquired: *transverse double-echo spin-echo (SE)* images, covering the entire brain (2000-2500/20-90) [TR msec/TE msec], 1 nex, 128×256 matrix, 23 cm field of view; 4-5 mm slice thickness with 10% intersection gap; *coronal turbo spin-echo (TSE) TW2* images (2300/100) [TR msec/TE msec], 4 nex, 256×256 matrix, 23 cm field of view, 3 mm-thick sections with 10 per cent intersection gap, turbo factor of 15; *coronal TSE fluid-attenuated inversion-recovery (FLAIR) T2W* sequence (6000/100/2000) [TR msec/TE msec/inversion time msec], 3 nex, 238 × 256 matrix, 23 cm field of view, 3 mm-thick sections with 10 per cent intersection gap, turbo factor of 15; *coronal TSE inversion recovery (IR) T1W* images (3000/20/400) [TR msec/TE msec/inversion time msec], 2 nex, 256 × 256 matrix, 23 cm field of view, 3 mm-thick sections with 20 per cent intersection gap, turbo factor of 4. The three coronal sequences were planned to image the frontal lobes completely. Transverse and coronal sections were acquired parallel and perpendicular to the bicommissural line, respectively. In most patients *3D volume FFE T1W* images were also acquired in the sagittal plane (30/4.6) [TR msec/TE msec], 30° flip angle, 1 nex, 512 × 512 matrix, 23 cm field of view, 1 mm-thick sections with 0 intersection gap, and source images were reformatted in transverse and coronal planes. When a lesion with blood-brain-barrier disruption was suspected on unenhanced images, T1W images were also obtained in different planes, both before and after intravenous contrast injection.

Eighteen patients had a tailored surgical resection after detailed electroclinical work-up to define the epileptogenic zone (EZ) identified as the area responsible for seizure generation. The pathological findings in surgical specimens were characteristic of cortical tubers (CTs) (n = 6), Taylor's focal cortical dysplasia (T-FCD) (n = 2), cytoarchitectural cortical dysplasia (C-CD) (n = 1), architectural cortical dysplasia (A-CD) (n = 2), polymicrogyria and periventricular nodular heterotopia (n = 1), dysembryoplastic neuroepithelial tumour (DNET) (n = 1), DNET combined with C-CD (n = 1), pilocytic astrocytoma (n = 2), ganglioglioma (n = 1), and cavernous haemangioma (n = 1).

To distinguish the different histologic subtypes of FCD we followed a new simplified neuropathological classification based on the most frequent observations in surgical specimens removed from our epileptic patients (Tassi *et al.*, 2002). Lesions were grouped as: (i) architectural dysplasia (A-CD) in which mild cortical dyslamination is generally associated with increased scattered neurons in the white matter; (ii) cytoarchitectural dysplasia (C-CD) characterized by disarray of the normal cortical architecture, associated with neuronal cytomegaly and spreading of ectopic neurons into the subcortical white matter; (iii) Taylor's focal cortical dysplasia (T-FCD), defined by complete loss of cortical lamination, and by the presence of cytomegalic and dysmorphic neurons variably associated with grotesque cells of uncertain lineage called 'balloon cells' (BC). Both abnormal neurons and BC were scattered in the deepest portions of the cortex and in the subcortical white matter.

CTs were histologically characterized by disruption of cortical lamination due to collections of both giant bizarre cells looking like dysmorphic, cytomegalic neurons, and of atypical astrocytes. Many of these cells were reminiscent of BC of T-FCD. A marked demyelination and cystic degeneration of the subcortical white matter were often observed as well as diffuse calcification of the tubers.

Results

Out of 24 patients studied by MR, images were considered positive in 19 cases (79 per cent) and negative in five cases. Visualized structural lesions included: three T-FCD, one A-CD, eight tuberous sclerosis with single cortical tuber in four cases and multifocal cortical tubers in four cases, two polymicrogyria with associated periventricular nodular heterotopia in one case, one DNET with associated cortical dysplasia, one ganglioglioma, one pilocytic astrocytoma, one glial tumour in the broadest sense, and one cavernous haemangioma.

The main MRI features of T-FCD were focal thickening of the cortical ribbon, blurring of the grey-white matter junction, increased signal on T2WI and decreased signal on T1WI of the subcortical white matter, variably tapering to the ventricle, with normal appearing cortical surface (Fig. 1) (Taylor & Falconer, 1971; Yagishita *et al.*, 1997; Colombo *et al.*, 2003).

Chapter 17 MRI in the diagnosis of frontal lobe epilepsy

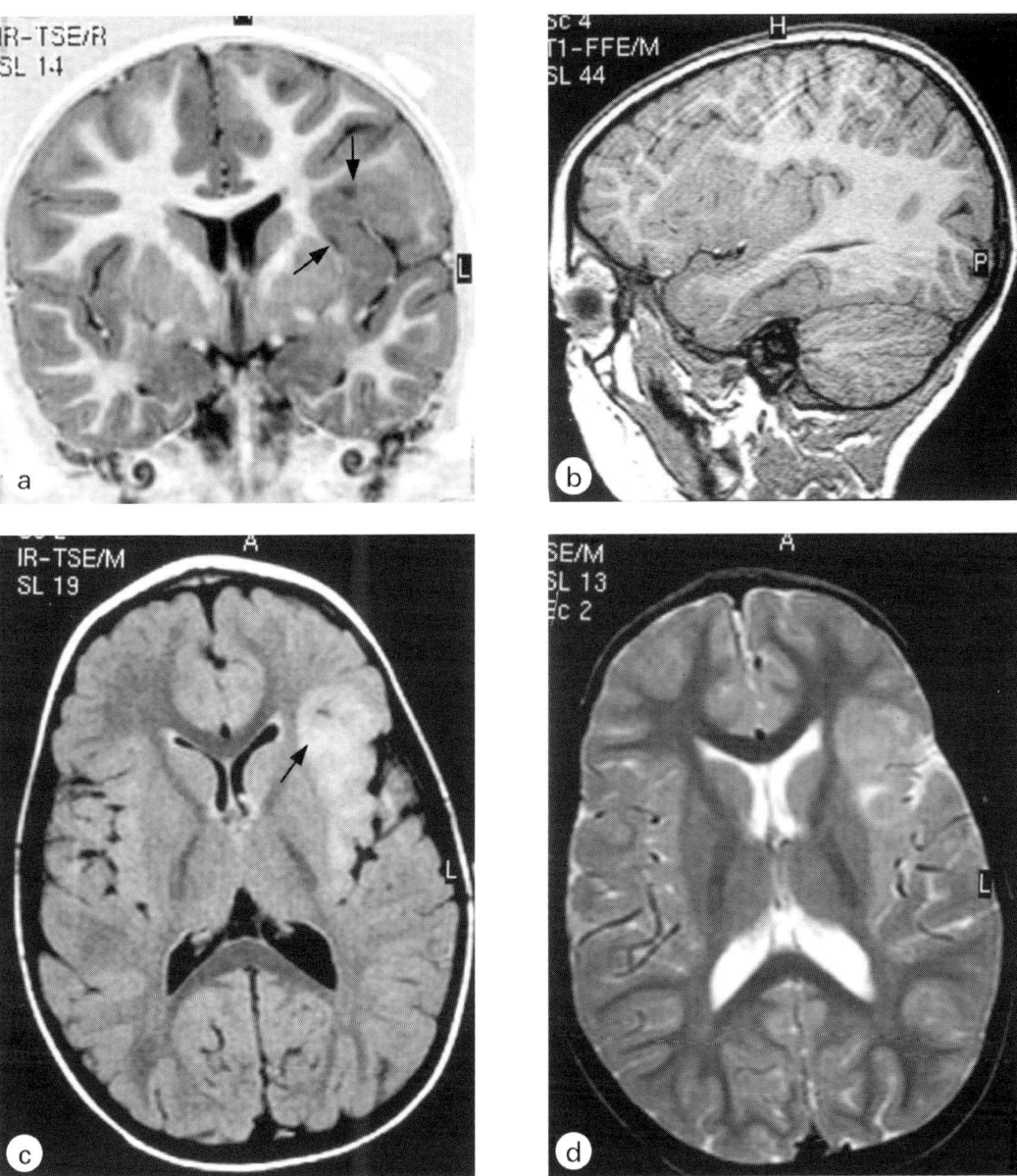

Fig. 1. Taylor's focal cortical dysplasia in a 4-year-old girl with intractable left fronto-central seizures since the age of 11 months. a) TSE IRT1W coronal image, b) FFE T1W sagittal image, 1 mm thick, from a 3D volume acquisition, c) TSE FLAIR T2W axial image, d) SE T2W axial image. Abnormal cortical thickening of the left insula and fronto-opercular region, with blurred demarcation between the grey and white matter and diffusely increased signal of the subcortical white matter on T2WI. More discrete foci of reduced signal on T1WI and increased signal on T2WI are observed beneath the cortex (arrows in a and c). Subarachnoid spaces overlying the dysplastic cortex are slightly enlarged compared to the contralateral side. (Surgically proven case.)

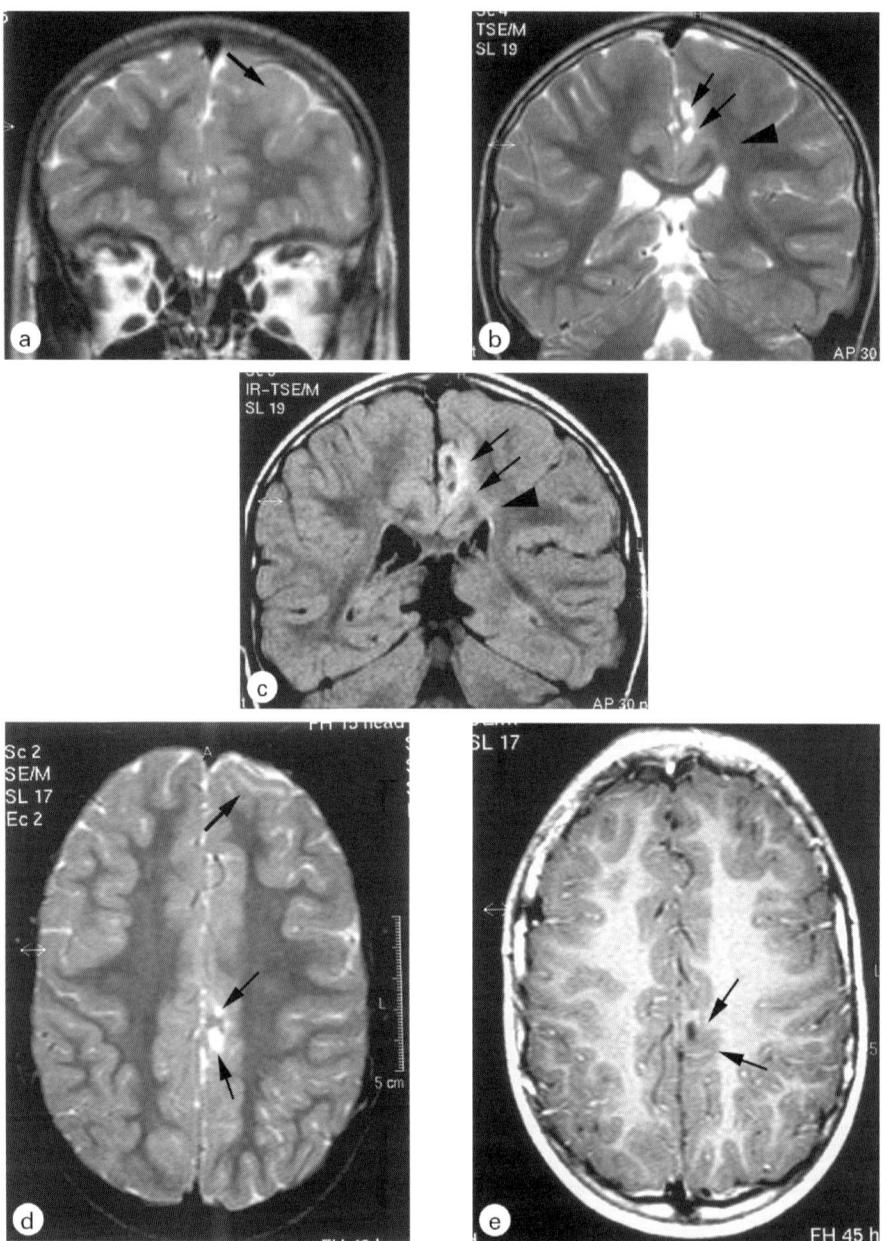

Fig. 2. Cortical tubers in a 9-year-old girl with daily fronto-central seizures since the age of 2 years. No other stigmata of tuberous sclerosis complex were present. a-b) SE T2W coronal images, c) TSE FLAIR T2W coronal image, d) SE T2W axial image, e) SE T1W axial image. Two cortical tubers involve the left superior frontal gyrus over the convexity more anteriorly (arrow in a and d), and the mesial aspect of the left superior frontal gyrus posteriorly (arrows in b-e). The involved gyri are enlarged. The peripheral portion of the lesions consists of thickened cortex, the central 'core' of abnormal white matter appearing of low signal intensity on T1W and FLAIR images (e, c) and of high signal intensity on T2W images (a, b, d). Note on coronal images (a-c) that the medial aspect of the tubers is poorly defined and a linear hyperintensity extends from the more posterior tuber to the superior profile of the left ventricular trigone (arrowhead in b and c). These lesions do not enhance after administration of intravenous contrast. The more posterior lesion was resected.

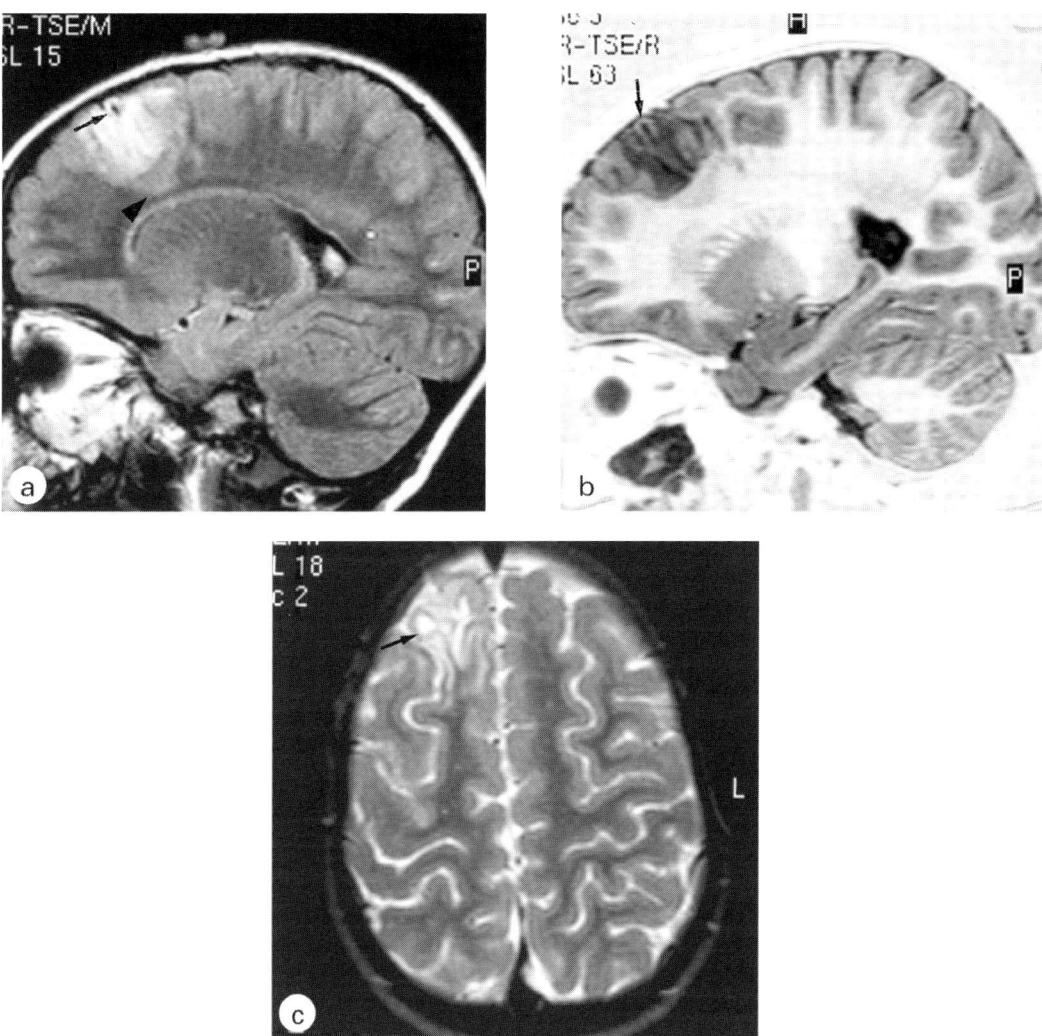

Fig. 3. DNET associated with cortical dysplasia in a 3-year-old boy with right mesial-frontal seizures since the age of 18 months. (Surgically proven case.) a) TSE FLAIR T2W sagittal image, b) TSE IRT1W sagittal image, c) SE T2W axial image. A slightly expansile lesion with cortical-subcortical extension is seen in the right superior frontal gyrus. The lesion consists of a cyst (arrow) included in enlarged gyri with pseudocystic aspect (gyriform pattern) exhibiting inhomogeneous decreased signal on IR and increased signal on T2W sequences. The cortex surrounding the tumour shows slightly increased signal on T2WI, deeply extending through the subcortical white matter to the ventricle (arrowhead in a), corresponding to the area of cytoarchitectural dysplasia in the surgical specimen.

A-CDs were diagnosed when MRI showed lobar/sublobar hypoplasia, with enlargement of the subarachnoid spaces overlying the cortex, and shrinkage of the local white matter with mild hypersignal on T2W images, without notable cortical thickening (Kuzniecky, 1996; Colombo et al., 1998; Choi et al., 1999; Mitchell et al., 1999; Colombo et al., 2003). CTs were characterized by enlarged gyri, with smooth or dimpled surface, and by increased thickness of the cortex clearly demarcated from the underlying white matter which was also involved by the lesion. CTs often appeared as cortical-subcortical masses, with peripheral cortex and a subcortical 'core' of abnormal white matter, with signal abnormalities changing with age. In neonates and children under 2 years of age the tuber was hyperintense compared to the adjacent unmyelinated white matter on T1WI and hypointense to white matter on T2WI. In older children they had a low signal intensity centre on T1WI changing to high signal intensity on T2WI (Fig. 2) (Barkovich, 1995; Nixon et al., 1989). Foci of calcification inside the CTs showed reduced signal in all pulse sequences. Inconstant contrast enhancement was observed. Diagnosis was facilitated in patients with multifocal lesions and coexisting subependymal nodules and/or giant cell astrocytomas, and white matter heterotopias which are characteristic of tuberous sclerosis complex. The DNET appeared as an intracortical lesion, with cystic and gyriform pattern, surrounded by cerebral tissue with 'dysplastic' features (Fig. 3) (Daumas-Duport et al., 1988; Daumas-Duport, 1996; Ostertun et al., 1996; Prayson et al., 1993; Koeller & Dillon, 1992).

The diagnostic criteria used to identify the other pathological conditions in our series have been extensively reported in the literature (Figs. 4, 5, 6) (Barkovich, 1999; Raybaud et al., 1996; Peretti-Vitton et al., 1991; Tampieri et al., 1991). In our series, MRI and histopathologic diagnosis were concordant in 13 of the 18 cases operated on (76 per cent) including: six CTs, two T-FCD, one DNET & C-CD, one polymicrogyria combined with periventricular nodular heterotopia, one ganglioglioma, one pilocytic astrocytoma, and one cavernous haemangioma. MRI diagnosis differed from the histopathologic results in five cases: one A-CD was not visualized on MR, one A-CD was misinterpreted as a Taylor type of FCD (Fig. 7), one cytoarchitectural-CD was misinterpreted as A-CD (Fig. 8), one pilocytic astrocytoma as a non-specific glioma, and one DNET as a cortical tuber (Table 1).

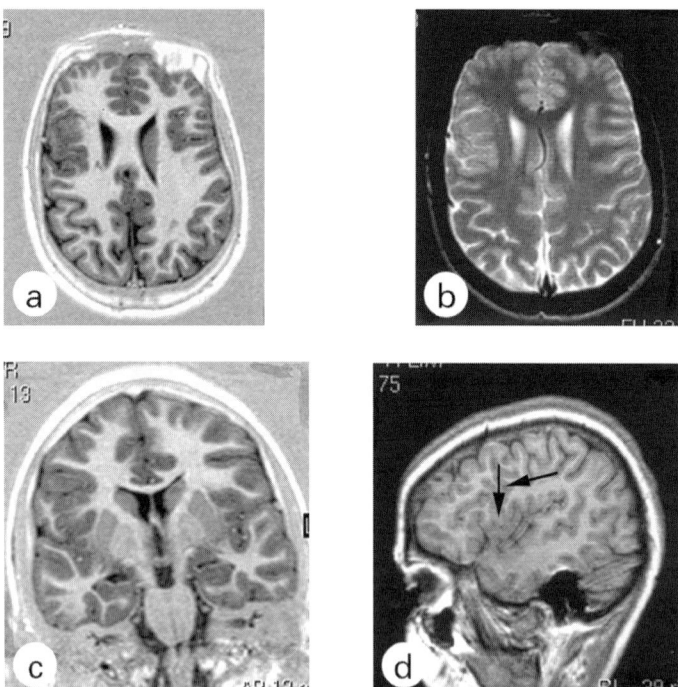

Fig. 4. Polymicrogyria in a 16-year-old girl with asymmetric axial spasms since the age of 6 months. a) TSE IRT1W axial image, 5 mm thickness, b) SE T2W axial image, 5 mm thickness, c) TSE IRT1W coronal image, 3 mm thickness, d) FFE T1W sagittal image, 1 mm thickness, from a 3D volume acquisition. Right fronto-opercular polymicrogyria is seen, simulating pachygyria on routine spin-echo images (a, b). Thin section (d) shows the multiple small gyri (arrow) and a tiny irregularity of the grey-white matter junction. Focal enlargement of the adjacent sulci containing a large draining vein is also present (a, b). Polymicrogyric cortex is isointense to normal cortex in all pulse sequences.

Table 1. Discrepancies between MR and histopathologic diagnosis in five patients

MR diagnosis	Histology
1 Negative	A-CD
1 T-FCD	A-CD
1 A-CD	C-CD
1 Glioma	Pilocytic astrocytoma
1 Cortical tuber	DNET

Abbreviations: A-CD = architectural dysplasia; C-CD = cytoarchitectural dysplasia; DNET = dysembryoplastic neuroepithelial tumour.

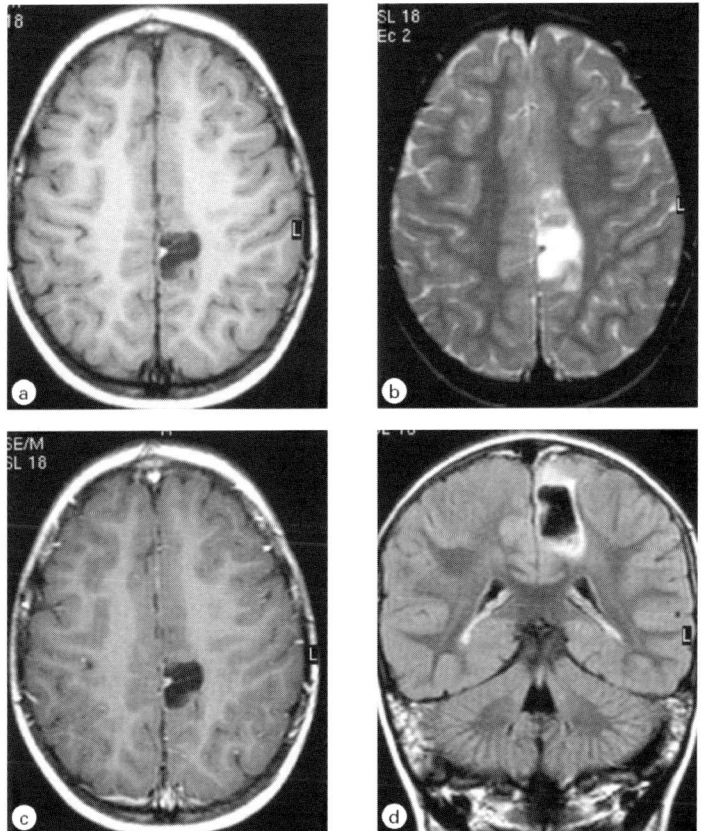

Fig. 5. Ganglioglioma in a 6-year-old boy with left central seizures from age 7 months. (Surgically proven case.) a) SE T1W axial image, b) SE T2W axial image, c) SE T1W axial image after contrast injection, d) TSE FLAIR T2W coronal image. A mass lesion of mixed signal intensity is seen in the mesial aspect of the left superior frontal gyrus posteriorly. The lesion, with cortical-subcortical extension, is cystic in the centre and solid at the periphery, where it exhibits hyperintense signal on T2WI (b, d). A small calcification is present along the mesial wall of the cyst, appearing hyperintense on T1W and hypointense on T2W images. There was no contrast enhancement.

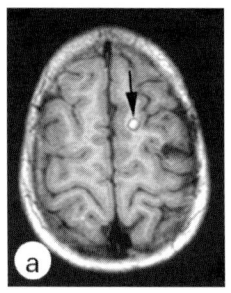 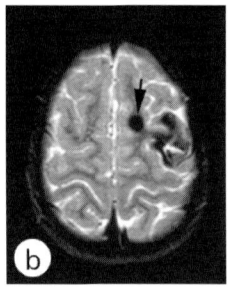

Fig. 6. Cavernous haemangioma in a 5-year-old boy. a) SE T1W axial image, b) SE T2W axial image. A small round lesion is seen in the left superior frontal gyrus with haemorrhagic content in the subacute-chronic stage, appearing hyperintense on T1WI and hypointense on T2WI (arrow). The diffuse hypointensity seen over the left frontal convexity on T2W images (b) represents haemosiderin deposition from previous bleeding.

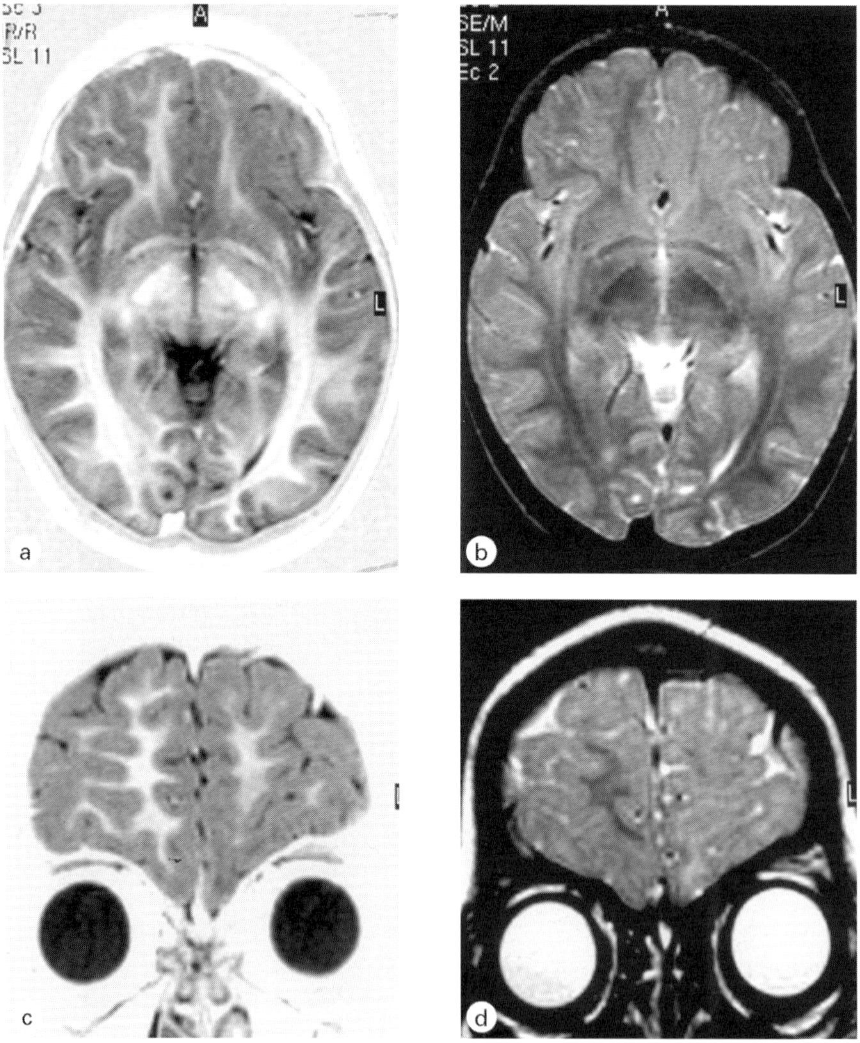

Fig. 7. Histologically proven architectural cortical dysplasia in a 2-year-old girl with several spasms per day since the age of 9 months. (Surgically proven case.) a) TSE IRT1W axial image, b) SE T2W axial image, c) TSE IRT1W coronal image, d) SE T2W coronal images. Slightly reduced volume of the left frontal pole with shrinkage of the white matter. The cortex is thickened, the cortical-subcortical junction is blurred and the subcortical white matter is diffusely hyperintense on T2W images (b, d). On MRI the dysplastic lesion was misinterpreted as a Taylor FCD.

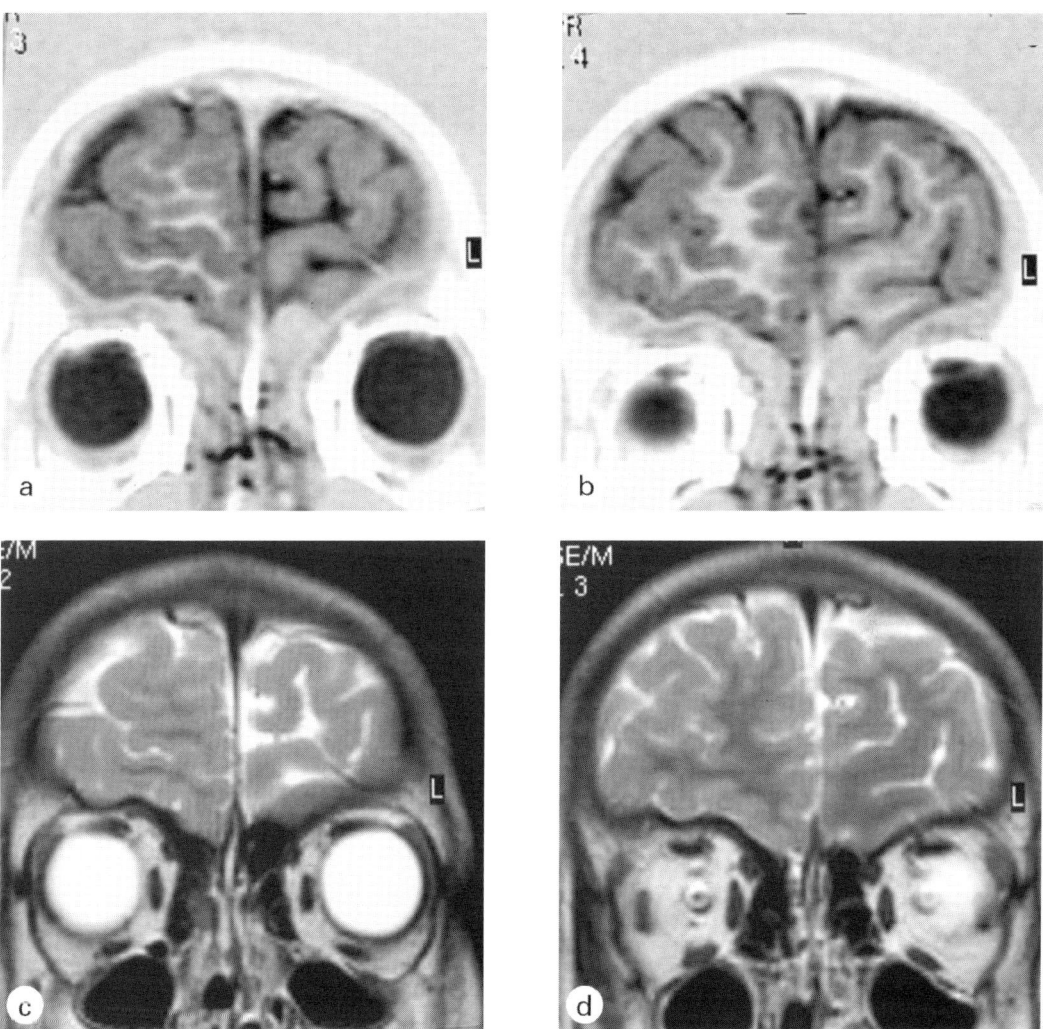

Fig. 8. Histologically proven cytoarchitectural cortical dysplasia in a 6-year-old boy with daily left fronto-central seizures since the age of 1 month. (Surgically proven case.) a), b) TSE-IRT1W contiguous coronal images ; c), d) SE-T2W coronal images at the same levels. Abnormal gyration and marked hypoplasia of the left frontal pole. No cortical thickening or signal alterations are noted in the lesion which was misinterpreted on imaging as an architectural type of dysplasia.

Among the six patients still waiting for surgery, MRI showed no structural lesion in four subjects, and showed polymicrogyria in one case and multiple cortical tubers in one. In the surgical group, 50 per cent of patients are seizure-free (Class Ia) (Engel, 1987) after more than 1 year of follow-up.

References

Barkovich, A.J. (1995): Disorders of neuronal migration and organization. In: *Magnetic resonance in epilepsy*, eds. R.I. Kuzniecky & G.D. Jackson, pp. 235–255. New York: Raven Press.

Barkovich, A.J. (1999): Neuroradiology of malformations of cortical development: band heterotopia, hemimegalencephaly, and polymicrogyria. In: *Abnormal cortical development and epilepsy*, eds. R. Spreafico, G. Avanzini & F. Andermann, pp. 161–170. Mariani Foundation Paediatric Neurology Series, vol. 7. London: John Libbey & Company.

Choi, D., Na, D.G., Byun, H.S., Suh, Y.L., Kim, S.E., Ro, D.W., Chung, II G., Hong, S.C. & Hong, S.B. (1999): White-matter change in mesial temporal sclerosis: correlation of MRI with PET, pathology and clinical features. *Epilepsia* **40** (11), 1634–1641.

Colombo, N., Tassi, L., Galli, C., Munari, C. & Scialfa, G. (1998): Malformations of cortical development: clinical-neuroradiologic correlations in 38 patients. *Boll. Lega Ital. Epil.* **102/103**, 17–28.

Colombo, N., Tassi, L., Galli, C, Citterio, A., Lo Russo, G., Scialfa, G., Spreafico, R. (2003): Focal cortical dysplasias: MR imaging, histopathologic, and clinical correlations in surgically treated patients with epilepsy. *A.J.N.R.* **24**, 724–733.

Daumas-Duport, C. (1996): Dysembryoplastic neuroepithelial tumours in epilepsy surgery. In: *Dysplasias of cerebral cortex and epilepsy*, eds. R. Guerrini, F. Andermann, R. Canapicchi, J. Roger, B.G. Zifkin & P. Pfanner, pp. 71–80. Philadelphia: Lippincott-Raven.

Daumas-Duport, C., Scheithauer, B.W., Chodkiewicz, J.P., Laws Jr, E.R., & Vedrenne, C. (1988): Dysembryoplastic neuroepithelial tumour: a surgically curable tumour of young patients with intractable partial seizures. Report of 39 cases. *Neurosurgery* **23**, 545–556.

Engel, J. Jr. (1987): Outcome with respect to epileptic seizures. In: *Surgical treatment of the epilepsies*, ed. J. Engel Jr, pp. 553–571. New York: Raven Press.

Koeller K.K., & Dillon P.W. (1992): Dysembryoplastic neuroepithelial tumours: MR appearance. *A.J.N.R.* **13**, 1319–1325.

Kuzniecky, R.I. (1996): MRI in focal cortical dysplasia. In: *Dysplasias of cerebral cortex and epilepsy*, eds. R. Guerrini, F. Andermann, R. Canapicchi, J. Roger, B.G. Zifkin & P. Pfanner, pp. 71–80. Philadelphia: Lippincott-Raven.

Kuzniecky, R.I. & Jackson, G.D. (1995): Frontal lobe epilepsy. In: *Magnetic resonance in epilepsy*, eds. R.I. Kuzniecky & G.D. Jackson, pp. 183–202. New York: Raven Press.

Mitchell, L.A., Jackson, G.D., Kalnins, R.M., Saling, M.M., Fitt, G.J., Ashpole, R.D. & Berkovic, S.F. (1999): Anterior temporal abnormality in temporal lobe epilepsy. A quantitative MRI and histopathologic study. *Neurology* **52**, 327–333.

Nixon, J.R., Houser, O.W., Gomez, M.R. & Okasaki H. (1989): Cerebral tuberous sclerosis: MR imaging. *Radiology* **170**, 869–873.

Ostertun, B., Wolf, H.K., Campos, M.G., Matus, C., Solymosi, L., Elger, C.E., Schramm, J. & Schild, H.H. (1996): Dysembryoplastic neuroepithelial tumours: MR and CT evaluation. *A.J.N.R.* **17**, 419–429.

Peretti-Vitton, P., Perez-Castillo, A.M., Raybaud, C., Grisoli, F., Bernard, F., Poncet, M. & Salamon, G. (1991): Magnetic resonance imaging in gangliogliomas and gangliocytomas of the nervous system. *J. Neuroradiol.* **18**, 189–199.

Prayson, R.A., Estes, M.L. & Morris, H.H. (1993): Coexistence of neoplasia and cortical dysplasia in patients presenting with seizures. *Epilepsia* **34**, 609–615.

Raybaud, C., Girard, N., Canto-Moreira, N. & Poncet, M. (1996): High-definition magnetic resonance imaging identification of cortical dysplasias: micropolygyria *vs* lissencephaly. In: *Dysplasias of cerebral cortex and epilepsy*, eds. R. Guerrini, F. Andermann, R. Canapicchi, J. Roger, B.G. Zifkin & P. Pfanner, pp. 131–143. Philadelphia: Lippincott-Raven.

Robitaille, Y., Rasmussen, T., Dubeau, F., Tampieri, D. & Kemball, K. (1992): Histopathology of non-neoplastic lesions in frontal lobe epilepsy. Review of 180 cases with recent MRI and PET correlations. In: *Advances in Neurology*, eds. P. Chauvel, A.V. Delgado-Escueta *et al.*, vol. 57, pp. 499–513. New York: Raven Press.

Tampieri, D., Moumdijan, R., Melanson, D. & Ethier, R. (1991): Intracerebral gangliogliomas in patient with partial complex seizures. *A.J.N.R.* **12**, 749–755.

Tassi, L., Colombo, N., Garbelli, R., Francione, S., Lo Russo, G., Mai, R., Cardinale, F., Cossu, M., Ferrario, A., Galli, C., Bramerio, M., Citterio, A. & Spreafico, R. (2002): Focal cortical dysplasia: neuropathological subtypes, EEG, neuroimaging and surgical outcome. *Brain* **125**, 1719–1732.

Taylor, D.C. & Falconer, M.A. (1971): Focal dysplasia of the cerebral cortex in epilepsy. *J. Neurol. Neurosurg. Psychiatr.* **34**, 369–387.

Yagishita, A., Arai, N., Maehara, T., Shimizu, H., Tokumaru, A.M. & Oda, M. (1997): Focal cortical dysplasia: appearance on MR images. *Radiology* **203**, 553–559.

Chapter 18

Electroclinical semeiology of frontal lobe seizures in infants and children: contribution of intracranial video EEG recording

Martine Fohlen, Claude Jalin and Olivier Delalande

*Neurosurgery Service, Fondation Ophtalmologique A. de Rothschild,
25, rue Marin, 75019 Paris, France*
mfohlen@fo-rothschild.fr

Summary

The purpose of this study is to investigate the relations between electroclinical patterns and anatomical origin of frontal lobe seizures in infants and children with cortical dysplastic lesions using intracranial video-EEG recording before epilepsy surgery.

Between 1992 and 2000, 12 patients (five girls and seven boys) aged 7 months to 14 years underwent intracranial intensive monitoring for intractable frontal lobe epilepsy due to cortical dysplasia. Intracranial recording with subdural and depth electrodes comprising 64 to 104 channels was performed. Electrodes were placed according to ictal and interictal scalp video-EEG, MRI and ictal SPECT. The mean duration of 24-hour video-EEG recording was 5 days (range 3 to 7 days). Seizures were recorded on a BMSI computer with 128 EEG channels using software (Stellate Systems, Montreal, Canada) for automatic detection of paroxysmal electrical events. Identification of the seizures or rhythmic discharges was made by medical staff and parents and by automatic detection.

From eight to 110 seizures were recorded in each patient. Clinical and EEG ictal patterns were evaluated, followed by electroclinical and anatomical correlation. Most seizures included a major motor component with ipsi- (six patients) or contra- (five patients) lateral deviation of head and eyes, and unilateral or bilateral tonic, clonic, or dystonic contraction of the limbs that always predominated on the side opposite the lesion. These could occur at seizure onset or later in its course. In the latter case, they were preceded by staring, modification of either gaze or behaviour, or by a sudden fall.

Some 'behavioural' seizures were not recognized by parents and medical staff but could be diagnosed by intracranial recording. This occurred in four patients: video monitoring showed inappropriate laughing or spasmodic crying, sudden arrest of crying, behavioural stereotypies, sudden agitation, or awakening when the seizure occurred during sleep.

Some seizures consisted of loss of contact with or without automatisms. Some ictal EEG activity had no evident clinical counterpart. Around 70 per cent of all types of seizures occurred during sleep.

The ictal EEGs showed several patterns. The most characteristic consisted of a high frequency (> 70 Hz) low amplitude discharge preceded by modification of the interictal spike activity in the epileptogenic focus (disappearance of spikes or slow waves, or synchronization with increased amplitude of interictal spikes or burst suppression). A second ictal pattern consisted of a sequence of irregular spikes or polyspikes, followed either by regular rhythmic spikes at 1 to 8 Hz or by decreasing frequency and increasing amplitude spikes. A third pattern consisted of flattening followed by rhythmic spikes.

Electroclinical and anatomical correlations: seizures with a motor component affected Brodmann areas 4 and 6, the supplementary motor area, the paracentral lobule. Behavioural seizures, absences and outwardly asymptomatic discharges involved frontopolar, orbital frontal and intermediary dorsolateral areas.

In conclusion, electroclinical patterns of frontal seizures in children have features similar to those described in adults by Penfield, and by Bancaud & Talairach. Nevertheless, behavioural seizures and epileptic stereotypies seem to be a particular feature of childhood epilepsy involving the most anterior and inferior part of the frontal lobe. Those seizures are usually misdiagnosed on scalp video-EEG because the epileptogenic zone is far from the brain convexity and because they are more often considered as behavioural manifestations in children with developmental delay and autistic features. When surgery is considered, intracranial EEG recording can identify these seizures and help determine the extent of brain resection.

The clinical patterns of frontal lobe seizures (FLSs) have been well documented in adults since the first reports by Penfield & Kristiansen (1951) and later those of Bancaud & Talairach (1992) whose depth electrode studies helped to determine the site of origin of seizures and established some electroclinical and anatomical correlations.

There are few reports of these events in infants and children. Nordli et al. (1997) emphasized the difficulty in determining whether a seizure in an infant is partial or generalized and, when partial, in determining the lateralization. Wyllie & Bass (1996) reported supplementary sensorimotor area seizures in children and adolescents and concluded that they do not differ from those seen in adults. Nevertheless there are no reports of the clinical patterns of FLSs in childhood originating from the other parts of the frontal lobe, and especially from the more anterior dorsolateral, frontobasal and orbitofrontal areas.

We have studied FLSs in 12 infants and children with frontal lobe epilepsy due to pathologically proven cortical dysplasia who became seizure-free after surgery. Focal cortical dysplasia (Taylor & Falconer, 1971) is a dysgenetic malformation of the cortex, and is the main cause of early onset symptomatic partial epilepsy in children. All patients in this series had intracranial EEG recording followed by tailored cortical resection of the epileptic zone. Intracranial recording provides an excellent opportunity to study EEG patterns and clinical signs, and to establish precise anatomical origin.

Material and methods

We retrospectively reviewed 27 patients with unilateral frontal lobe epilepsy, operated on after intracranial investigation between 1992 and 2000, and selected 12 patients (five girls and seven boys), based on the following criteria: (i) age at surgery under 15 years; (ii) total relief from seizures after surgery (Engel class Ia); (iii) pathologically confirmed cortical dysplasia.

Mean age of seizure onset was 15 months (range 8 days to 11 years; before 9 months in 10 patients). Mean duration of epilepsy was 4.3 years (range 6.5 months to 9 years) and mean age at intracranial recording and surgery was 5.1 years (range 6.5 months to 14 years).

Neurologic examination showed mild contralateral hemiparesis in three patients, contralateral hand neglect in two, and no deficit for the seven others. Neuropsychological evaluation (Brunet-Lezine or WISC-R) showed that IQ was normal in two patients, between 50 and 80 in eight with memory defects and frontal lobe syndrome, and under 50 in two. The four most impaired patients also had autistic features.

At the time of surgery, all patients had partial motor seizures (ipsi- or contralateral turning of head and eyes and/or unilateral or asymmetrical tonic or clonic limb movements). Seizure frequency was weekly (one patient), daily (Bancaud & Talairach, 1992) or several times a day (Munari et al.,

1995). At least four antiepileptic drugs had been used in each patient. Three patients had previous hemispasms combined in two cases with hypsarrhythmia and in one case with suppression bursts, and were controlled with corticosteroids and/or vigabatrin. All 12 patients underwent prolonged video-EEG evaluation two or three times, most recently in our department less than 6 months before surgery. Scalp EEG recordings showed continuous paroxysmal spike and slow wave activity, more or less localized to the frontal or fronto-Rolandic areas. Recorded seizures identified the affected side in all cases. The location of intracranial electrodes was thus determined by scalp video-EEG results in order to define the boundaries of the brain resection and to perform functional mapping when onset of the seizures was close to the sensorimotor and speech area.

MRI was performed at least twice in all patients: repeated imaging with T1, T2 fluid attenuation inversion recovery (FLAIR) and inversion recovery sequences, with general anaesthesia in the younger or mentally retarded patients, helped identify subtle abnormalities. In all cases, MRI demonstrated a structural lesion involving frontobasal (three cases), fronto-Rolandic (four cases), opercular (one case), or premotor (two cases) areas, or the whole frontal lobe (three cases). The most indicative signs of focal cortical dysplasia were blurring of the grey-white matter border and broad gyri. A cyst within the lesion in one case suggested a dysembryoplastic neuroepithelial tumour which was confirmed on histology.

Areas of interictal hypoperfusion (seven patients) and ictal hyperperfusion (two patients) found by single photon emission computed tomography (SPECT) were consistent with the epileptogenic area determined by intracranial recording.

Intracranial recordings

All 12 patients had intracranial recording with subdural electrode arrays and depth electrodes. Subdural electrodes consisted of 3 mm stainless steel contacts 1 cm apart embedded in a 1.5 mm thick Silastic sheet. Platinum depth electrodes were 3 mm in diameter with 5 to 7 mm between contacts. Grids covered the epileptogenic area defined by scalp recording and the neighbouring functional areas. After craniotomy, depth electrode insertion was guided by ultrasound into and around the lesion, and into the mesial structures of the hemisphere that cannot be easily covered with grids. From 64 to 104 channels were recorded in each patient. Monitoring was continuous for 3 to 7 days (mean 5). Seizures were recorded on a BMSI computer with 128 EEG channels using software (Stellate Systems, Montreal, Canada) for automatic detection of paroxysmal electrical events. One parent and a nurse were with the child at all times. Seizures were identified by medical staff and parents, and by computer detection. Interpretation of recordings included the analysis of clinical signs, EEG patterns, and electroclinical and anatomical site of onset and early propagation of the seizures. Seizures were analysed at least twice by one physician at a time. Functional mapping of the motor strip and language area was performed according to the method of Jayakar (Jayakar *et al.*, 1992). Tailored cortical resection was performed 5 to 9 days (mean 7) following craniotomy and consisted of removing the area of seizure onset and early propagation, while sparing the functional areas disclosed by mapping. In three patients, a cortical transection of motor strip was also performed as described by Morrell (Morrell *et al.*, 1989).

Neuropathological findings were consistent with cortical dysplasia in 11 cases and with the combination of dysplasia with dysembryoplastic tumour in one patient. Antiepileptic medication was stopped in seven cases and decreased in five with a mean follow-up of 4 years and 5 months.

Results

We recorded 14 to 110 seizures in each patient. Seizures were classified according to their anatomical origin within the frontal lobe using Bancaud's classification (1982) (see Fig. 1 p. 68).

Orbitofrontal and prefrontal cortex

Seizures originated in the orbitofrontal cortex in five patients and from the frontopolar cortex in one.

Different seizure types were seen in each patient and a single patient could have several seizure types depending on the level of vigilance.

Most seizures were recorded during sleep and consisted of brief arousals sometimes associated with mumbling, turning onto one side, or suddenly sitting up in bed.

During wakefulness, seizures consisted of changes in behaviour such as: (i) stereotyped movements such as clapping the hands in two patients, hiding one eye in two patients, tapping a toy in one patient and hiding the face in the pillow in another child; (ii) sudden mood changes such as inappropriate laughing in one case and spasmodic crying in another; (iii) subtle changes in behaviour such as becoming quieter or less alert, a decrease in motor or social activities or staring in three patients (Fig. 1).

Seizure duration ranged from 30 seconds to 18 minutes for the longest one.

Many electroencephalographic seizures in sleep and wakefulness seemed to have no clinical accompaniment.

Discharges spread posteriorly to the premotor and motor cortex in less than 10 per cent of the seizures. In these cases, motor features occurred and seizures were recognized easily. All other seizures were initially only recognized by automatic seizure detection algorithm. Most of them were unrecognized by staff and parents, and others were considered as abnormal behaviour. We refer to these as behavioural seizures.

The intracranial EEG tracing showed several different patterns: (i) flattening followed by rhythmic sharp waves with progressive increase in amplitude, followed by synchronous rhythmic spikes and waves of decreased frequency; (ii) synchronous rhythmic spike-wave sequences; (iii) sequence of low-amplitude beta activity ending with a brief cluster of spikes.

Dorsolateral cortex

Six patients had seizures originating from dorsolateral frontal cortex which consisted of: (i) mood changes: in one case the child looked uncomfortable and restless, with an unpleasant spasmodic crying, remained restless and irritable. The EEG showed high-amplitude spikes and polyspikes that were more or less regular and localized over the most anterior and superior dorso-lateral electrodes without spreading: this seizure lasted 18 minutes; (ii) awakening and raising the head: as the discharge spread posteriorly, there was contralateral deviation of the head and eyes (Fig. 2); (iii) initial anarchic movements of the limbs and trunk followed by automatisms such as handling clothes, anxious gaze and incomprehensible words: awareness was preserved at onset and when discharge spread to the premotor cortex, the boy had contralateral hypertonia of the upper limb with ipsilateral deviation of head and eyes; (iv) others included changes in respiratory rhythm, and motor arrest followed by motor activity when the discharge spread posteriorly: motor activity means epileptic motor manifestations such as lateral deviation of head and eyes, unilateral or bilateral tonic, clonic, or dystonic contraction of the limbs and asymmetrical hypertonia of upper limbs; (v) initial staring

Chapter 18 Electroclinical semeiology of frontal lobe seizures in infants and children

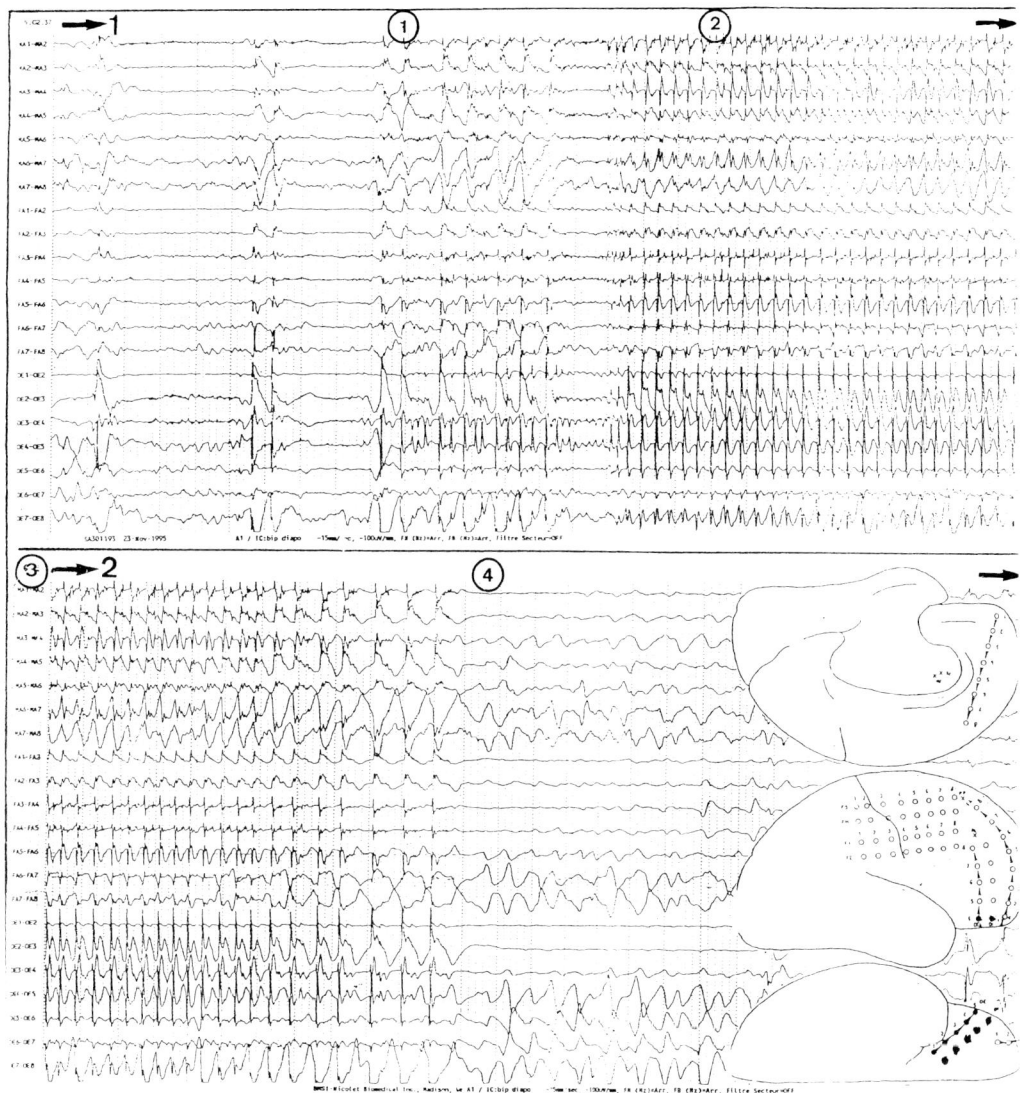

Fig. 1. Orbital frontal seizure recorded with subdural elecrodes in a boy aged 3 years: Clinical signs: ①: decrease of motor activity, ② and ③: clapping hands, ④: stop clapping and returning to normal social and motor activity. Electrical signs (see dark circles on the figure): ①: bursts of polyspikes followed by a flattening with low amplitude spikes over orbitofrontal electrodes (OE1 to OE 4), ② and ③: spike and wave discharges with higher amplitude over orbitofrontal electrodes, ④: end of discharge and slow waves or flattening of EEG.

followed by contralateral deviation of the head and eyes, tonic abduction, and clonic movements of the contralateral upper limb; (vi) there were many subclinical discharges during sleep and wakefulness lasting from a few seconds to several minutes: the longest subclinical event was 80 seconds long.

These are very similar to the seizures originating from prefrontal and orbitofrontal areas but motor signs occur early in these dorsolateral seizures probably because of spread to the nearby motor and premotor cortex.

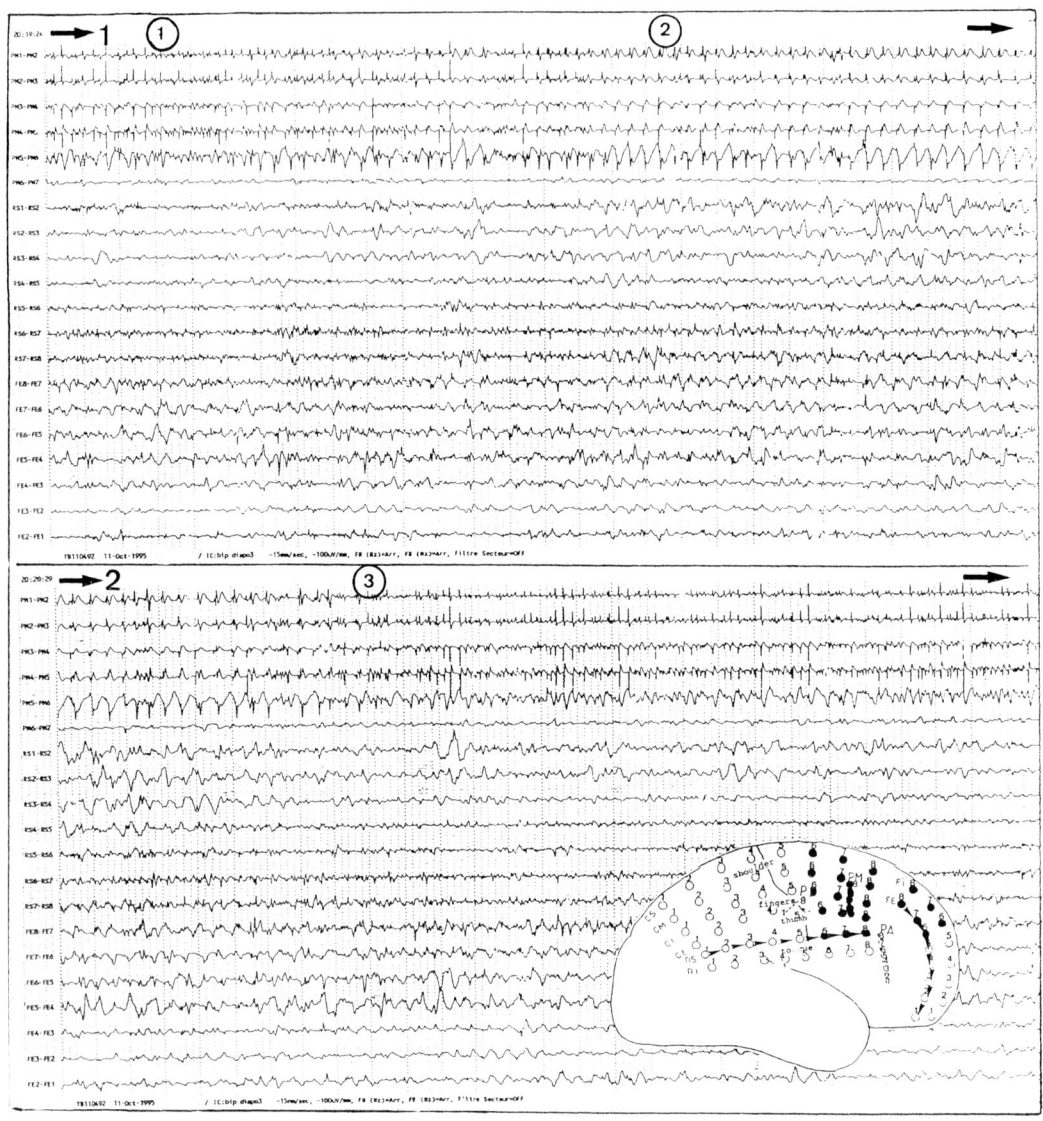

Fig. 2. Dorsolateral seizure recorded with subdural electrodes in a boy aged 4 years. Clinical signs ①: the child appears restless and uncomfortable; ② unpleasant spasmodic crying lasting about 18 minutes; ③ stops crying and recovering of usual behaviour. EEG (see dark circles): ① irregular spikes and polyspikes over dorsolateral area; ② more regular spike and wave rhythmic discharge; ③ end of the discharge.

Supplementary motor area (area 6)

One patient had seizures coming from the supplementary motor area (SMA). These occurred during sleep: the child awakened and had asymmetric hypertonia of the upper limbs and trunk with vocalization. The seizure lasted 12 seconds: the EEG showed several asynchronous foci of decreasing frequency low-amplitude spikes from the mesial part of area 6.

Motor cortex (area 4)

Seizures originating from area 4 in one patient consisted of clonic movements of the contralateral thumb with Jacksonian march to the hand and proximal arm with preservation of consciousness. Intracranial EEG showed rhythmic and fast spikes over the primary motor strip.

Another child had vibratory hypertonia or jerks of the contralateral side, followed by clonic movements of the contralateral limbs and eyelids of both sides. The intracranial EEG showed flattening with rapid rhythms followed by low-amplitude repetitive spike-waves alternating with sequences of synchronous high-amplitude rhythmical spike-wave activity over mesial and external parts of areas 6 and 4. The latter were associated with clonic movements. Seizures lasted about 1 minute.

Opercular

The seizures recorded in one patient began with clonic movements of the tongue, hypersalivation, isolated slow protrusion of the tongue and apnoea, eyelid blinking, and clonic movements of the right arm when the discharge spread to the left motor strip. Consciousness seemed intact. He would remain quiet or run towards his mother. Intracranial EEG showed rapid rhythmic spikes over motor opercular electrodes whose precise location was assessed by cortical stimulation. The mean duration of seizures was 40 seconds.

Conclusions

Frontal epileptic seizures are very similar in children and adults. Penfield defined three different groups: (i) SMA seizures with tonic posturing at onset; (ii) focal motor seizures, with tonic or clonic limb movements or contraversion of the head and eyes; (iii) complex partial seizures (CPSs) with unresponsiveness and complex motor automatisms.

This classification can be applied to infants and children, but frontal lobe CPSs in children can be more varied and subtle. CPSs in eight of our patients arose from several areas over much of the frontal lobe including frontopolar, orbital-frontal and dorsolateral cortex. There is a wide variety of clinical manifestations. Some consist of subtle changes in awareness or vigilance; others which are very frequent and occur during sleep look almost like a normal arousal, others consist of a change in mood such as crying, laughing or smiling; and others consist of complex motor automatisms that we referred to as stereotypies. Most of those seizures were overlooked, some because they were considered as behavioural events in children with cognitive impairment and autistic features, and some because they appeared to be simple arousals from nocturnal sleep. When surgery is considered, intracranial EEG monitoring associated with seizure detection equipment can document these seizures which can otherwise easily be overlooked in children. Awareness of such seizures should increase the index of suspicion in interpreting prolonged scalp video-EEGs.

References

Bancaud, J. & Talairach, J. (1992): Clinical semiology of frontal lobe seizures. In: *Advances in Neurology*, eds. P. Chauvel, A.V. Delgado-Escueta *et al.*, vol. 57, pp. 3–34. New York: Raven Press.

Fogarasi, A., Janszki, J., Faveret, E., Pieper, T. & Tuxhorn, I. (2001): A detailed analysis of frontal lobe seizure semiology in children younger than 7 years. *Epilepsia* **42** (1), 80–85.

Geier, S., Bancaud, J., Talairach, J., Bonis, A., Enjelvin, M. & Hossard-Bouchaud, H. (1976): Automatisms during frontal lobe epileptic seizures. *Brain* **99**, 447–458.

Harvey, A.S., Hopkins, I.J., Bowe, J.M., Cook, D.J., Shield, L.K. & Berkovic, S.F. (1993): Frontal lobe epilepsy: clinical seizure characteristcs and localization with ictal 99m Tc-HMPAO SPECT. *Neurology* **43**, 1966–1980.

Jayakar, P., Alvarez, L.A., Duchowny, M.S. & Resnick, T.J. (1992): A safe and effective paradigm to functionally map the cortex in childhood. *J. Clin. Neurophysiol.* **9**, 288–293.

Kotagal, P., Rothner, A.D., Erenberg, G., Cruse, R.P. & Wyllie, E. (1987): Complex partial seizures of childhood onset. A five-year follow up study. *Arch. Neurol.* **44**, 1177–1180.

Ludwig, B., Ajmone Marsan, C. & Van Buren, J. (1975): Cerebral seizures of probable orbitofrontal origin. *Epilepsia* **16**, 142–158.

Manford, M., Fish, D.R. & Shorvon, S.D. (1996): An analysis of clinical seizure patterns and their localizing value in frontal and temporal lobe epilepsies. *Brain* **119**, 17–40.

Morrell, F., Whisler, W.W. & Bleck, T.P. (1989): Multiple subpial transection: a new approach to the surgical treatment of focal epilepsy. *J. Neurosurg.* **71** (4), 629–630.

Munari, C., Tassi, L., Di Leo, M. *et al.* (1995): Video-stereo-electroencephalographic investigation of orbitofrontal cortex. Ictal electroclinical patterns. *Adv. Neurol.* **66**, 273–295.

Munari, C. & Bancaud, J. (1992): Electroclinical symptomatology of partial seizures of orbital frontal origin. In: *Advances in Neurology*, eds. P. Chauvel, A.V. Delgado-Escueta, *et al.*, vol. 57, pp. 257–265. New York: Raven Press.

Nordly, D.R., Bazil, C.W., Scheuer, M.L. & Pedley, T.A. (1997): Recognition and classification of seizures in infants. *Epilepsia* **38**, 553–560.

Penfield, W. & Kristiansen, K. (1951): *Epileptic seizure patterns. A study of the localizing value of initial phenomena in focal cortical seizures.* Springfield IL: Charles C. Thomas.

Quesney, L.F., Constain, M. & Rasmussen, T. (1992): Seizures from the dorsolateral frontal lobe. In: *Advances in Neurology*, eds. P. Chauvel, A.V. Delgado-Escueta *et al.*, vol. 57, pp. 233–308. New York: Raven Press.

Salanova, V., Morris, H.H., Van Ness, P., Kotagal, P., Wyllie, E. & Lüders, H. (1995): Frontal lobe seizures: electroclinical syndromes. *Epilepsia* **36** (1), 16–24.

Talairach, J., Bancaud, J., Bonis, A., Szikla, G., Trottier, S., Vignal, J.P., Chauvel, P., Munari, C. & Chodkieviecz, J.P. (1992): Surgical therapy for frontal epilepsies. In: *Advances in Neurology*, eds. P. Chauvel, A.V. Delgado-Escueta *et al.*, vol. 57, pp. 707–732. New York: Raven Press.

Taylor, D.C. & Falconer, M.A. (1971): Focal dysplasia of the cerebral cortex in epilepsy. *J. Neurol. Neurosurg. Psychiatry* **34**, 369–387.

Wyllie, E. & Bass, N.E. (1996): Supplementary sensorimotor area seizures in children and adolescents. In: *Advances in Neurology*, vol. 70: *Supplementary sensorimotor area*, ed. Hans O. Lüders. Philadelphia: Lippincott Raven Press.

Chapter 19

Secondary bilateral synchrony: significant EEG pattern in frontal lobe seizures

Anne Beaumanoir and Laura Mira

Fondazione Pierfranco e Luisa Mariani, viale Bianca Maria 28, 20129 Milan, Italy
Annebeaum@aol.com

Summary

The EEG pattern of secondary bilateral synchrony (SBS) was described by Jasper at the 2nd International Congress of EEG held in Paris in 1947, but the relevant report was published only in 1951. In 1951 Jasper, in collaboration with Pertuiset & Flamigan, described SBS in connection with generalized spike and wave discharges possibly related to a temporal focus and some temporal lobe seizures. His later paper with Tükel (1952), describing the EEG in parasagittal lesions, still stands out as a reference for describing SBS.
As Tükel & Jasper pointed out in 1952 and as Blume & Pillay defined it in 1985, SBS corresponds to a sequence of spikes, polyspikes or spike and wave complexes, more rarely slow waves, immediately followed by a burst of bilateral, synchronous and symmetrical spike and wave activity widely distributed over both hemispheres. Spencer *et al.* (1985) refined this definition introducing the notion of an interval between onset of the focal discharge (primary discharge) and the first element of the secondary bilateral discharge.
The primary focus is significantly more frequent in the pre-Rolandic than in the post-Rolandic regions. In most cases it is frontal.
Within the SBS paroxysm, the morphology of the primary focal discharge differs from that of the SBS. On the contrary, the components of the focal discharge are often identical to those of the focus, if there is only one, or the most active focus – which is usually taken as the primary focus – if the inter-ictal epileptiform abnormalities are multifocal.
SBS is always related to an epilepsy which is severe and cryptogenic or to a worsening of the ictal and inter-ictal symptoms in less severe cases or in cases of idiopathic partial epilepsy (IPE).
We review and discuss the different physiopathogenetic hypotheses and we discuss the restrictive use of terminology related to SBS.

Jasper described the secondary bilateral synchrony (SBS) for the first time at the 2nd International congress of EEG held in Paris in 1949 but the official reports were published in 1951, when he, together with Pertuiset & Flamigan, went back to the issue in connection with generalized spike and wave discharges related to a temporal focus. These antecedents notwithstanding, his paper published in 1952 in collaboration with Tückel, describing the EEG in parasagittal lesions, stands out as the reference work for the characterization of SBS. In the following decade several papers, both clinical and experimental, discussed SBS, including those by Dell & Hécaen (1951), Odgen *et al.* (1956), Bates *et al.* (1956), Ralston (1961), Niedermeyer (1968, 1972), Gabor & Ajmone Marsan (1969), Marcus & Watson (1966, 1968) and Bancaud (1969). They compared SBS

195

with the discharges of rhythmic, apparently synchronous and symmetrical spike and wave activity (primary bilateral synchrony, PBS), considered typical of *Petit Mal* absences. But as early as 1951, Dell & Hécaen pointed out that some versive seizures manifest themselves in the EEG 'by generalized spike and wave discharges with onset in one hemisphere, most often in the frontal region'. Lennox & Robinson (1952) attributed to the anterior cingulate region the origin of seizures 'similar to *Petit Mal* absences but with different EEG expression, consisting of asymmetrical spike and wave activity, repeating with a rhythm slower than 3/s. These old data show that the study of SBS, after many years, still has a place in the discussion of frontal seizures and epilepsies.

General features

By *synchrony* we mean the simultaneous onset of identical waves in several electrodes over the same hemisphere. We speak of *bilateral synchrony* (BS) when identical waves appear simultaneously over homologous areas of both hemispheres.

Blume & Pillay (1985) refined the definition of SBS: it is an EEG pattern consisting of a sequence of spikes, polyspikes, or spike and wave complexes, more rarely slow waves, immediately followed by a burst of bilateral, synchronous and symmetrical spike and wave activity widely distributed over both hemispheres. Spencer *et al.* (1985) better specified this definition and introduced the notion of an interval between onset of the triggering focal discharge and the first element of the secondary bilateral discharge. Blume & Pillay applied the term SBS strictly to bursts of the primary discharge followed by bilateral discharge, which recur identically at least twice during the same short recording.

SBS should thus not be mistaken either for spike and wave discharges beginning in one hemisphere or for the generalized asynchronous spike and slow wave discharges (*'Petit Mal Variant'*) that are most often associated with progressive or stable epileptogenic encephalopathies. It should also be differentiated from the generalized discharges of spike and wave activity or polyspike and wave activity which can occur in some EEG recordings showing an epileptic focus. The association between one or more epileptogenic zones, responsible for partial seizures, and spike and wave discharges typical of primary bilateral synchrony (PBS) provides evidence of a genetically low threshold for convulsions in an individual with partial epilepsy (PE). It is no surprise that this is notably more frequent in idiopathic partial epilepsy (IPE), whereas SBS is found in symptomatic and cryptogenic or IPE as well.

Description of secondary bilateral synchrony

The primary discharge

Morphology

The focal inter-ictal spikes or spike and wave activity triggering the bilateral discharge are identical to those not triggering it, recorded in the same EEG. However, their morphology is different from that of paroxysmal elements constituting the SBS discharge.

Topography

Gabor & Ajmone Marsan pointed out in 1969, and all authors have confirmed, that the focus of origin of SBS is most often frontal. Blume & Pillay (1985) compared the EEG recordings of a group of epileptic patients whose EEG focus triggered SBS to those of a comparable group without SBS and demonstrated that the number of frontal foci is significantly higher in the group with SBS (51 per cent *vs* 30 per cent), whereas temporal foci are less often associated with SBS (28 per cent vs 40 per cent). The difference is even greater for other localizations. However, SBS is facilitated by the presence of multiple foci. Blume & Pillay reported that 96 per cent of cases with SBS had at least 2 foci. The most active focus in the inter-ictal period was responsible for the SBS in 91 per cent of cases. The presence and localization of focal slow waves associated with the spikes was the best indicator of the primary focus.

The SBS discharge

Morphology

The BS discharge consists of a sequence of stereotyped spike and wave complexes. The bilateral discharge is different from the focal activity that triggers it, although in some cases and especially when the focus is anterior, recruited focal spikes and spike and wave activity can lead to the SBS.

Amplitude

The SBS elements are of higher amplitude than those of the focus. They may be asymmetric. Amplitude is usually lower on the side of the triggering discharge in the case of a lesional epilepsy.

Frequency

The frequency of repetition of the spike and wave activity is usually around 2-2.5 c/s. Exceptionally it may reach 3-4 c/s.

Beginning and end

The first element of the SBS paroxysm occurs abruptly but its end may be gradual, in which case the last spike and wave complexes of the discharge or the following slow waves usually occur on the side of the focus which triggered the BS. Blume & Pillay (1985) reported this in 96 per cent of their cases (Fig. 1).

Interval between the primary discharge and onset of the generalized discharge

This is very brief and can be difficult to discern in routine EEG recordings. It is longer than the mean callosal transmission time and it must be less than 80 ms (Spencer et al., 1985).

Synchrony

The time difference (TD) between the bilateral spike and wave complexes, calculated by different procedures (Gotman, 1981; Kobayashi et al., 1992, 1994), is variable and higher than the minimal TD of any PBS that may be present. Kobayashi et al. (1994) claim that a TD higher than 9 ms (the time of callosal transmission according to Amassian & Cracco, 1987) is the hallmark of SBS and can reach 40 ms. In some cases the longer TD is seen at onset of the discharge, although the spike and wave complexes may be asymmetric, but then the TD diminishes as the discharge continues, while synchrony takes place. The SBS discharge then resembles PBS (Yoshinaga et al., 1996). Since the synchrony is not perfect, there is no *synmorphism* as defined by Petsche & Rappelsberger (1973) (Fig. 2).

Topography

All authors report that the BS discharge is more or less diffuse over the two hemispheres, but it most often predominates over the frontal regions (among others Tükel & Jasper, 1952; Bancaud, 1969; Gabor & Ajmone Marsan, 1969; Blume & Pillay, 1985; Gobbi et al., 1989; Tinuper et al., 1998).

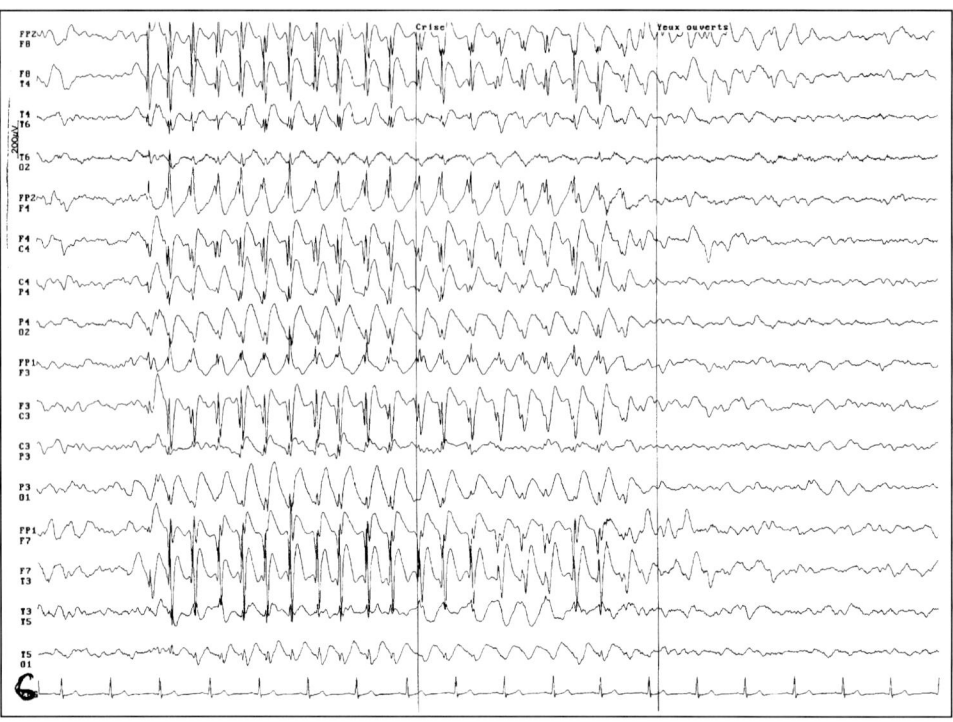

Fig. 1. Bilateral fronto-temporal focus: the right focus is more anterior than the left. Right fronto-temporal slow after-discharge. [Dr. Jallon, Geneva.]

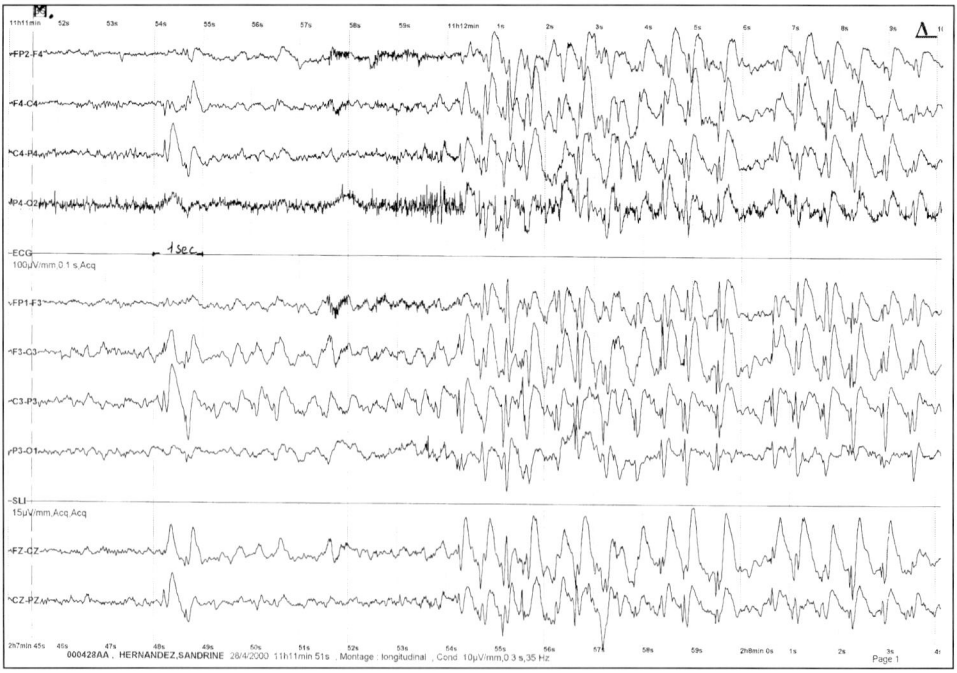

Fig. 2. Left fronto-central focus: bilateral fronto-central discharge, beginning on the left and then generalized SW discharge, initially asynchronous and then synchronous. [Dr. Daquin, Marseille.]

Facilitation

Hyperventilation increases the chance of recording SBS in 43 per cent of cases (Blume & Pillay, 1985), but intermittent photic stimulation is ineffective. In almost 80 per cent of cases sleep facilitates or causes SBS. Some drugs may have the same result. The effect of carbamazepine (CBZ) has been recognized since its introduction (Gobbi *et al.*, 1989; Capizzi *et al.*, 1995) in patients with PE and in the wake recordings of subjects with continuous spike and wave activity during sleep (CSWS) (Dalla Bernardina *et al.*, 1989; Beaumanoir, 1995). High dose polytherapy with antiepileptic drugs has also been suspected as a cause of SBS in CSWS (Beaumanoir, 1995; Deonna, 1995; Van Lierde, 1995; Pratts *et al.*, 1994; Kobayashi *et al.*, 1994), in Lennox-Gastaut-like syndromes (Beaumanoir *et al.*, 1979; Beaumanoir, 1982; Dravet & Roger, 1988; Gastaut & Zifkin, 1988) and in non-convulsive status epilepticus in PE (Ohtsuka *et al.*, 1999). Dalla Bernardina *et al.* (1989) showed that SBS is equally often seen in cryptogenic and IPE.

This review of EEG studies suggests that SBS requires a primary discharge, originating from the same focus in the case of multiple foci, which triggers a discharge of generalized or widely distributed slow spike and wave activity. In some patients and not in others their topography and synchrony could show a difference between the two hemispheres which could or could not disappear in the course of the discharge.

These data result from traditional EEG recordings. It is obvious that paroxysms of symmetrical and apparently synchronous spike and wave complexes can be triggered by focal discharges inaccessible to scalp EEG.

Incidence and prevalence

Only Blume & Pillay (1985) investigated the percentage of EEG recordings showing SBS, which ranged from 0.5 per cent to 0.7 per cent in their subjects, who had a mean age of 19 years. There are no studies evaluating explicitly the number of EEG recordings with SBS in a general epileptic population. This has however been studied in specific epileptic syndromes (see *Clinical correlations*).

Age

SBS can occur at any age, although a tendency to BS seems greater in young subjects, as already pointed out by Niedermeyer in 1968. It may be facilitated at some relatively late maturational stages of the cerebral commissures, particularly of the corpus callosum (CC).

Delay of occurrence

Except for Bureau & Maton (1998), the reported latency, without any further specification, between the finding of one or more foci and the occurrence of SBS is in the range of years. Gobbi *et al.* (1989) reported a latency of 3 to 12 years (mean 9 years).

Duration

No study took this into account. BS can be transient, for example if it is iatrogenic (Beaumanoir, 1982). It can disappear, independently from therapy, in children with IPE.

Clinical correlations

- *Seizures*. Few studies have adequately described clinical correlations. Seizures are predominantly absence, tonic versive, atonic or tonic-clonic attacks (Huck *et al.*, 1980). All these seizures point to the frontal cortex. Tinuper *et al.* (1998) reported that 74 per cent of cases with ictal falls were related to SBS, generated by a frontal focus in 22 cases out of 31. Atonic falls were remarkably frequent in patients with atypical Lennox-Gastaut syndrome (LGS) and SBS, reported in 22.5 per cent (Gastaut

& Zifkin, 1988) and in 40 per cent of cases with CSWS and SBS (Beaumanoir, 1995). Eighty per cent of the patients studied by Blume & Pillay (1985) had multiple generalized seizure types, among which tonic-clonic seizures, exceptional in other studies, are not rare. Simple partial motor seizures, hemiclonic seizures and tonic versive seizures represent 90 per cent of the partial ictal semiology of atypical LGS with SBS studied by Gastaut & Zifkin (1988). They are less frequent in less selected populations, found in 25 per cent and 23 per cent of those studied by Gabor & Ajmone Marsan (1969) and by Niedermeyer (1972) respectively.

- *Interictal signs.* According to Huck *et al.* (1980), inter-ictal signs consist essentially of attention disturbances. Mental retardation is reported in 52 per cent of cases by Tinuper (1998) and in 56 per cent by Blume & Pillay (1985). Cognitive deficits are obviously present in Lennox-Gastaut syndrome as well as in CSWS, in which cases SBS pertains to EEG semiology. The inter-ictal semiology as well as the ictal signs suggest frontal lobe involvement.

- *Epileptic syndromes.* SBS was present in 36 per cent of children studied by Bureau & Maton (1998), who had an adverse course of their symptomatic or cryptogenic PE, and in 17 per cent of patients studied by Gobbi *et al.* (1989) with severe PE. Tassi *et al.* (1998) reported SBS in five of 16 children (31 per cent) evaluated for surgery for intractable symptomatic or cryptogenic epilepsy. SBS was found in only 9 per cent of cases of lesional PE of childhood studied by Bourgeois *et al.* (1998). It is present in 77 per cent of the subjects with a hemispheric epilepsy reported by Blume (1998). The proportion of EEG recordings with SBS ranges from 33 per cent (Ohtahara, 1995) to 75 per cent (Gastaut & Zifkin, 1988) in borderline or atypical LGS. According to Tassinari *et al.* (1992), Dalla Bernardina *et al.* (1989), Beaumanoir (1995), Deonna (1995), and Kobayashi (1994), it represents the most significant sign in the waking state EEG recording of subjects with CSWS. SBS is more frequent in cryptogenic than in symptomatic epilepsies. It is equally often found in cryptogenic and idiopathic epilepsies of childhood (Dalla Bernardina *et al.*, 1989).

Prognostic features

Cibula & Gilmore (1997) note that SBS may appear before the occurrence of multiple epileptiform EEG foci, while others claim that SBS appears when multiple foci are already present. No longitudinal studies with repeated recordings have been carried out to clarify the issue. Several authors such as Tinuper (1998), Bureau & Maton (1998) and Rougier *et al.* (1997), report that the appearance of SBS is a bad prognostic sign but others claim that the occurrence of SBS does not imply any worsening of the ictal symptomatology (Roger *et al.*, 1991; Oguni *et al.*, 1994). It seems likely that its impact on the course of epilepsy depends on the functional and structural nature, progressive or stable, of the focus or foci causing it.

Physiopathogenetic aspects

The positive effects of cortical excision on SBS, when indicated, confirm the triggering role of the primary epileptogenic zone, formerly assessed pre-surgically by intracarotid amytal-pentyletetrazol testing (Gloor *et al.*, 1976) or by intravenous thiopenthal (Lombroso & Erba, 1970). Data are sparse in the case of multifocal discharges, which are now considered a negative factor in evaluation for possible surgery.

To explain the effect of the ablation of the primary focus on the SBS, Cibula & Gilmore (1997) introduced the notion of dependent secondary focus, corresponding to the first stages of formation of the mirror focus described by Morrell (1985).

The effects of commissurotomy on EEG are difficult to interpret because of different methods of analysis of SBS. Anterior callosotomy always affects SBS; there may be lengthening of the interval between the triggering discharge and the secondary bilateral discharge or even suppression of the bilateral discharge, without any change or with enhancement in the primary focus (Huck et al., 1980; Gates et al., 1984; Spencer et al., 1993; Andermann et al., 1988; Oguni et al., 1994; Matzuka et al., 1999).

According to Kobayashi et al. (1992) and Yoshinaga et al. (1996), the SBS spike and wave complexes are asynchronous and asymmetrical at the beginning of the discharge, but in some patients they may become synchronous and symmetrical in the course of the discharge, an observation which suggests that the potential fields generated by deep structures are identical in PBS and SBS.

The electrophysiological data and the variable effects of callosotomy could be related to different neurophysiological mechanisms that experimenters have tried to clarify.

Studies in cats and in monkeys by Marcus & Watson (1966, 1968) confirmed the role of cortico-cortical transcallosal connections for discharge synchronization, especially when the experimental foci are bilateral and frontal. This model, however, only partially explains the mechanism of BS with one primary focus, since in this case the discharges can be asymmetrical or only ipsilateral to the focus.

PBS models also provide some insight into SBS mechanisms. The PBS generalized spike and wave complexes typical of the EEG of feline generalized penicillin epilepsy (FGPE) are suppressed by spreading depression of the cortex, thereby confirming the role of the cortex in their production (Avoli & Gloor, 1994). In the same animal, corpus callosum (CC) section abolishes discharge synchronization (Musgrave & Gloor, 1980), a finding which attributes a major role to the CC. The Strasbourg school has shown that the hemicortical spreading depression also abolishes the spike and wave discharges of the Genetic Absence Epilepsy of the Rat from Strasbourg (GAERS) (Marescaux et al., 1984; Vergnes & Marescaux, 1994) in the transiently excluded cortex, but also in the ipsilateral thalamic structures, without affecting the spike and wave activity in the intact hemisphere, therefore confirming that the functional cortico-thalamo-cortical circuit is necessary for the production of generalized spike and wave activity. The resumption of rhythmic spike and wave discharges cannot occur until the cortex has recovered its normal activity, which emphasizes that the thalamus alone cannot produce the discharge by itself. A lesion of the lateral thalamus, involving the reticular nucleus, suppresses the spike and wave activity. A cortex deprived of thalamic afferents is unable to produce generalized spike and wave complexes.

In GAERS, CC section abolishes discharge synchrony. Spike and wave complexes can appear independently in the two hemispheres or start on one side, reaching the other hemisphere only after an interval of more than 50 ms. The discharge, in similar experiments, can continue unchanged without any modification of synchrony. These findings show that the CC plays a complex role in the processes of bisynchrony which themselves must depend on multiple factors.

The separation of the two thalami by midline nuclei lesions does not affect the spike and wave discharge. After a callosotomy in this preparation, spike and wave complexes can appear independently in the two hemispheres or occur bilaterally, but in the latter case they are asynchronous.

Thalamic stimulation gives rise to rhythmic spike and wave complexes at 2.5 c/s in the rhesus monkey with epileptogenic alumina cream lesions in both pre-motor areas (David et al., 1982). Avanzini et al. (1993) were able to slow permanently the rhythm of spike and wave discharges in

GAERS ipsilateral to previously lesioned thalamic reticular nuclei. These findings prove the primary role of the fluctuations of the thalamo-cortical circuit for the production of spike and wave complexes and that of thalamic nuclei for their rhythm.

CC maturation is slow and ends late, similar to frontal maturation. Grigonis & Murphy (1994) showed that the epileptic focus of the immature brain contributes to hinder synaptogenesis of the inter-hemispheric connections, which could explain the preferential age of onset of SBS, particularly in IPE due to maturational abnormalities. It has been suggested that the production of bilateral synchrony is related to the maturation of the thalamo-cortical systems (Avanzini et al., 1999).

On the basis of experimental results, several physiopathogenic hypotheses can be advanced.

The CC is responsible for the transmission of the discharges from the damaged hemisphere to the other. It is still an open question whether it is a matter of the primary discharge or of the first elements of the discharge of the rhythmic spike and wave activity, ipsilateral to the cortical lesion.

The first postulated mechanism is that the dominant discharge can be transmitted to the homologous contralateral region; the situation studied by Marcus & Watson (1968) and by David et al. (1982) then occurs, and a slow spike and wave discharge can be triggered. In another proposed mechanism, a thalamic volley provokes a spike and wave discharge in the damaged cortex which is transmitted to the contralateral cortex. In this case the spike and wave discharge is not strictly bisynchronous, but it can become so with the participation of thalamic synchronizing networks.

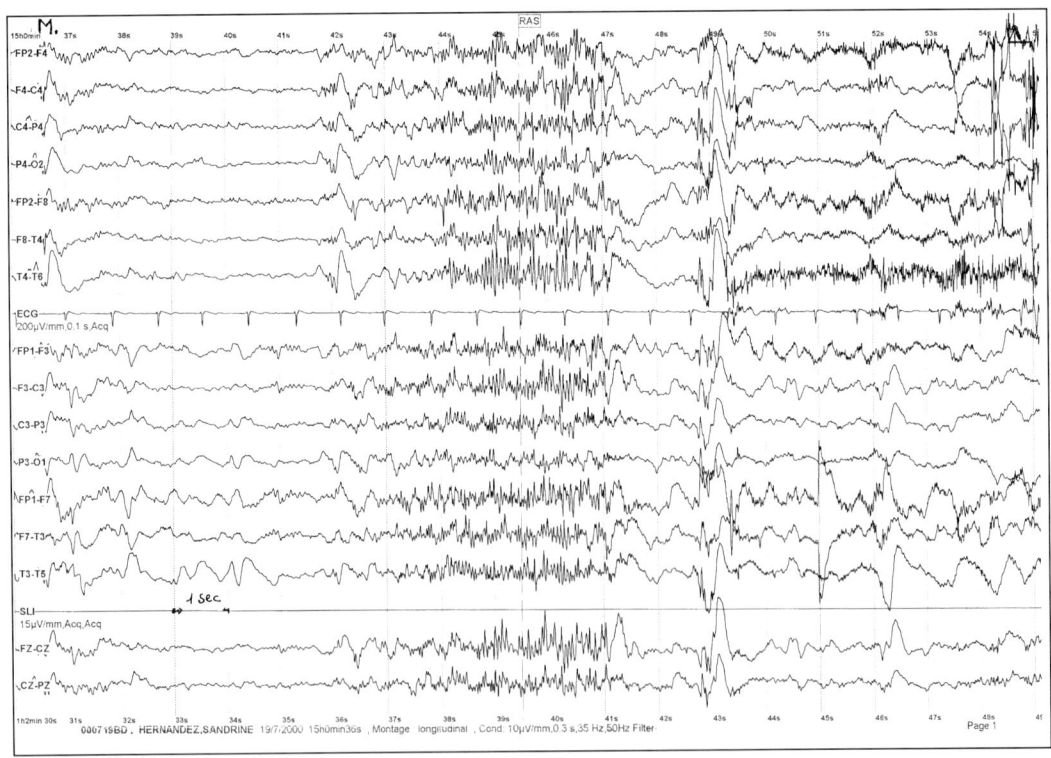

Fig. 3. Same patient as in Fig. 2. Rapid discharge, beginning on the left, becoming bilateral and then bisynchronous.

Conclusions

At the time of writing, several questions remain unanswered. Therefore, it does not seem too restrictive to speak of SBS only when the secondary generalized discharge consists of spike and wave complexes. Other EEG patterns characterized by more complex elements or by fast rhythms (FR) widely distributed over the scalp, apparently triggered by a spike, a spike and wave complex or a focal discharge of fast rhythm may presumably be attributed to a process of secondary bisynchrony (Fig. 3). The FR discharge is accompanied by tonic manifestations, whereas in BS with spike and wave complexes seizures are dialeptic and motor seizures are atonic.

The structures responsible for the secondary spike and wave complexes or FR discharges must be different, but located in the brainstem or involving different thalamic nuclei with similarly different, although pre-Rolandic, cortical projections: to motor areas in the case of FR, and to integrative and inhibitory areas in the case of slow spike and wave complexes.

Is it justified to label as synchrony an EEG pattern in which slow spike and wave activity at the beginning of the secondary generalized discharge is clearly asynchronous? For the sake of a better understanding of the process, would it not be preferable to speak of immediate or primary SBS and delayed SBS, and further defining the morphology of the elements, i.e. spike and wave complexes, FR or both?

References

Amassian, V.E., & Cracco, R.Q. (1987): Human cerebral responses to contralateral transcranial stimulation. *Neurosurgery* **20**, 148–155.

Andermann, F., Olivier, A., Gotman, J. & Sergent, J. (1988): Callosotomy for the treatment of patients with intractable epilepsy and the Lennox-Gastaut syndrome. In: *The Lennox-Gastaut syndrome*, eds. E. Niedermeyer & R. Degen, pp. 361–376. New York: Alan R. Liss, Inc.

Avanzini, G., Vergnes, M., Spreafico, R. & Marescaux, C. (1993): Calcium-dependent regulation of genetically determined spikes and waves by the reticular thalamic nucleus of rats. *Epilepsia* **34**, 1–7.

Avanzini, G., Sancini, G., Canafoglia, L. & Franceschetti, S. (1999): Maturation of cortical physiological properties relevant to epileptogenesis. In: *Abnormal cortical development and epilepsy*, eds. R. Spreafico, G. Avanzini & F. Andermann, pp. 63–76. Mariani Foundation Paediatric Neurology Series, vol. 7. London: John Libbey & Company.

Avoli, M. & Gloor, P. (1994): Physiopathogenesis of feline generalized penicillin epilepsy: the role of thalamocortical mechanisms. In: *Idiopathic generalized epilepsies*, eds. A. Malafosse, P. Genton, E. Hirsch, C. Marescaux, D. Broglin & R. Bernasconi, pp. 111–121. London: John Libbey & Company.

Bancaud, J. (1969): Physiopathogenesis of generalized epilepsies in organic nature. In: *The physiopathogenesis of the epilepsies*, eds. H. Gastaut, H. Jasper, J. Bancaud & A. Waltregny. Springfield: Charles Thomas.

Bates, J.V., Cobb, W. & Willams, D.J. (1956): A verified case of secondary bilateral synchrony. *Electroencephal. Clin. Neurophysiol.* **8**, 161–166.

Beaumanoir, A. (1982): The Lennox-Gastaut syndrome: a personal study. *EEG Clin. Neurophysiol.* **34** (Suppl. 35), 85–89.

Beaumanoir, A. (1995): EEG data. In: *Continuous spikes and waves during slow sleep, electrical status epilepticus during slow sleep. Acquired epileptic aphasia and related conditions*, eds. A. Beaumanoir, M. Bureau, T. Deonna, L. Mira & C.A. Tassinari, pp. 217–223. Mariani Foundation Paediatric Neurology Series, vol. 3. London: John Libbey & Company.

Beaumanoir, A., De Castro, R., Nahory, A. & Zagury S. (1979): A follow up study of four cases of subacute anti-epileptic drugs encephalopathy. *Abstract 11th Epilepsy Int. Symp.* Florence, p. 234.

Blume, W.T. (1998): Hemispheric epilepsy. *Brain* **10**, 1937–1949.

Blume, W.T. & Pillay, N. (1985): Electrographic and clinical correlates of secondary bilateral synchrony. *Epilepsia* **26**, 636–641.

Bourgeois, M., Sainte Rose, C., Lellouch-Tubiana, A., Brunelle, F., Charron, B., Laroussine, F. & Salefranque, F. (1998): Epilepsie et lésions focales chez l'enfant: intérêt des exérèses lésionnelles. In: *Épilepsies partielles graves pharmaco-résistantes de l'enfant: stratégies diagnostiques et traitements chirurgicaux*, eds. M. Bureau, P. Kahane & C. Munari, pp. 212–226. Paris: John Libbey Eurotext.

Bureau, M. & Maton, B. (1998): Valeur de l'EEG dans le pronostic précoce des épilepsies partielles non idiopathiques de l'enfant. In: *Épilepsies partielles graves pharmaco-résistantes de l'enfant: stratégies diagnostiques et traitements chirurgicaux*, eds. M. Bureau, P. Kahane & C. Munari, pp. 67–77. Paris: John Libbey Eurotext.

Capizzi, G., Costa, P., Grioni, D., Mira, L., Valseriati, D., Vigliano, P. & Van Lierde, A. (1995): The influence of antiepileptic drugs on the behaviour of functional spikes in partial idiopathic epilepsy. In: *Continuous spikes and waves during slow sleep, electrical status epilepticus during slow sleep. Acquired epileptic aphasia and related conditions*, eds. A. Beaumanoir, M. Bureau, T. Deonna, L. Mira & C.A. Tassinari, pp. 165–167. Mariani Foundation Paediatric Neurology Series, vol. 3. London: John Libbey & Company.

Cibula, J.E. & Gilmore, R.L. (1997): Secondary epileptogenesis in humans. *J. Clin. Neurophysiol.* **14**, 111–127.

Dalla Bernardina, B., Fontana, E., Michelezza, B., Colamaria, V. & Tassinari, C.A. (1989): Partial epilepsies of childhood, bilateral synchronisation, continuous spike-wave during slow sleep. In: *Advances in epileptology*, vol. 17, pp. 295–302. New York: Raven Press.

David, J., Marathe, S.B., Patil, S.D. & Grewal, R.S. (1982): Behavioural and electrical correlates of absence seizures induced by thalamic stimulation in juvenile rhesus monkeys with frontal aluminium hydroxide implants: a pharmacological evaluation. *J. Pharmacol. Toxicol. Methods* **7**, 219–229.

Dell, M.B. & Hécaen, H. (1951): Complexes pointe-ondes à début unilatéral et épilepsies giratoires. *Rev. Neurol.* **84**, 656–659.

Deonna, T. (1995): Are continuous spike-wave discharges during slow sleep an iatrogenic condition? *Dev. Med. Child Neurol.* **37**, 280.

Dravet, C. & Roger, J. (1988): The Lennox-Gastaut syndrome: historical aspects from 1966 to 1997. In: *The Lennox-Gastaut syndrome*, eds. E. Niedermeyer & R. Degen, pp. 9–23. New York: Alan R. Liss, Inc.

Gabor, A. & Ajmone Marsan, C. (1969): Coexistence of focal and bilateral diffuse paroxysmal discharges in epileptics. *Epilepsia* **10**, 453–472.

Gastaut, H. & Zifkin, B. G. (1988): Secondary bilateral synchrony and Lennox-Gastaut syndrome In: *The Lennox-Gastaut syndrome*, eds. E. Niedermeyer & R. Degen, pp. 221–242. New York: Alan R. Liss, Inc.

Gates, J.R., Leppik, I.E., Yap, J. & Gumnit, R.J. (1984): Corpus callosotomy: clinical and electroencephalographic effects. *Epilepsia* **25**, 309–316.

Gloor, P., Rasmussen, T., Altuzarra, A. & Garretson, H. (1976): Role of the intracarotid amobarbital-pentylenetetrazol EEG test in the diagnosis and surgical treatment of patients with complex seizure problems. *Epilepsia* **17**, 15–31.

Gobbi, G., Tassinari, C.A., Roger, J., Bureau, M., Dravet, C. & Salas Puig, X. (1989): Particularités électroencéphalographiques des épilepsies partielles symptomatiques de l'enfant. *Neurol. Physiol. Clin.* **19**, 209–218.

Gotman, J. (1981): Interhemispheric relations during bilateral spike and wave activity. *Epilepsia* **22**, 453–466.

Grigonis, A.M. & Murphy, E.H. (1994): The effect of epileptic cortical activity on the development of callosal projections. *Dev. Brain Res.* **77**, 251–257.

Huck, F.R., Radvany, J., Avila, S.D., Pires de Carmago, C.H., Ragazzo, P.C., Riva, D. & Arlant, P. (1980): Anterior callosotomy in epileptics with multiform seizures and bilateral synchronous spike and wave EEG pattern. *Acta Neurochir. Suppl.* **10**, 127–135.

Jasper, H. (1951): Etude anatomo-physiologique des épilepsies. *Electroencephalogr. Clin. Neurophysiol.* **3** (Suppl. 2), 99–111.

Jasper, H., Pertuiset, B. & Flamigan, H. (1951): EEG and cortical electrogram in patients with temporal lobe seizures. *Acta Neurol. Psychiatry* **65**, 272–292.

Kobayashi, K., Otsuka, Y & Ohtahara, S. (1992): Primary and secondary bilateral synchrony in epilepsy: differentiation by estimation of interhemispheric small time differences during short spike-wave activity. *Electroencephalogr. Clin. Neurophysiol.* **83**, 93–103.

Kobayashi, K., Nishibayashi, N., Otsuka, Y., Oka, E. & Ohtahara, S. (1994): Epilepsy with electrical status epilepticus during slow sleep and secondary bilateral synchrony. *Epilepsia* **35**, 1097–1103.

Lennox, M.A. & Robinson, P. (1952): Cingulate-cerebellar mechanisms in the physiological pathogenesis of epilepsy. *Electroencephalogr. Clin. Neurophysiol.* **4**, 197–205.

Lombroso, C.T. & Erba, G. (1970): Primary and secondary bilateral synchrony in epilepsy. *Arch. Neurol.* **22**, 321–334.

Marcus, E.M. & Watson, C.W. (1966): Bilateral synchronous spike wave electrographic patterns in the cat. Interaction of bilateral cortical foci in the intact, the bilateral cortical-callosal and adiencephalic preparation. *Arch. Neurol.* **14**, 601–610.

Marcus, E.M. & Watson, C.W. (1968): Symmetrical epileptogenic foci in monkey cerebral cortex. *Arch. Neurol.* **19**, 99–116.

Marescaux, C., Micheletti, G., Vergnes, M., Depaukis, A., Rumbach, L. & Warter, J.M. (1984): A model of chronic spontaneous Petit Mal like seizures in rat: comparison with pentylenetetrazol-induced seizures. *Epilepsia* **25**, 326–331.

Matsuzaka, T., Ono, K., Baba, H., Matsuo, M., Tanaka, S., Kamimura, N. & Tsuji, Y. (1999): Quantitative EEG analysis and surgical outcome after corpus callosotomy. *Epilepsia* **40**, 1269–1278.

Morrell, F. (1985): Secondary epileptogenic lesions. *Epilepsia* **26**, 538–569.

Musgrave, J. & Gloor, P. (1980): The role of the corpus callosum in bilateral interhemispheric synchrony of spike and wave discharge in feline generalized penicillin epilepsy. *Epilepsia* **21**, 369–378.

Niedermeyer, E. (1968): The occurrence of generalized (centrencephalic) and focal seizure patterns in some patients. *Johns Hopkins Med. J.* **112**, 11–25.

Niedermeyer, E. (1972): *The generalized epilepsies, a clinical electroencephalographic study.* Springfield, Illinois: Ch. Thomas.

Odgen, T.E., Aird, R.B. & Garoutte, J. (1956): The nature of bilateral and synchronous spiking. *Acta Psychiatr. Neurol. Scand.* **31**, 273–284.

Oguni, H., Andermann, F., Gotman, J. & Olivier, A. (1994): Effect of anterior callosotomy on bilaterally synchronous spike and wave and other EEG discharges. *Epilepsia* **35**, 505–513.

Ohtahara, S., Otsuka, Y. & Kobayashi, K. (1995): Lennox Gastaut syndrome: a new vista. *Psychiatry Clin. Neurosci.* **49**, 179–183.

Ohtsuka, Y., Sato, M. & Oka, E. (1999): Non convulsive status epilepticus in childhood localization-related epilepsy. *Epilepsia* **40**, 1003–1010.

Petsche, H. & Rappelsberger, P. (1973): The problem of synchronisation in the spread of epileptic discharges leading in seizures in man. In: *Epilepsy: its phenomenon in man*, ed. M. Brazier, pp. 1121–1151. New York: Academic Press.

Pratts, J.M., Garaizar, C., Zuaco, E. & Madoz, P. (1994): Are continuous spikes and waves discharges during slow sleep an iatrogenic condition? *Dev. Med. Child Neurol.* **36**, 1026–1027.

Ralston, B. (1961): Cingulate epilepsy and secondary bilateral synchrony. *Electroencephal. Clin. Neurophysiol.* **13**, 591–598.

Roger, J., Bureau, M., Gobbi, G., Tassinari, C.A. & Dravet, C. (1991): Les épilepsies partielles sévères de l'enfant. *Epilepsies* **2**, 191–198.

Rougier, A., Claverie, B., Pedespan, J.M., Marchal, C. & Loiseau, P. (1997): Callosotomy for intractable epilepsy: overall outcome. *J. Neurosurg. Sci.* **4**, 51–57.

Spencer, S., Spencer, D.D., Williamson, P.D. & Watson, C.W. (1985): Effect of corpus callosum section on secondary bilateral synchronous interictal EEG discharges. *Neurology* **35**, 1089–1094.

Spencer, S.S., Katz, A., Ebersole, J., Novotny, E. & Mattson, R. (1993): Ictal EEG changes with corpus callosum section. *Epilepsia* **34**, 568–573.

Tassi, L., Mai, R., Kahane, P., Minotti, L., Francione, S., Garrel, S. & Munari, C. (1998): Valeur et utilité de l'EEG de scalp critique chez les enfants candidats à un traitement chirurgical de leur épilepsie. In: *Epilepsies partielles graves pharmaco-résistantes de l'enfant: stratégies diagnostiques et traitements chirurgicaux*, eds. M. Bureau, P. Kahane & C. Munari, pp. 113–134. Paris: John Libbey Eurotext.

Tassinari, C.A., Bureau, M., Dravet, C., Dalla Bernardina, B. & Roger, J. (1992): Epilepsy with continuous spikes and waves during slow sleep. In: *Epileptic syndromes in infancy, childhood and adolescence*, eds. J. Roger, M. Bureau, C. Dravet, F.E. Dreifuss, A. Perret & P. Wolf, pp. 245–246. London: John Libbey & Company.

Tinuper, P., Cerullo, A., Marini, C., Avoni, P., Riva, R., Baruzzi, A. & Lugaresi, E. (1998): Epileptic drop attacks in partial epilepsy: clinical features, evolution, and prognosis. *J. Neurol. Neurosurg. Psychiatry* **64**, 231–237.

Tükel, K. & Jasper, H. (1952): The EEG in parasagittal lesions. *Electroencephalogr. Clin. Neurophysiol.* **4**, 481–494.

Van Lierde, A. (1995): Therapeutic data. In: *Continuous spikes and waves during slow sleep, electrical status epilepticus during slow sleep*, eds. A. Beaumanoir, M. Bureau, T. Deonna, L. Mira & C.A. Tassinari, pp. 225–227. Mariani Foundation Paediatric Neurology Series, vol. 3. London: John Libbey & Company.

Vergnes, M. & Marescaux, C. (1994): Pathophysiological mechanisms underlying genetic absence epilepsy in rats. In: *Idiopathic generalized epilepsies*, eds. A. Malafosse, P. Genton, E. Hirsch, C. Marescaux, D. Broglin & R. Bernasconi, pp. 151–168. London: John Libbey & Company.

Yoshinaga, H., Kobayashi, K., Sato, M., Oka, E. & Ohtahara, S. (1996): Investigation of bilateral synchronous spike-wave discharge by EEG topography. *Brain Topogr.* **8**, 255–260.

Chapter 20

Medical treatment of frontal lobe seizures in children

Paola Costa, Daniela Valseriati[1], Andréa Van Lierde[2],
Pierangelo Veggiotti[3] and Piernanda Vigliano[4]

Department of Child Neuropsychiatry, Ospedale Burlo Garofalo, via dell'Istria 65/1, 34137 Trieste, Italy
1. Spedali Civili, P. le Spedali Civili 1, 25125 Brescia, Italy
2. First Paediatric Clinic, University of Milan, Italy
3. Department of Child Neuropsychiatry, University of Pavia, Italy
4. Department of Child Neuropsychiatry, University of Torino, Italy
costa@burlo.trieste.it

Summary

The anatomical and physiological characteristics of the frontal lobe account for the complex electroclinical manifestations of frontal epilepsy. Clinical presentation, prognosis and drug sensitivity are heterogeneous, especially in the child, whose symptoms are also related to maturation of the nervous system. The aetiology of frontal lobe epilepsy is varied and includes clear-cut genetic syndromes and symptomatic lesional epilepsies. Ictal signs include focal motor seizures and supplementary motor area seizures, which can occur in sequence, with a variable tendency to secondary generalization. Ictal and interictal EEG patterns are also variable.
Therefore there is no single first-choice therapy in frontal lobe epilepsy. Only in nocturnal frontal lobe epilepsy is the selective efficacy of carbamazepine (CBZ), as already shown by clinical experience, apparently confirmed at the molecular level. Another exception concerns secondary bilateral synchrony, where it is advisable to avoid drugs such as CBZ and phenobarbital which can facilitate hypersynchrony and lead to clinical deterioration.
Based on published data and our personal experience, we suggest reserving long-term polytherapy for carefully selected children with frontal lobe seizures, while remaining alert to the possible adverse effects of medications and drug interactions on cognitive performance and behaviour at different ages.

Electroclinical manifestations of frontal lobe epilepsy (FLE) are heterogeneous; this is due to the size and multiple functions of the frontal lobe and its rich intra and inter-cortical connections. Ictal semiology varies according to the localization of seizure onset within the frontal lobe and the pattern of seizure spread. In infants, observable ictal symptoms may be concentrated on the major motor manifestations while other seizures clinically appear as behavioural disturbances that are difficult to explain. An analogous variability is found both in ictal and inter-ictal EEG. These features can delay identification of the main epileptic focus and accurate syndromic diagnosis, with resulting difficulty in the choice of treatment. This choice should take into account relevant differences between adults and children at different ages and developmental stages, including the effects of maturation on the epileptic disorder.

Functional maturation of the frontal lobe can be thought of as a non-linear multistage process. Progressive functional maturation of the frontal lobes, age at onset of seizures, seizure frequency, epileptiform discharges, brain pathology, genetic factors and antiepileptic drugs interact and can have a significant impact on cognitive function.

Partial seizures arising from the frontal lobe differ in many ways from those of temporal origin. Therefore, medications having different mechanisms of action should have distinct efficacy for these different partial epilepsy types. However, it has been observed that 'some selectivity might be expected to exist in the response to different antiepileptic drugs for seizures arising in frontal or extra-temporal *vs* temporal areas, but experimental data are not available to make such a distinction' (Mattson, 1992).

The following review of the literature should not be regarded as exhaustive, but focuses on two issues relevant to drug treatment: nocturnal FLE and the EEG pattern of secondary bilateral synchrony.

Nocturnal frontal lobe epilepsy

Several published reports show that carbamazepine (CBZ) is particularly effective in nocturnal FLE. Vigevano *et al.* (1993) reported 10 children with a stereotyped pattern of repetitive tonic partial postural seizures, mainly during sleep. Age at onset of seizures ranged from 6 to 12 years. All had normal psychomotor development and normal neurological examinations. In six patients CBZ treatment was used after unsuccessful attempts with other antiepileptic drugs. In all patients seizures were promptly stopped by CBZ. When described, irritability and apathy disappeared soon after institution of the treatment. In half of the patients, seizures recurred after suspension or reduction of CBZ. Sheffer *et al.* (1995) described five families containing 47 individuals with nocturnal FLE. The age of onset ranged from 2 months to 52 years. The patients were all of normal intellect with no abnormalities on neurological examination. Fifteen were on CBZ treatment alone and 12 were well controlled. Eleven of the more severely affected individuals were on more than one medication. CBZ produced good seizure control in many of the patients but all required long-term medication. Cessation of CBZ in adult life was followed by seizure recurrence. Sodium valproate was generally not effective in controlling seizures but substituting CBZ led to dramatic improvement in seizure control. Provini *et al.* (1999) reviewed 100 consecutive cases of nocturnal FLE. The seizures began in infancy and adolescence; 80 patients received CBZ in monotherapy (59 cases) or polytherapy (21 cases). Based on their earlier experience CBZ was the drug of choice. In 20 per cent, CBZ controlled the nocturnal seizures completely, in 24 per cent it reduced nocturnal seizures by at least 75 per cent and reduced occasional diurnal seizures by half. In 32 per cent CBZ did not modify seizure frequency. An analysis of the resistant cases showed that most had more than 25 seizures per month. Phenytoin, clobazam and valproic acid were not effective. In the authors' opinion, nocturnal FLE does not typically remit spontaneously. In the cases responding to treatment, withdrawal was always followed by the reappearance of seizures. Ito *et al.* (2000) described a Japanese family with autosomal dominant FLE. The onset of seizures in children was in infancy or early childhood. Three children showed hyperactivity and two had mild mental retardation. The children's seizures did not respond to antiepileptic drugs but the adults' seizures disappeared spontaneously or were easily controlled by CBZ.

The efficacy of CBZ in FLE shown in clinical studies has been evaluated with more recent experimental work. Genetic and pharmacologic studies of autosomal dominant nocturnal FLE (ADNFLE) are leading to a better understanding of the molecular pathogenesis of this epileptic phenotype, allowing also a further comprehension of the action mechanisms of antiepileptic drugs and the design of new drugs.

A linkage between the genetically transmissible form of nocturnal FLE (ADNFLE) and mutations within the alpha4 and beta2 subunits of neuronal nicotinic acetylcholine receptors (nAChRs) has been proven (Steinlein et al., 1995; De Fusco et al., 2000). The linkage illustrated for the first time the role that neuronal nAChRs may have in brain dysfunction and raises the question of the specific action of this receptor in epileptogenesis.

NAChRs are integral membrane proteins which result from the assembly of five subunits and form both a ligand-binding domain in the extracellular part of the protein sequence and a ionic pore in the centre of the pentamer. Acetylcholine (ACh) determines the opening of the channel. The mutations described in ADNFLE are located within the wall of the ionic pore and cause an overall modification of function with changes in the permeability of the receptor channel and the duration of desensitization.

In view of the high sensitivity of ADNFLE to CBZ, Picard et al. (1999) studied the effects of this drug on the human alpha4beta2 nAChR and its mutations. ACh-evoked currents at the human alpha4beta2 receptors are readily and reversibly inhibited at pharmacologic concentrations of CBZ. The drug probably acts as a non-competitive inhibitor of nAChRs, entering the channel and blocking it by steric hindrance. Dose-response inhibition curves studied in normal receptors and in ADNFLE mutant receptors showed a greater sensitivity of the mutants to CBZ, with about a threefold higher sensitivity. In contrast, valproate has nearly no effect on control or mutant nAChRs. This is consistent with the lesser efficacy of valproate in clinical reports of ADNFLE.

Genetic polymorphism of an integral membrane protein, of which nAChR mutations in ADNFLE are an example, can thus cause different responses to antiepileptic drugs in clinical use. Picard et al. suggest that this can explain individual specific sensitivity to a drug.

Secondary bilateral synchrony

In clinical practice, the choice of an antiepileptic drug is based upon the evaluation of several specific clinical and electroencephalographic conditions. Some epileptic syndromes can be particularly sensitive to facilitation of secondary bilateral synchrony by certain drugs. Syndromes more at risk include FLE, childhood absence epilepsy, Lennox-Gastaut syndrome and severe myoclonic epilepsy of infancy.

In frontal lobe epilepsies, a variety of interictal and ictal EEG patterns can be seen. The interictal scalp EEG can be normal or show spikes, sharp waves, spike and wave complexes, multiple spike and wave bursts, periodic sharp and slow wave complexes, low-voltage fast rhythms, or paroxysmal fast activity. Ictal discharges can also be complex and variable. As with the interictal discharges, the ictal discharges may be bilaterally synchronous or secondarily generalized (Westmoreland, 1998).

Mechanisms equivalent to secondary bilateral synchrony are found in epilepsy with electrical status epilepticus during slow wave sleep, and in non-convulsive status epilepticus with atypical absences, brief atonic seizures, and the myoclonic seizures observed in the course of some partial epilepsies of childhood (Gastaut et al., 1987; Dalla Bernardina et al., 1989; Beaumanoir et al., 1992; Kobayashi et al., 1994).

Even if multiple drug treatment is more prone to cause electroclinical deterioration, a specific paradoxical effect of CBZ has been suggested, linked to its tendency to potentiate generalized epileptiform discharges.

In the population retrospectively studied by Horn *et al.* (1986), the largest group of patients adversely affected by CBZ had absence epilepsy. The second largest group had FLE. Blume & Pillay (1985), in their review of secondary bilateral synchrony, found that 51 per cent of their patients had a frontal lobe focus.

Snead & Hosey (1985) suggest that CBZ should be avoided in the presence of generalized, synchronous spike and wave discharges of 2.5-3 Hz. This EEG pattern appears to be a risk factor for the induction of absences by CBZ. A slower frequency of the discharges (1-2 Hz) is associated with the risk of inducing generalized convulsive seizures. In a review of the paradoxical ability of antiepileptic drugs to precipitate or exacerbate seizures, Perrucca *et al.* (1998) recommend using CBZ with caution, or not at all, in patients with generalized bilaterally synchronous spike and wave discharges. However, the authors note that the underlying mechanisms are poorly understood and that further studies are required to evaluate the prevalence of this phenomenon, to investigate its mechanisms in greater detail and to characterize additional prognostic factors in order to identify situations at risk.

The choice of a drug should take into account its efficacy in animal models and the growing knowledge of its action on cell membranes. Many animal seizure models are available. The maximal electroshock test (MES) in rodents and the pentylenetetrazol (PTZ) test in mice have been carefully standardized. The MES model has identified drugs that are functionally similar to phenytoin and most of these compounds inactivate voltage-dependent Na^+ channels in a use-dependent fashion. These drugs suppress sustained repetitive firing in cultured neurons. Activity in this model seems highly predictive of the ability to protect against partial and secondarily generalized tonic-clonic seizures. CBZ and several newer agents such as felbamate, gabapentin, lamotrigine and topiramate fit this model of activity (Rho *et al.*, 1999).

The PTZ model is a good predictor of clinical efficacy against generalized spike and wave epilepsies of the absence type. Compounds that suppress Ca^{++} conductance across low-threshold T-type channels, such as trimethadione, ethosuximide and valproic acid, seem to be active in this model.

Newer *in vivo* models are being introduced that incorporate known genetic defects which more closely resemble human epilepsy. Among these are the Genetic Absence Epileptic Rat of Strasbourg (GAERS) and the lethargic *(lh/lh)* mutant mouse. The lethargic *(lh/lh)* mutant mouse has spontaneous spike and wave discharges that are blocked by drugs found to be clinically effective in reducing spike and wave activity such as benzodiazepines, ethosuximide, valproic acid and lamotrigine. Paradoxical effects of CBZ and phenytoin have also been observed in animal models of generalized epilepsies (Rho *et al.*, 1999).

In their work on non-convulsive status epilepticus in childhood localization-related epilepsy, Ohtsuka *et al.* (1999) support the opinion that this condition is an age-dependent, transient electroclinical condition. It is known that this condition, like the enhancement of absences, myoclonic, and atonic seizures, is provoked or worsened by carbamazepine and other antiepileptic drugs, but in the experience of the authors CBZ is not the only cause. Their patients became free of these seizures after rationalization of drug regimens, and they believe that it is more likely that polytherapy can exacerbate the seizures.

CBZ and complex polytherapy can also exert a negative effect on cognitive function, favouring generalized epileptiform clinical and subclinical discharges. Moreover, prolonged electrical discharges with involvement of frontocentral regions seem to be related to cognitive impairment (Aarts *et al.*, 1984).

Finally, secondary bilateral synchrony can be an age-dependent, transient pattern in the course of some childhood epilepsies. In these situations a correct syndromic diagnosis and a search for specific prognostic factors are very important. Careful follow-up with particular attention to the relation between the course of the epilepsy and maturation may suggest therapeutic restraint despite apparently troubling electroclinical situations. Very aggressive treatment is not always effective and can have paradoxical or deleterious effects.

We retrospectively reviewed 42 patients with a clinical diagnosis of FLE to compare the drug treatment proposed and the response to specific drugs with particular regard to these issues.

Material and methods

The study population consisted of patients collected in Brescia, Pavia, Torino and Trieste Epilepsy Centres. There were 42 patients (21 girls and 21 boys). Mean age at seizure onset was 5.6 years. (range 2 months to 13 years). Mean follow-up was 6.2 years (range 14 months to 18 years). Because of electroclinical variability and consequent difficulty in localizing diagnosis in younger children, we arbitrarily decided to evaluate the epilepsy history at 2 years 6 months even in those cases in which the first seizure occurred in the first year of life.

Results

We classified our population into three groups according to treatment response.

Group A consisted of patients with a complete response to the first drug. Group B obtained seizure control only after other drugs were used. Group C consisted of pharmacoresistant patients. At the time of data analysis, 71.4 per cent of patients were seizure-free and 28.6 per cent were drug-resistant.

The three groups were evaluated according to the mean age at seizure onset (Table 1).

Table 1. Age at seizure onset

	Range	Medium
Group A	12 mo-9 yrs 9 mo	4 yrs 9 mo
Group B	9 mo-12 yrs 4 mo	6 yrs 3 mo
Group C	2 mo-13 yrs	4 yrs 8 mo

They were also studied with respect to successful therapy (in the first two groups), presence of only one or more than one seizure type, circadian distribution of seizures, EEG patterns, and cognitive development (Table 2). We defined clinical seizure semiology derived from Lüders' classification (Lüders *et al.*, 1998) (Table 3). We then considered which drugs were more effective with respect to the clinical seizure pattern and EEG pattern (Table 4).

Discussion

The age at onset of seizures is not clearly different in the three groups. Patients within Group A do not differ substantially according to seizure type and electrical pattern. The same is true for patients in Group C. The subjects with more than one seizure type were all pharmacoresistant patients (Group C). In Group C, patients had cognitive deficits and hyperactivity which could be made worse by multiple drug treatment. EEG patterns of generalized discharges or of secondary bilateral synchrony were more frequent in Group C. Successful drug treatment varied. Efficacy was related to the EEG pattern, similar to what was observed in experimental models.

Table 2. Electroclinical characteristics of each group

		Group A (10 pts) No. pts	Group B (20 pts) No. pts	Group C (12 pts) No. pts
Effective therapy	One drug	10	12	
	Two drugs		8	
	Polytherapy			
Seizure type	One	9	18	5
	Two	1	2	5
	Three			2
Circadian distribution	Awake	3	9	4
	Awake/sleep	4	7	7
	Sleep	3	4	1
EEG pattern	Normal		2	
	Focal anomalies	5	12	4
	Focal + generalized	3	1	2
	Focal + SBS	2	5	6
Cognitive development	Normal	10	14	5(3*)
	Mild delay		5 (1*)	3 (1*)
	Moderate delay		1	2
	Severe delay			2 (1*)

* Hyperactivity.

Table 3. Seizure type

	Group A (10 pts) No. pts	Group B (20 pts) No. pts	Group C (12 pts) No. pts
Seizures			
Dialeptic	3	4	
Simple motor	4	9	5 (1*)
Hypermotor	2	3	
Autonomic		2	
Dialeptic + partial motor	1	1	5
Partial motor + autonomic		1	
Dialeptic + partial motor + autonomic			2

* Clonic and tonic versive.

Table 4. Effective drugs in different EEG patterns

		Group A (10 pts) No. pts	Group B (20 pts) No. pts
EEG	Drug		
Focal	CBZ	4	6
	VPA	1	1
	TPM		1
	LTG		1
	VPA + Clob		2
	VPA + CBZ		1
Focal + generalized	CBZ	1	
	VPA	2	
	LTG		1
Focal + SBS	VPA	2	
	PB		1
	VPA + ETS		1
	VPA + LTG		1
	VPA + Clob		1
	LTG + CBZ		1
Normal	CBZ		1
	ETS + FBM		1

Abbreviations: CBZ: carbamazepine, Clob: clobazam, ETS: ethosuximide, FBM: felbamate, LTG: lamotrigine, PB: phenobarbital, TPM: topiramate, VPA: valproate.

Conclusions

The retrospective analysis of our cases confirms that CBZ was the first choice and most efficacious drug for nocturnal FLE.

In other cases the electrical pattern can suggest the correct choice of antiepileptic drug. If focal EEG abnormality is recorded, drugs such as CBZ, phenytoin, topiramate and benzodiazepines can be prescribed. With secondary bilateral synchrony, we found that valproate, ethosuximide, lamotrigine and benzodiazepines were the drugs of choice.

References

Aarts, J.H.P., Binnie, C.D. & Smit, A.M. (1984): Selective cognitive impairment during focal and generalized epileptiform EEG activity. *Brain* **107**, 293–308.

Beaumanoir, A. & Dravet, C. (1992): The Lennox-Gastaut syndrome. In: *Epileptic syndromes in infancy, childhood and adolescence*, 2nd ed., eds. J. Roger, M. Bureau, C. Dravet, F.E. Dreifuss, A. Perret & P. Wolf, pp. 115–132. London: John Libbey & Company.

Bertrand, D. (1999): Neural nicotinic acetylcholine receptors: their properties and alteration in autosomal dominant nocturnal frontal lobe epilepsy. *Rev. Neurol.* **155**, 6–7, 457–462.

Dalla Bernardina, B., Fontana, E., Michelizza, B., Colamaria, V., Capovilla, G. & Tassinari, C.A. (1989): Partial epilepsies of childhood, bilateral synchronization, continuous spike-waves during slow sleep. In: *Advances in epileptology: XVIIth Epilepsy International Symposium*, eds. J. Manelis, E. Bental, J.N. Loeber & F.E. Dreifuss, pp. 295–302. New York: Raven Press.

De Fusco, M., Becchetti, A., Patrignani, A., Annesi, G., Gambardella, A., Quattrone, A., Ballabio, A., Wanke, E. & Casari, G. (2000): The nicotinic receptor beta2 subunit is mutant in nocturnal frontal lobe epilepsy. *Nature Genet.* **26**, 275–276.

Gastaut, H., Zifkin, B., Magaudda, A. & Mariani, E. (1987): Symptomatic partial epilepsies with secondary bilateral synchrony: differentiation from symptomatic generalized epilepsies of the Lennox-Gastaut type. In: *Presurgical evaluation of epileptics*, eds. H.G. Wieser & C.E. Elger, pp. 308–316. Berlin: Springer Verlag.

Hirose, S., Iwata, H., Akiyoshi, H., Kobayashi, K., Ito, M., Wada, K., Kaneko, S. & Mitsudome, A. (1999): A novel mutation of CHRNA4 responsible for autosomal dominant nocturnal frontal lobe epilepsy. *Neurology* **53** (8), 1749–1753.

Horn, C.S., Ater, S.B. & Hurst, D.L. (1986): Carbamazepine-exacerbated epilepsy in children and adolescents. *Pediatr. Neurol.* **2**, 340–345.

Ito, M., Kobayashi, K., Fuji, T., Okuno, T., Hirose, S., Iwata, H., Mitsudome, A. & Kaneko, S. (2000): Electroclinical picture of autosomal dominant nocturnal frontal lobe epilepsy in a Japanese family. *Epilepsia* **41** (1), 52–58.

Luders, H., Acharia, J., Baumgartner, C., Benbadis, S., Bleasel, A., Burgess, R., Dinner, D. S., Ebner, A., Foldvary, N., Geller, E., Hamer, H., Holthausen, H., Kotagal, P., Morris, H., Meencke, H.J., Noachtar, S., Rosenow, F., Sakamoto, A., Steinhoff, B.J., Tuxhorn, I. & Wyllie, E. (1998): Semeiological seizure classification. *Epilepsia* **39** (9), 1006–10013.

Mattson, R.H. (1992): Drug treatment of partial epilepsy. *Adv. Neurol.* **57**, 643–650.

Meldrum, B.S. (1992): Novel antiepileptic drugs: relations with neurotransmitter mechanisms underlying frontal epilepsies. *Adv. Neurol.* **57**, 635–641.

Perrucca, E., Gram, L., Avanzini, G. & Dulac, O. (1998): Antiepileptic drugs as a cause of worsening seizures. *Epilepsia* **39** (1), 5–17.

Picard, F., Bertrand, S., Steinlein, O.K. & Bertrand, D. (1999): Mutated nicotinic receptors responsible for autosomal dominant nocturnal frontal lobe epilepsy are more sensitive to carbamazepine. *Epilepsia* **40** (9), 1198–1209.

Provini, F., Plazzi, G., Tinuper, P., Vandi, S., Lugaresi, E. & Montagna, P. (1999): Nocturnal frontal lobe epilepsy. A clinical and polygraphic overview of 100 consecutive cases. *Brain* **122**, 1017–1103.

Rho, J.M. & Sankar, R. (1999): The pharmacologic basis of antiepileptic drug action. *Epilepsia* **40** (11), 1471–1483.

Sachdeo, R. & Chokroverty, S. (1986): Carbamazepine and EEG epileptiform activity. *Electroenceph. Clin. Neurophysiol.* **58**, 47–48.

Sheffer, I.E. (2000): Autosomal dominant nocturnal frontal lobe epilepsy. *Epilepsia* **41** (8), 1059–1061.

Sheffer, I., Bhatia, K., Lopes-Cendes, I., Fish, D.R., Marsden C.D., Andermann, E., Andermann, F., Desbiens, R., Keene, D., Cendes F., Manson, J.I., Constantinou, J.E.C., McIntosh, A. & Berkovic, S.F. (1995): Autosomal dominant nocturnal frontal lobe epilepsy. A distinctive clinical disorder. *Brain* **118**, 61–73.

Snead, O.C. & Hosey, L.C. (1985): Exacerbation of seizures in children by carbamazepine. *N. Engl. J. Med.* **313**, 916–921.

Steinlein, O.K., Mulley, J.C., Propping, P., Wallace, R.H., Phillips, H.A., Sutherland, G.R., Scheffer, I.E. & Berkovic, S.F. (1995): A missense mutation in the neuronal nicotinic acetylcholine receptor alpha4 subunit is associated with autosomal dominant nocturnal frontal lobe epilepsy. *Nat. Genet.* **11**, 201–203.

Steinlein, O.K., Magnusson, A., Stoodt, J., Bertrand, S., Weiland, S., Berkovic, S.F., Nakken, K.O., Propping, P. & Bertrand, D. (1997): An insertion mutation of the CHRNA 4 gene in a family with autosomal dominant nocturnal frontal lobe epilepsy. *Hum. Mol. Genet.* **6**, 943–947.

Talwar, D., Arora, M.S. & Sher, P.K. (1994): EEG changes and seizures: exacerbation in young children treated with carbamazepine. *Epilepsia* **35**, 1154–1159.

Vigevano, F. & Fusco, L. (1993): Hypnic tonic postural seizures in healthy children provide evidence for a partial epileptic syndrome of frontal lobe origin. *Epilepsia* **34**, 1100–1199.

Westmoreland, B. (1998): The EEG findings in extratemporal seizures. *Epilepsia* **39** (Suppl. 4), S1–S8.

Poster 1

Neuropsychological aspects of frontal lobe epilepsy

Francesca Maria Battaglia, Maria Giuseppina Baglietto, Roberto Gaggero, Maria Cirrincione, Eleonora Garbarino and Edvige Veneselli

Child Neuropsychiatric Unit, Istituto Giannina Gaslini, Largo Gaslini 5, 16147 Genova, Italy
Department of Neurosciences, Ophthalmology and Genetics, University of Genova, via De Toni 5, 16132 Genova, Italy
piabaglietto@ospedale-gaslini.ge.it

Neuropsychological studies in adults with frontal lobe lesions suggested that these were associated with impairments of attention, praxis organization, concept formation and behaviour planning for novel tasks (Shallice & Evans, 1978; Shallice, 1982; Smith & Milner, 1984; Stuss & Benson, 1986; Shallice, 1988). It is still debated whether a lateralized lesion causes specific cognitive deficits (Stuss & Benson, 1986). Other studies on patients with frontal lobe epilepsy, with or without evident lesions, showed significant attention deficit, difficulty in concept formation, and emotional control disorders (Milner, 1964; Smith & Milner, 1984). The presence of memory impairments and their differentiation from those observed in patients with temporal lobe epilepsy are still debated topics (Delaney *et al.*, 1980; Kemper *et al.*, 1992).

The few studies carried out in children on the association of 'frontal syndrome' with epileptiform EEG activity showed neuropsychological disorders similar to those observed in adults, as well as possible neuropsychological dysfunctions due to functional epileptiform activity in non-lesional cases (Boone *et al.*, 1988; Jambaqué & Dulac, 1989; Gaggero *et al.*, 1990).

This study evaluates the possible correlation between frontal paroxysmal EEG activity and disturbances of several functions controlled by mechanisms that can be localised to the frontal lobes, and reports the clinical histories and data of three patients with frontal partial epilepsy, with results of specific neuropsychological tests.

Neuropsychological testing

Cognitive functions were assessed with the revised Wechsler intelligence scale for children (WISC-R) and with standardized test batteries for the evaluation of more specific functions (Deutsch-Lezak, 1995):

- *Attention:* Trail making test, Cancellation task of letters, numbers and geometric figures, Stroop test.
- *Memory:* verbal short-term memory (Digit span) and non-verbal short-term memory (Corsi's block tapping test), verbal long-term memory (Luria learning test word lists, Story immediate and delayed recall) and non-verbal long-term memory (Benton visual retention test, Rey-Osterreith complex figure)
- *Speech:* Token test, Boston naming test and semantic/phonological fluency, Peabody picture vocabulary test.
- *Visuomotor abilities:* Bender visual motor gestalt test.
- *Spatial abilities:* Ghent-Poppelreuter's test, Street's gestalt completion test, Judgement of line orientation.

R.G., male, age 8 years 5 months

Family and clinical history: negative. Seizure onset: at 8 years of age. Seizure type: complex partial. Seizure frequency: weekly. Standard EEG: bilateral frontal focus. CT/MRI: negative. Treatment: sodium valproate.

Neuropsychological data are summarised below according to the different functions:

- *Intelligence tests:* WISC-R did not show any discrepancies between Verbal IQ and Performance IQ. However, with Bannantyne's subtest recategorization, lower scores were observed in the 'conceptual' and 'sequential' categories with respect to the 'spatial' category. The low scores obtained in the coding and labyrinth tests are significant.
- *Attention:* form B of Trail making test required a longer execution time. Focused attention was impaired.
- *Memory:* difficulties in verbal and visuospatial short-term memory. Both verbal and visuospatial long-term memories were satisfactory.
- *Language:* semantic verbal fluency was appropriate for chronological age, while phonological verbal fluency was at the low end of the normal range.
- *Visuomotor abilities:* poor.
- *Visuospatial perception:* normal.
- *Emotional and behavioural aspects:* attention deficit, hyperactivity, fatiguability.

B.A., male, age 10 years 8 months

Family history: negative. Clinical history: prematurity, respiratory distress, signs of dysmaturity on neurologic examination. Seizure onset: 10 years of age. Seizure type: complex partial. Seizure frequency: daily. Standard EEG: bilateral frontal focus. CT/MRI: negative. Treatment: carbamazepine.

Neuropsychological data are illustrated below:

- *Intelligence tests:* WISC-R did not show any discrepancy between Verbal IQ and Performance IQ. With reference to Bannantyne's subtest recategorization, sequential category scores were at the low end of the normal range. Lower scores were observed in the following subtests: comprehension, figure memory, figure completion, coding and labyrinth tests.
- *Attention:* forms A and B of the Trail making test required a longer execution time, and a large number of errors was observed in the Cancellation test. Focused attention was poor.

- *Memory:* deficits in verbal and visuospatial short-term memory. Poor verbal memory and normal visuospatial long-term memory.
- *Language:* poor phonological verbal fluency.
- *Visuomotor abilities:* poor.
- *Visuospatial perception:* normal.
- *Emotional and behavioural aspects:* strong inhibition and tendency to withdraw in the face of difficulties.

R.F., male, age 12 years 10 months

Family history: negative. Clinical history: signs of dysmaturity on neurologic examination. Seizure onset: at 3 years 3 months of age. Seizure type: complex partial in wakefulness and tonic-postural in sleep. Seizure frequency: weekly. Standard EEG: bilateral frontal focus, more marked on the left. CT/MRI: negative. Therapy: carbamazepine, vigabatrin.

Neuropsychological data are illustrated below according to the different functions:

- *Intelligence tests:* WISC-R showed no discrepancy between Verbal IQ and Performance IQ. Considering Bannantyne's subtest recategorization, lower scores were observed in the conceptual and sequential categories compared to the spatial category. Low scores were also observed in the following subtests: comprehension, figure memory, coding and labyrinth tests.
- *Attention:* forms A and B of Trail making test and the Cancellation test required longer execution time. Deficits in focused attention.
- *Memory:* verbal and visuospatial short-term memory impairment. Poor verbal long-term memory.
- *Language:* deficits in semantic and phonologic verbal fluency.
- *Visuomotor abilities:* not appropriate for chronological age.
- *Visuospatial perception:* normal.
- *Emotional and behavioural aspects:* strong inhibition and fatiguability.

Conclusions

The role of the frontal lobes in childhood is still debated. In the few reported cases of frontal lobe lesions in children and adolescents, lesion-induced dysfunctions included: attention deficit, hyperactivity, poor concept formation, reduced short-term memory, slight impairment of movement velocity, inadequate social adaptation, aggressiveness, and affective lability (Stelling *et al.*, 1986; Mac Donald *et al.*, 1984). In these studies, the neuropsychological evaluation did not include tests of frontal lobe functions commonly used in adults (Wisconsin card sorting test, Trail making test, Stroop test, Labyrinths, Finger tapping, Verbal fluency).

Neuropsychological aspects of the frontal syndrome have rarely been evaluated in children with frontal lobe epilepsy, especially in the presence of interictal paroxysmal EEG activity (Boone *et al.*, 1988; Jambaqué & Dulac, 1989; Gaggero *et al.*, 1990).

The patients reported in this study underwent a battery of neuropsychological tests. The results confirm much of the reported data, and in these three patients we could observe some specific deficits of the frontal syndrome.

With reference to Bannantyne's classification of WISC-R categories (1974), two of the three patients had lower scores in the sequential and conceptual categories compared to the spatial category. In all three, planning and simulation abilities were significantly deficient. Attention deficit, reduced phonologic verbal fluency, and reduced ability to inhibit a response in favour of another (Stroop test) were documented in the three patients. Poor performance was also observed in both verbal and spatial span tests, suggesting frontal lobe involvement in working memory, as hypothesised by other authors (Baddeley & Hitch, 1974; Baddeley, 1983). Therefore, even though the temporal lobes play the most important role in retention of new information, there is also frontal lobe involvement in serial memory tasks, which require planning and organisation strategies (Jambaqué et al., 1993).

As to behaviour disorders, one patient showed variable and hyperactive behaviour, while two patients presented a component of inhibition.

These results suggest that children with frontal lobe dysfunction can have the same types of cognitive and behavioural disturbances as do adults. In addition, these data underline that interictal paroxysmal activity can cause neuropsychological deficits typical of the frontal syndrome, without evident lesions.

Acknowledgments: The authors thank Anna Capurro for her help in revising the text.

References

Baddeley, A.D. (1983): Working memory. *Phil. Trans. R. Soc.* **302**, 311–324.

Baddeley, A.D. & Hitch, G.J. (1974): Working memory. In: *The psychology of learning and motivation. Advances in research and theory*, ed. G.H. Bower, vol. **8**, pp. 47–89. New York: Academic Press.

Bannantyne, A. (1974): Diagnostic: a note on a recategorization of the WISC scores. *J. Learn. Disab.* **7**, 272–273.

Boone, K.B., Miller, M.D., Rosenberg, L., Durazo, A., McIntyre, H. & Weil, M. (1988): Neuropsychological and behavioral abnormalities in an adolescent with frontal lobe seizures. *Neurology* **38**, 583–586.

Delaney, R.C., Rosen, A.J., Mattson, R.H. & Novelly, R.A. (1980): Memory function in focal epilepsy: a comparison of non-surgical, unilateral temporal lobe and frontal lobe samples. *Cortex* **16**, 103–117.

Deutsch-Lezak, M. (1995): *Neuropsychological assessments.* London: Oxford University Press.

Gaggero, R., Boragno, F., Baglietto, M.G., Cirrincione, M. & De Negri, M. (1990): L'epilessia del lobo frontale nell'età evolutiva: aspetti clinici e neuropsicologici. *G. Neuropsi. Età Evolutiva* **10**, 4, 301–308.

Jambaqué, I. & Dulac, O. (1989): Syndrome frontal réversible et épilepsie chez un enfant de 8 ans. *Arch. Fr. Pediatr.* **46**, 525–529.

Jambaqué, I., Dellatolas, G., Dulac, O., Ponsot, G. & Signoret, J.L. (1993): Verbal and visual memory impairment in children with epilepsy. *Neuropsychologia* **31**, 1321–1337.

Kemper, B., Helmstaedter, C. & Elger, C.E. (1992): Kognitive Profile von prächirurgischen Patienten mit Frontal- und Temporallappenepilepsie. In: *Epilepsie'91*, ed. D. Scheffner, pp. 345–350. Reinbeck: Einhorn Presse Verlag.

Mac Donald, J.T., Stauffer, A.E. & Heitoff, K. (1984): Adrenoleukodystrophy: early frontal lobe involvement on computed tomography. *J. Comput. Assist. Tomogr.* **8**, 128–130.

Milner, B. (1964): Some effects of frontal lobectomy in man. In: *The frontal granular cortex*, eds. J.M. Warren & K. Akert, pp. 313–334. New York: McGraw-Hill.

Shallice, T. (1982): Specific impairments of planning. *Phil. Trans. R. Soc. London* **B 298**, 199–209.

Shallice, T. (1988): *From neuropsychology to mental structure.* Cambridge: University Press.

Shallice, T. & Evans, M.E. (1978): The involvement of the frontal lobes in cognitive estimation. *Cortex* **14**, 294–303.

Smith, M. & Milne, B. (1984): Differential effects of frontal lobe lesions on cognitive estimation and spatial memory. *Neuropsychologia* **22**, 697–770.

Stelling, M.W., McKay, S.E., Carr, W.A., Walsh, J.W. & Baumann, R.J. (1986): Frontal lobe lesions and cognitive function in craniopharyngioma survivors. *Am. J. Dis. Child.* **140**, 710–714.

Stuss, T.D. & Benson, T. (1986): *The frontal lobes.* New York: Raven Press.

Poster 2

Genetics of autosomal dominant nocturnal frontal lobe epilepsy

Maria Teresa Bonati, Rosanna Asselta, Stefano Duga, Romina Combi,
Massimo Malcovati, Luigi Ferini-Strambi*, Marco Zucconi*, Alessandro Oldani*,
Maria Luisa Tenchini and Leda Dalprà

Department of Biology and Genetics for Medical Sciences, University of Milan, via Viotti 3/5, 20133 Milan, Italy
* Centre for Sleep Disorders, Faculty of Medicine, University of Milan, Istituto Scientifico H San Raffaele,
via Prinetti 29, 20127 Milan, Italy
mt.bonati@auxologico.it

Summary

Autosomal dominant nocturnal frontal lobe epilepsy (ADNFLE, MIM 600513) is a familial partial epilepsy with reduced penetrance (70–80 per cent). Clinical symptoms include clusters of motor seizures occurring mostly during light sleep and developing within the first two decades.
Three different mutations in the CHRNA4 gene on chromosome 20q13.2, coding for the $\alpha 4$ subunit of the neuronal nicotinic acetylcholine receptor (nAChR), have been reported. Linkage of ADNFLE to 15q24 region has been reported; this region contains the *CHRNA5/A3/B4* cluster, coding for $\alpha 3$, $\alpha 5$ and $\beta 4$ subunits of the neuronal nAChR.
We performed segregation and linkage analyses to both chromosome 20q13.2 and 15q24 regions on 14 ADNFLE families. No linkage of ADNFLE to both regions was found in 12 (20q13.2) and 10 (15q24) families by means of a multi-point analysis. Sequencing of the genes mapped in these regions and coding for subunits of the neuronal nAChRs, in families showing some evidence of linkage, did not reveal the presence of mutations in these genes. These data strongly suggest that the neuronal nAChR $\alpha 3$, $\alpha 4$, $\alpha 5$ and $\beta 4$ subunits are not involved in the pathogenesis of ADNFLE in the analysed families. Exclusion of linkage to both 20q13.2 and 15q24 chromosomal regions demonstrates the existence of at least three loci responsible for ADNFLE, thus confirming locus heterogeneity for this disease. Linkage analysis of ADNFLE to genes coding for additional subunits of the neuronal nAChR is in progress.

Autosomal dominant nocturnal frontal lobe epilepsy (ADNFLE, MIM 600513) is an idiopathic partial epilepsy with autosomal dominant inheritance and reduced penetrance (70–80 per cent). Clinical symptoms include clusters of motor seizures occurring mostly during light sleep, developing within the first two decades. These seizures originate from a specific focus in the frontal lobes (Scheffer *et al.*, 1995; Oldani *et al.*, 1998).

In five unrelated ADNFLE kindreds, three different mutations responsible for ADNFLE have been identified in the neuronal nicotinic acetylcholine receptor $\alpha 4$ subunit gene (CHRNA4), mapped to chromosome 20q13.2 (Steinlein *et al.*, 1995, 1997; Hirose *et al.*, 1999). All these mutations are located in the exon 5 region coding for the second transmembrane domain (M2) of the CHRNA4. The first is a missense mutation replacing serine with phenylalanine (Ser252Phe), the second is a GCT insertion (776Ins3) introducing a leucine in the M2 domain, and the last one is a missense mutation replacing a serine with a leucine (Ser256Leu).

Several authors have reported locus heterogeneity of ADNFLE. Recently a second locus at 15q24, containing the *CHRNA5/A3/B4* cluster, has been reported, but neither the gene nor the mutation involved have been identified (Phillips *et al.*, 1998).

We performed segregation and linkage analyses for chromosome 20q13.2 and 15q24 regions in 14 ADNFLE families. Sequence analyses of candidate genes were carried out in families showing some evidence of linkage to one of these regions.

Segregation and linkage analyses to chromosome 20q13.2

Segregation analysis between ADNFLE and *CHRNA4* has been performed by haplotyping all available individuals belonging to 14 compliant Italian families (Fig. 1) for a total of nine polymorphisms, seven intragenic and two extragenic.

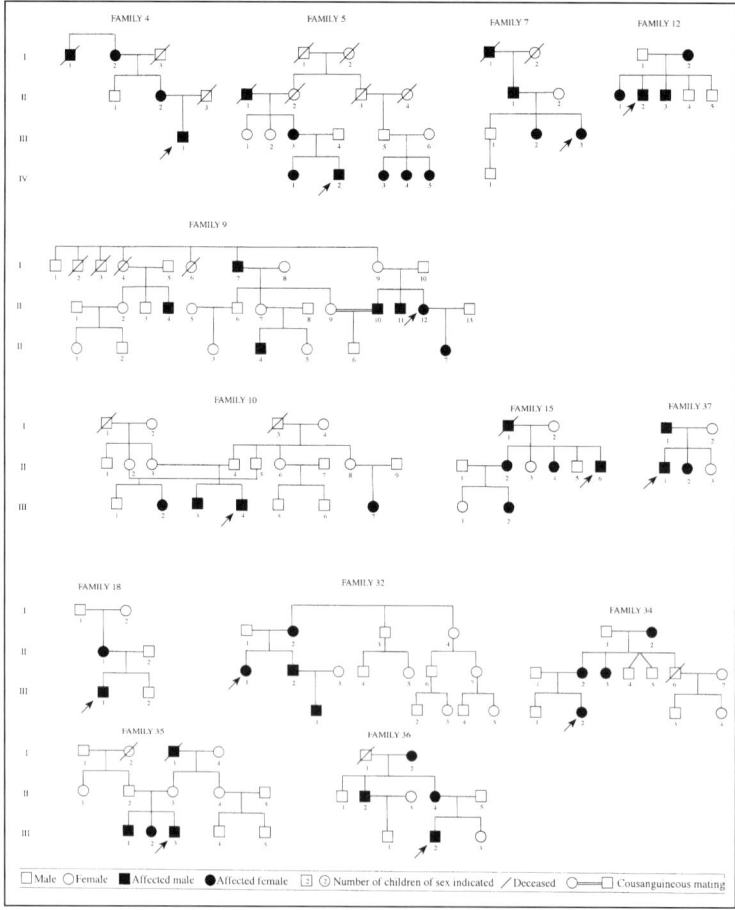

Fig. 1.

We thus excluded linkage of ADNFLE to *CHRNA4* in 12 families out of 14 (#5, left branch and right branch, 7, 9, 10, 12, 15, 18, 34, 35, 36, 37).

Two criteria have been considered for linkage exclusion:

- affected offspring inherited different alleles of the analysed chromosomal region from their affected parent;
- affected individual/s of the third generation did not receive any of the analysed chromosomal region from the affected grandparent.

Two families (#4 and 32) showed suggestive evidence for linkage of ADNFLE to CHRNA4.

LOD scores between ADNFLE and 2 intragenic markers (STR and 555) and an extragenic one (D20S20) were calculated by Mlink & Genehunter, considering a penetrance of 80 per cent. LOD scores are reported beside each pedigree.

CHRNA4 mutation analysis

We performed *CHRNA4* sequence analysis on the probands belonging to families showing evidence of linkage between ADNFLE and *CHRNA4* (families #4 and 32). In particular, we sequenced all the exons including exon/intron boundaries. This study, however, did not show any mutations in this gene.

Segregation and linkage analyses to chromosome 15q24

We performed linkage analysis between ADNFLE and the 15q24 region, containing the CHRNA5/CHRNA3/CHRNB4 gene cluster, in the same 14 families by haplotyping familial subjects for 16 STRs spanning a region of 10.7 cM (Généthon linkage map).

We thus excluded linkage of ADNFLE to CHRN-cluster genes in 10 families out of 14 (#4, 5 right branch, 9, 10, 15, 18, 32, 34, 36, 37). Criteria for linkage exclusion are the same as those reported for *CHRNA4* segregation analyses.

The other four families (left branch of #5, 7, 12, 35) showed suggestive evidence for linkage at segregation analysis, but none had significantly positive LOD score values. These families were also studied for *CHRNA5/A3/B4* intragenic polymorphisms. The same intragenic polymorphisms were also typed in families showing crossing-over in the region (#4, 5 right branch, 7, 9, 10, 15, 34). Comprehensive haplotype analysis in informative families (#4, 5 right branch, 7, 9, 15) allowed us to restrict the localization of the CHRN-cluster to an interval of 0.6 cM, between STRs D15S1027 and D15S1005 (data not shown; Bonati *et al.*, 2000).

LOD scores between ADNFLE and markers from the Généthon linkage map were calculated by MLINK and GENEHUNTER, considering a penetrance value of 80 per cent. LOD scores are reported beside each pedigree.

CHRNA5/A3/B4 mutation analysis

We performed *CHRNA5/A3/B4* genes sequence analysis on the probands belonging to families showing evidence of linkage between ADNFLE and the 15q24-CHRN cluster region (#5 left branch, 7, 12, 35). In particular, we sequenced all the exons including exon/intron boundaries. This study did not reveal the presence of mutations in these genes in family 5, 7, 12 and 35.

Conclusions

We have shown that 14 families with ADNFLE are not linked to the CHRNA4 locus and that 12 (#4, 5 right and left branch, 9, 10, 15, 18, 32, 34, 35, 36, 37) of the same 14 families are not linked to markers on chromosome 15q24, containing the CHRNA5/CHRNA3/CHRNB4 gene cluster.

We have therefore demonstrated locus heterogeneity of the disease. Exclusion of linkage to 20q13.2 and 15q24 chromosomal regions in several families demonstrates the existence of at least three loci responsible for ADNFLE, in agreement with Phillips *et al.* (1998).

Additional neuronal nicotinic acetylcholine receptor subunits not linked to candidate loci on chromosomes 20q13.2 and 15q24 are potential candidates as the cause of epilepsy in our families. Known locations of other subunits expressed in brain are 1q21 ($\beta2$), 8p11.2 ($\beta3$), 8p21 ($\alpha2$) and 15q14 ($\alpha7$) (Anand & Lindstrom, 1992).

References

Anand, R. & Lindstrom, J. (1992): Chromosomal localization of seven neuronal nicotinic acetylcholine receptor subunit genes in humans. *Genomics* **13**, 962–967.

Bonati, M.T., Asselta, R., Duga, S., Ferini-Strambi, L., Oldani, A., Zucconi, M., Malcovati, M., Dalprà, L. & Tenchini, M.L. (2000): Refined mapping of CHRNA3/A5/B4 gene cluster and its implications in ADNFLE. *NeuroReport* **11** (10), 2097–2101.

Hirose, S., Iwata, H., Akiyoshi, H., Kobayashi, K., Ito, M., Wada, K., Kaneko, S. & Mitsudome, A. (1999): A novel mutation of CHRNA4 responsible for autosomal dominant nocturnal frontal lobe epilepsy. *Neurology* **53**, 1749–1753.

Oldani, A., Zucconi, M., Asselta, R., Modugno, M., Bonati, M.T., Dalprà, L., Malcovati, M., Tenchini, M.L., Smirne, S. & Ferini-Strambi, L. (1998): Autosomal dominant nocturnal frontal lobe epilepsy: a video-polysomnographic and genetic appraisal of 40 patients and delineation of the epileptic syndrome. *Brain* **121**, 205–223.

Phillips, H.A., Scheffer, I.E., Crossland, K.M., Bhatia, K.P., Fish, D. R., Marsden, C.D., Howell, S.J.L., Stephenson, J.B.P., Tolmie, J., Plazzi, G., Eeg-Olofsson, O., Singh, R., Lopes-Cendes, I., Andermann, E., Andermann, F., Berkovic, S.F. & Mulley, C. (1998): Autosomal dominant nocturnal frontal lobe epilepsy: genetic heterogeneity and evidence for a second locus at 15q24. *Am. J. Hum. Genet.* **63**, 1108–1116.

Scheffer, I.E., Bhatia, K.P., Lopes-Cendes, I., Fish, D.R., Marsden, C.D., Andermann, E., Andermann, F., Desbiens, R., Keene, D., Cendes, F., Manson, J.I., Constantinou, J.E.C., McIntosh, A. & Berkovic, S.F. (1995): Autosomal dominant nocturnal frontal lobe epilepsy: a distinctive clinical disorder. *Brain* **118**, 61–73.

Steinlein, O.K., Mulley, J.C., Propping, P., Wallace, R.H., Phillips, H.A., Sutherland, G.R., Scheffer, I.E. & Berkovic, S.F. (1995): A missense mutation in the neuronal nicotinic acetylcholine receptor $\alpha4$ subunit is associated with autosomal dominant nocturnal frontal lobe epilepsy. *Nat. Genet.* **11**, 201–203.

Steinlein, O.K., Magnusson, A., Stoodt, J., Bertrand, S., Weiland, S., Berkovic, S.F., Nakken, K.O., Propping, P. & Bertrand, D. (1997): An insertion mutation of the CHRNA4 gene in a family with autosomal dominant nocturnal frontal lobe epilepsy. *Hum. Mol. Genet.* **6**, 943–947.

Poster 3

Continuous spike and wave activity during slow sleep and acquired epileptic frontal syndrome: long-term follow-up in two patients

Stefania Maria Bova, Elisa Granocchio, Cristiano Termine, Cristina Tebaldi, Pierangelo Veggiotti and Giovanni Lanzi

Fondazione 'Istituto Neurologico Casimiro Mondino', IRCCS, via Palestro 20, 27100 Pavia, Italy
stefania.bova@mondino.it

Continuous spike and wave activity during slow wave sleep (CSWS) is a well known EEG pattern (Patry *et al.*, 1971; Veggiotti *et al.*, 1999). Some children with CSWS develop a pattern of cognitive and behavioural disturbances, called acquired epileptic frontal syndrome, which is similar to that observed in adults with frontal damage (Roulet-Perez *et al.*, 1993). Very few studies have been concerned with follow-up of children with acquired epileptic frontal syndrome (Roulet-Perez *et al.*, 1993; Hommet *et al.*, 2000).

We report the long-term clinical, neuropsychological and EEG follow-up of two such patients. Outcome at age 19 and 16 was very similar in both.

Patient 1

We first saw this patient at our Institute at age 6 years. At age 4 this previously healthy boy had developed complex partial seizures with secondary generalization, typical and atypical absences, and atonic seizures only partially controlled by valproate and phenobarbital. At 5 years and 6 months, cognitive deterioration and language regression occurred with rapid deterioration, complete loss of speech and almost complete loss of verbal comprehension. This was followed by hyperactivity, irritability, enuresis and insomnia. On admission his EEG showed CSWS.

Following the initiation of steroid therapy, serial EEG recordings showed fluctuating CSWS associated with a reduction in seizure frequency. Over the succeeding 3 to 4 months he began using single words and then two-word sentences. His behaviour did not improve significantly.

By the age of 10 years, secure seizure control had been achieved with ethosuximide and valproate. The CSWS disappeared slowly, background activity normalized, and sporadic anterior spike and spike and wave activity with secondary bisynchrony developed. During this time his interest in the environment increased, although he was still markedly hyperactive. Language also improved; by age 10 there was no phonological or syntactic deficit, but naming was deficient with frequent semantic paraphasias and neologisms, and verbal perseveration became evident. Abstract reasoning was deficient, as shown by poor performance on Raven's progressive matrices at age 10 (score 47; < 5th percentile).

He had no seizures from age 10 to 19 but the EEG showed bilateral frontal abnormalities, while his complex cognitive impairment associated with behavioural disturbances (apathy, passivity and deficient social skills) became more marked.

Patient 2

This boy came to our attention at age 11 years 8 months. Early psychomotor development was apparently normal, except for slightly delayed language development with later learning difficulties which were attributed to social and attentional problems rather than to cognitive deficits. At 8 years he developed tonic generalized seizures, not controlled by valproate. At 8 years 4 months, absences became evident and increased in frequency. This was followed by progressive behavioural and cognitive deterioration leading to an autistic-like syndrome. At this time CSWS was noted, but subsequently he was lost to follow-up because of family problems. His behavioural disturbances and family problems were so severe that he was institutionalized at age 10.

We first evaluated him about a year later; CSWS was again documented. Following initiation of steroid therapy his absences disappeared and the generalized tonic seizures became less frequent. Subsequent EEGs showed fragmentation of the CSWS, a frontal epileptic focus with secondary bilateral synchrony, and normalization of background activity. Very soon after the initiation of steroids his behaviour changed surprisingly; for the first time in at least two years he became interested in his environment, manifested curiosity and tried to communicate with others. He could not express himself verbally but could understand simple sentences. Stereotypies and hyperactivity declined markedly.

Over the following 16 months (age 12-13 years), seizures were completely controlled. CSWS disappeared but secondary bilateral synchrony was present. He became able to dress himself and attend to personal hygiene. Expressive language progressively reappeared, and he began to repeat words and to ask the names of objects. However, only simple dialogue at a very concrete level was possible and abstract reasoning remained lacking, as documented by his very poor performance on the Leiter intelligence scale at age 13 (IQ 32; age equivalent 45 months).

At the most recent follow-up at age 16, he was seizure-free and continuing on valproate. From the behavioural and cognitive point of view, he had an obvious frontal lobe syndrome.

Outcome: acquired epileptic frontal syndrome

At the latest clinical assessment, both patients were seizure-free but their EEGs showed sporadic frontal spikes. The reading and writing abilities of these patients are typical of children in the first 2 years of primary school. Behaviour is characterized by social inhibition and apathy in patient 1, and by restlessness and lack of inhibition in patient 2. Both patients had complete neuropsychological assessments:

General intelligence was deficient with relative sparing of language, more evident in patient 1 (Full scale IQ (FIQ): 63; Verbal IQ (VIQ): 70; Performance IQ (PIQ): 61) than in patient 2 (FIQ: 41;

VIQ: 49; PIQ: 45). Language comprehension was fairly normal; phonology and morpho-syntax were intact, but language content and naming remained poor. Sustained and selective attention, and memory were deficient. Visual perception and visuomotor integration were normal when copying simple geometric figures. However, when copying complex geometric figures both patients showed many graphical perseverations, and planning difficulties were evident. Performance on 'frontal tests' (verbal fluency tests, Wisconsin card sorting test, Conners continuous performance test, and coding and maze of the Wechsler) were very poor. Attention was deficient and neither patient was able to plan activities or find strategies to solve problems. They tended to perseveration and inflexibility. Categorical and phonemic verbal fluency was very impaired.

Conclusions

In both cases the clinical history began with polymorphic seizures, followed by rapid cognitive, linguistic and behavioural deterioration. Following initiation of appropriate treatment the CSWS began to fluctuate and eventually disappeared, although frontal lobe EEG abnormalities persist even after several years of follow-up. The EEG improvement was associated with improved language and behaviour. Mild signs of frontal dysfunction were present at first, although frank cognitive deficits consistent with a frontal syndrome became evident only in adolescence.

Our follow-up data in these two patients support the supposition that long-term outcome in CSWS can be influenced by the location of the main epileptogenic focus and the maturity of the affected brain areas at CSWS onset. Thus, persistent frontal EEG abnormalities, as found in our patients, should be considered a sign of frontal lobe damage, either pre-existent or secondary to CSWS. Prolonged CSWS at an early age interferes with the development of frontal neural networks, while the rapid recovery of language and its relative sparing at most recent follow-up indicate that functions subsumed by structures already mature at the onset of CSWS may recover.

References

Hommet, C., Billard, C., Barthez, M.A., Gillet, P., Perrier, D., Lucas, B., de Toffol, B. & Autret, A. (2000): Continuous spikes and waves during slow sleep (CSWS): outcome in adulthood. *Epileptic Disord.* **2**, 107–112.

Patry, G., Lyagoubi, S. & Tassinari, C.A. (1971): Subclinical electrical status epilepticus induced by sleep in children: a clinical and electroencephalographic study of six cases. *Arch. Neurol.* **24**, 242–252.

Roulet-Perez, E., Davidoff, V., Despland, P.A., & Deonna, T. (1993): Mental and behavioural deterioration with epilepsy and CSWS: acquired epileptic frontal syndrome. *Dev. Med. Child. Neurol.* **8**, 661–674.

Veggiotti, P., Beccaria, F., Guerrini, R., Capovilla, G. & Lanzi, G. (1999): Continuous spikes-and-waves during slow-wave sleep: syndrome or EEG pattern? *Epilepsia* **40** (11), 1593–1601.

Poster 4

Neuropsychological profile in children with frontal lobe epilepsy

Michele Roccella and Marco Bonanno*

Department of Psychology, University of Palermo, viale delle Scienze, Edificio 15, 90128 Palermo, Italy
* Institute of Psychiatry, Polyclinic A. Gemelli, Largo Gemelli 8, 00168 Rome, Italy
bonanno_marco@libero.it

Early studies of the influence of epilepsy on cognitive functions mainly evaluated global deficit as dependent on epilepsy and its causes (Addi, 1987; ILAE Proposal, 1989; Ladavas *et al.*, 1979; Stores, 1978). More recently, some authors have described specific neuropsychological deficits in epileptic patients with a normal IQ, also showing relations between different forms of epilepsy and the nature of the deficits. We investigated neuropsychological functions in children with frontal lobe epilepsy (FLE) (Cardaci *et al.*, 1997; Lenti, 1995; Roulet-Perez *et al.*, 1993).

Materials and methods

We studied eight subjects, five boys and three girls aged between 8 and 11 years (average age 9 years 8 months), with FLE. Four of them had a left frontal focus and the other four a right frontal focus. Seizures were classified according to the 1989 ILAE proposal. We selected subjects with no neurological, cognitive, visual or auditory deficits, and normal imaging with CT and MRI. EEGs all showed a focal frontal abnormality and all subjects were taking a single antiepileptic drug with levels in the therapeutic range; they had all been treated for at least 4 months at the time of evaluation. All were seizure-free and were in regular classes.

The battery of tests included the WISC-R (all 12 subtests), Raven's progressive matrices, Zazzo's 'deux barrages' test, Benton's D-form of visual retention test, Frostig's development of visual perception test, Bender's test, Rey's complex figure test (B-form) and Goodenough's human figure test. We performed the same tests on a control group without epilepsy, matched for sex, age and economic situation, randomised in a school.

Results

Student's t, and the Mann-Whitney U test showed no significant differences between the performance of both groups. The statistic comparison of the scores attained by the epileptic subjects does

Table 1. WISC-R: verbal

	Information	Resemblances	Arithmetic	Vocabulary	Comprehension	Memory of number
L mean	7,74	7,20	8,62	7,65	7,34	8,15
SD	3,78	3,00	2,76	2,78	3,41	2,58
R mean	8,86	7,68	10,11	9,68	6,44	7,67
SD	3,78	3,44	2,00	4,22	3,72	2,78
t test	0,78	−0,30	−1,34	−1,42	0,78	0,32
P	0,20	0,33	0,07	0,06	0,21	0,34

(L mean: left frontal focus; SD: standard deviation; R mean: right frontal focus; t test: 't' of Student; P: score.)

Table 2. WISC-R: performance

	Completion of figures	Figurative histories	Cubes	Object reconstruction	Code	Labyrinth
L mean	7,20	8,21	8,00	8,52	6,22	10,20
SD	2,82	2,42	2,30	2,06	3,20	2,49
R mean	7,10	8,45	8,20	7,43	7,15	10,06
SD	2,22	2,60	2,06	2,40	3,18	4,70
t test	0,02	0,00	−0,32	0,52	0,71	0,10
P	0,45	0,48	0,32	0,21	0,19	0,42

Table 3. Benton

	Exact position errors	Omissions	Distortions	Perseverations	Rotations	Wrong collocation	Error of dimension	Left	Right	Total error
L mean	6,59	2,50	3,21	0,68	0,64	1,34	0,06	3,36	4,28	9,02
SD	2,30	2,28	3,18	1,10	1,08	1,44	0,22	2,44	2,80	5,60
R mean	4,38	2,58	3,44	1,04	1,04	1,68	0,01	3,74	5,40	10,02
SD	2,22	3,60	3,58	1,20	1,08	1,60	0,00	2,44	3,20	5,68
t test	0,32	−0,08	−0,36	−0,46	−0,42	−0,44	1,00	−0,30	−0,82	−0,44
P	0,36	0,44	0,40	0,30	0,28	0,14	0,15	0,33		0,31

not turn out meaningful, in relation to the variable left frontal focus *vs* right frontal focus. Some data are summarized in Tables 1 to 4.

Discussion and conclusions

Patients with epilepsy and cerebral damage have been reported to have reduced intelligence; those with idiopathic epilepsy have a normal IQ, but they tend to lie near the lower limit of the normal range (Alpherts & Aldenkamp, 1990; Roccella, 1998).

Several studies investigated the correlation between focal subclinical electroencephalographic activity and cortical functions, and showed a selective interest of focal cortical functions in that part of brain where paroxysmal activity is recorded (Powell et al., 1997; Roccella & Calamoneri, 1994).

The utilization of more selective and specific tests than common intelligence scales made these observations possible, related to studies of hemispheric functional specialization. There seems to be

Table 4. Test des deux barrages

	Velocity and performance index			
	V1	V2	R1	R2
L average	120,60	52,40	138,10	126,02
SD	50,02	26,02	64,03	58,06
R average	126,68	62,57	142,20	134,70
SD	40,84	20,40	50,40	82,28
t test	−0,74	−0,82	−0,14	−0,11
P	0,20	0,16	0,42	0,40
	Inaccuracy index and quotients			
	In1	In2	QV	QR
L average	0,13	0,24	0,89	1,00
SD	0,24	0,18	0,16	0,84
R average	0,14	0,22	0,86	0,68
SD	0,12	0,14	0,16	0,18
t test	0,10	−0,30	−0,62	1,10
P	0,40	0,32	0,22	0,12

(L average: left frontal focus; SD: standard deviation; R average: right frontal focus; t test: 't' of Student; P: score; V: velocity; R: performance; In: inaccuracy; Q: quotients.)

a precise connection between the type of epilepsy and the neuropsychological deficits: in subjects with generalized epilepsy, there seems to be a reduction of attention and an increase in reaction time. Patients with localization-related partial epilepsy have more specific deficits. With left temporal foci, these involve learning and verbal memory tasks, and right temporal foci affect visuo-spatial function, attention and pre-verbal aspects of communication.

In FLE, deficits seem to be related mostly to temporal orientation, verbal and non-verbal reasoning, learning of new information, operation and problem solving, comprehension of abstract verbal concepts, categorization, and language including reading and writing (Bianchi & Severi, 1989; Helmstaedter et al., 1998; Helmstaedter et al., 1996; Roccella, 1998).

Our study showed no significant difference in performance of the two groups of subjects with right and left FLE, and the control group without epilepsy. This can be due to the selection criteria; we excluded patients with evident focal injuries, and those with intractable and early-onset epilepsy.

References

Addi, D.P. (1987): Cognitive function in children with epilepsy. *Dev. Med. Child Neurol.* **29**, 394–404.

Alpherts, W.C.J. & Aldenkamp, A.P. (1990): Computerized neuropsychological aspects of learning disabilities in epilepsy. *Epilepsia* **31** (Suppl. 4), S9–S20.

Bianchi, A. & Severi, S. (1989): Validity of some neuropsychological tests in the study of frontal epilepsy. *Boll. Lega It. Epil.* **66/67**, 131–134.

Cardaci, M., Chifari, A., Gangemi, A., Ottaviano, S. & Roccella, M. (1997): Valutazione delle abilità logico-operatorie in bambini con epilessia parziale attraverso la somministrazione di un sistema multimediale (M.A.R.E.). Atti XVII Congr. Nazionale S.I.N.P.I., Assisi 22-25 October 1997, **2**, 865–869.

Commission on classification and terminology of the International League Against Epilepsy. Proposal for revised classification of epilepsies and epileptic syndromes (1989). *Epilepsia* **30** (4), 389–399.

Helmstaedter, C., Gleibner, U., Zentner, J. & Elger, C.E. (1998): Neuropsychological consequences of epilepsy surgery in frontal lobe epilepsy. *Neuropsychologia* **36** (4), 333–341.

Halmstaedter, C., Kemper, B. & Elger, C.E. (1996): Neuropsychological aspects of frontal lobe epilepsy. *Neuropsychologia* **34** (5), 399–406.

Ladavas, E., Umiltà, C. & Provinciali, L. (1979): Hemisphere-dependent cognitive performances in epileptic patients. *Epilepsia* **20**, 493–502.

Lenti, C. (1995): *Neuropsicologia e funzioni mentali dell'epilessia in età evolutiva.* Milano: Franco Angeli.

Powell, A.L., Yudd, A., Zee, P. & Mandelbaum, D.E. (1997): Attention deficit hyperactivity disorder associated with orbitofrontal epilepsy in a father and son. *Neuropsychiatry Neuropsychol. Behav. Neurol.* **10** (2), 151–154.

Roccella, M. (1998): Neuropsychologic follow-up in subjects with partial atypical benign epilepsy of childhood. *Int. J. Psychophysiol.* **30** (1-2), 254–255.

Roccella, M. & Calamoneri, F. (1994): Profili neuropsicologici in soggetti con epilessia parziale; dati preliminari. Atti XVI Congr. Nazionale S.I.N.P.I., Brescia, 21-24 September 1994, **1**, 227–230.

Roccella, M. (1999): *Epilessie e funzioni cognitive in età evolutiva.* Palermo: Carbone Editore.

Roulet-Perez, E., Davidoff, V., Despland, P.A. & Deonna, T. (1993): Mental and behavioural deterioration of children with epilepsy and CSWS; acquired epileptic frontal syndrome. *Dev. Med. Child Neurol.* **35**, 661–674.

Stores, G. (1978): School-children with epilepsy at risk for learning and behaviour problems. *Dev. Med. Child Neurol.* **20**, 502–508.

Achevé d'imprimer par Corlet, Imprimeur, S.A.
14110 Condé-sur-Noireau
N° d'Imprimeur : 70651 - Dépôt légal : octobre 2003
Imprimé en France